LBS

LEAN BODY

SOLUTIONS

BY

JASON SHEA, M.S.

LBS

LEAN BODY
SOLUTIONS

BY

JASON SHEA, M.S.

Table of Contents

Acknowledgements

Back in 2007 one of my greatest inspirations was born. Feeling rejuvenated, with motivation to spare and my inspiration sitting on my lap, I began outlining a book aimed at the question I had written on a piece of paper that day: does the human metabolism automatically slow down with age. From here I dedicated myself to reading book after book and journal article after journal article. Eventually, I was able to put some of what I had learned into writing.

As this topic is so broad, the book kept expanding. Just when I thought one section or chapter was complete, a new line of thinking crept in, and the course slowly veered in yet another direction. Soon I became frustrated with writers block and put the book on the back burner, directing my energies toward The In Season Training Manual.

It was in the late summer and fall of 2010 that I got my ass back in gear. Sparked with some renewed motivation, it was time to get this project off my plate. Dedicating myself for months to waking at 4:30 every morning to ensure I had quiet time to write before my son awoke, the end was soon in sight. I can still remember putting on the earphones every morning and dialing into my son's favorite song at the time, Viva La Vida by Colplay, for a little jolt of inspiration. And with that the writing was done and soon began, the long, arduous task of editing, re-editing, and then some more editing.

And now to thank a few very important people in my life.

First, I would like to give a big thank you to my brother Jeremy. Without him I would never have been able to gather the necessary amount of research and scientific literature to make this book a reality.

Next I would like to give another big thank you to my wife Wendy and my mother in law Nora, for the tremendous amount of effort they put forth in the initial editorial process. I thank you from the bottom of my heart for your tremendous generosity and support.

I would like to thank the tremendous community at APECS and CrossFit Tri-Valley for their constant encouragement and contagious enthusiasm. I would especially like to thank the women of the morning class, as you truly are an inspiration to me!

I would like to thank Laurie Warren and Dr. Erin Thomas for their expert insight and feedback on the initial drafts. Thank you. I would like to thank my great friends Jeff Dufficy, Paul Dipillo, Andy Kurtz, Mike Regan, and Tony Sirianni. Jeff for your inspiration and for your brilliant idea for the title. Paul for the work you put in in helping to bring this to fruition. Andy and Mike for your constant support, loyalty, and friendship. Tony, for constantly pushing and challenging me to do and be better. It's all about HEART.

I would like to thank my editor-in-chief Elyse Brightman for your guidance, professionalism and support throughout the editorial process. I would also like to thank TJ Leland for your uncanny ability to proofread, final edit, and find the most minute of mistakes. Thank you both for helping this book to become a reality.

I would also like to give a great thank you to the books figure model star, Rory Cellucci. Rory, thank you for all of your support over the years. You have been a great friend to us and inspiration to all those around you. Thank you.

Of course, I want to thank the staff at APECS. It is both a tremendous honor and pleasure to work side by side with you guys. Your support, loyalty and friendships mean more than you know.

I would like to give a special thank you to my Aunt Carol, Uncle David, Luc, Lacie, and Mac for your unbelievable support, inspiration, and for always being there when we needed you☺

An extra special thank you to my parents for constantly believing in me throughout my life and teaching me to walk tall, be strong and persevere through any challenges. You have given me both root and wings! I love you guys. Thank you!

Lastly, I would like to give another extra, extra special thank you to my absolute inspirations, Ayden, Bryn, and Wendy. Thank you for your support and understanding when "Daddy" was working on weekends. Ayden and Bryn you are the lights of my life. Wendy, you have been my inspiration since the day we met.

Thank you all.

Sincerely,

Jason

It seems that life begins to catch up with us when the biological clock hits 40. Past transgressions against our better judgment and health come back to haunt us. The old, I'll do "this" now because I won't feel the effects until I am "older" mindset. This attitude permeates amongst many teenagers and twentysomethings, not realizing that one day, we must "pay the piper". Whether it is fat gain, hormonal changes, sickness, weakened immune function, autoimmune disease, or even loss of enjoyment of the simple pleasures of life, the decisions we make regarding our health can have a lasting effect throughout our lives.

Why the age of forty? This is more of an arbitrary number, symbolic of our passing from youth to adulthood (for some, anyway). Family, work, and commitments take precedence, and it seems our health becomes second fiddle. Before we know it, attitudes like "I'll get to the gym tomorrow" or "diet starts Monday" begin to creep in slowly. From the initial slip, it becomes easier and easier to continue sliding down the slippery slope, leading to a ripple effect of fat gain and its related negative health complications.

Besides the changing attitude, it is about this age (give or take, of course) when those previously mentioned "past transgressions" can begin to take their toll on our bodies. From toxic buildup over a lifetime to compromised digestive processes due to lifelong poor nutritional habits, the human body is very durable, but it can only take so much abuse. Culprits such as alcohol, stress and environmental toxin exposures can have lasting effects on our body's ability to function properly.

This book explores many of the factors that may compromise our body's ability to "battle the bulge" and maintain our youthful vitality. This is not a diet or exercise book, but rather a functional analysis and introduction to many of the reasons why it becomes increasingly difficult to lose weight/body fat and maintain our youthful energy over a lifetime. Once you understand what may be causing your weight loss and health issues, it may become easier to look at the complete picture and find a suitable action plan to finally break through these plateaus.

CHAPTER 1

THE MILLION DOLLAR QUESTION?

Does the metabolism of the human organism (species) automatically slow down with age? What is metabolism? Metabolism is basically how the body absorbs/ingests calories, breaks them down into usable components, and converts those ingested calories into energy, while excreting the rest as waste products. There is a general assumption that our metabolism just slows down with age, and we are doomed to accept the accumulation of fat cells everywhere on our body, along with decreased energy levels and vitality. But what if this weren't the case? What if we do not have to accept our banishment to the land of lipogenesis, where fast food restaurants and smelly sunken couch seats are the norm? What if we can keep our metabolic rate up as we age, capable of fending off many of the negative effects associated with obesity?

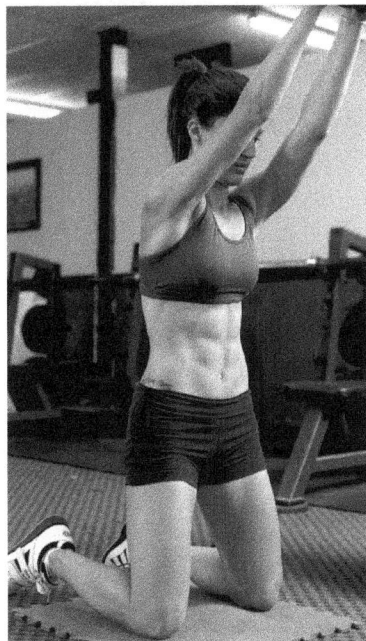

Studies have shown that the cards are stacked against us in the battle of the bulge and maintenance of metabolism. For instance, with lack of physical activity, specifically weight training, lean tissue (muscle) may be lost (10, 34), and with this loss of muscle comes a decrease in ones working and resting metabolism (10,24,30). Environmental toxin accumulation has been shown to affect our body's ability to mobilize fat cells (20,31) and impair proper endocrine functioning (3,15). Hormones including leptin (39), insulin (7,27,35) thyroid , testosterone, estrogen and sex hormone binding globulin (41) and growth hormone (IGF1) (6,11,21) all play key roles in maintenance of a healthy metabolism.

A study conducted at the University of Glasgow looked at the basal metabolic rate and fat free mass of 22 physically active subjects all around the age of 62. The researchers then re-measured those same biomarkers six years later and found minimal or insignificant changes in metabolic rate and fat free mass. The researchers concluded that by remaining physically active, these 22 men maintained their health and fat free mass, even at the age of almost 70 (30).

> In 2009, at the ripe age of 74, Sri Chinmoy overhead pressed two dumbbells totalling 740lbs (335.66kg)

Oxidative Stress

Oxidative stress, or the stress on the cells, can have profound effect on our body's ability to remain young and vibrant while still maintaining optimal health. Oxidative stress has been shown in studies to be a primary component in human aging [5,16] as well as human health. The easiest way to begin a discussion about oxidative stress and antioxidants is to first delve into the actual root meaning of the term "antioxidant".

Anti: from the Greek word for against, opposed to, or preventive

Oxidants (otherwise known as "free radicals"): substances created through bodily processes requiring oxygen, as well as external environmental stressors, that may lead to negative effects including cellular damage, gaining weight, and chronic disease.

Basically, the human body undergoes millions of chemical reactions and processes throughout the day, each of which requires oxygen. Oxidation inside the human body, when left unchecked by "antioxidants", can create a breakdown in cellular tissue, leading to the generation of free radicals. Oxidation is not all bad as it also helps protect the body from toxins, viruses and bacteria. This process decreases the potential for more serious health consequences from typical "bugs" such as the common cold and flu.

It is the accumulation or overproduction of these oxidants that we need to be concerned with, especially when there is a lack of antioxidants present.

Free radicals are extremely unstable atoms or groups of atoms with an unpaired number of electrons that have the ability to react/attack other molecules. By attacking the powerhouse of our cells, the mitochondria, free radicals can destroy our DNA (or RNA). They basically steal an electron from a susceptible molecule, and then transform that molecule into a free radical itself. The new free radical then seeks out other susceptible molecules, starting a chain of events, eventually leading to cell death or disruption.

Think of the effects oxygen has on food that is left out or on metallic substances that develop rust. The free radical creation is similar to this process in that immune function is disrupted, leading to a wide array of negative health consequences, including neurodegenerative diseases, cancer, heart and cardiovascular disease, and many forms of autoimmune disease.

For instance, the oxidation of "bad" LDL (low density lipoproteins) cholesterol can lead to the buildup of fatty deposits inside the arteries, causing strokes and/or heart attacks. Contrary to popular belief, it is not the presence of the LDL alone that is causing this blockage of the internal plumbing, but rather the oxidation of the LDL, that often leads to dangerous plaque buildups.

> A 2009 study found that of 137,000 patients, more than 75% of those hospitalized for heart attacks had cholesterol levels that would indicate they weren't at high risk.

So, what can we do to prevent this damage to our cells from oxidation? This is where antioxidants come in. Antioxidants are molecules that scavenge or react/bind with free radicals. This process neutralizes their negative effects, thereby stopping the chain reaction that leads to cellular death/disruption.

Antioxidants can come from many sources, both external and internal, as the human body does have its own free radical defense system. The human body produces what is regarded as antioxidant enzymes as its primary defense against cellular damage. The three major ones are Glutathione, Superoxide Dismutase, and Catalase.

Glutathione, one of the most important antioxidants in the human body, is synthesized from the amino acids glycine, L-glutamic acid, and L-cysteine. It is a major detoxifying agent, readily donating an electron to free radicals or toxic substances making them less harmful and packaged for excretion. Besides its role in free radical scavenging and detoxification, glutathione also plays a major role in immune health and DNA/cellular function and repair.

Superoxide Dismutase is a class of enzymes primarily responsible for the breakdown or dismantling of oxidants/free radicals into the less harmful hydrogen peroxide. This extremely potent antioxidant is composed of zinc, copper, manganese, iron, and nickel, each of which plays a crucial role in the protective properties of this enzyme/antioxidant.

Catalase gets to do its work after superoxide dismutase has broken down the oxidant/free radicals into hydrogen peroxide. Catalase breaks down the hydrogen peroxide into oxygen and water.

So there you have the simplified version of the human anti-oxidation system. A system in which oxidants/free radicals are bonded to, broken down into less harmful substances, and then excreted. Though this is an extremely efficient system, problems may occur when it becomes overburdened, losing effectiveness and decreasing efficiency. At this point natural external antioxidants come into play.

> A 2003 study found that during the 6-month preseason, 50% of the triathlete subjects sustained an injury due to overuse.

Have you ever noticed that the more endurance exercise you seem to partake in over periods of time, the more susceptible you become to stuffy noses and cold symptoms? Excessive endurance training can lead to an increased accumulation of free radicals [4]. In order to keep these molecules under control and prevent them from damaging the body, antioxidants are needed to counteract their effects [1,4,5,28].

Because the body cannot manufacture certain micronutrients containing valuable antioxidants, they must be supplied through the diet. Of major importance are Vitamin E, Vitamin C, beta-carotene, CoQ10, Selenium, and Alpha Lipoic Acid. World-renowned antioxidant expert, Dr. Lester Packer, refers to these nutrients as the Network Antioxidants. These highly important antioxidants work in conjunction with each other, magnifying the body's antioxidant effects in combating oxidative stress [9,17,22,25,26,28]. Let's take a look at each of these:

Alpha Lipoic Acid:

> Alpha lipoic acid has been used to treat diabetic neuropathy for years over in Europe. In fact studies have shown that dosages of 600mg per day were most effective in treating the chief symptoms of diabetic polyneruopathy. (Ziegler 2004).

Alpha Lipoic acid has been proven to play a major role in the metabolism and generation of the body's most potent naturally occurring antioxidant, glutathione (9,33). Along with its ability to decrease oxidative stress (29), studies show that Alpha Lipoic Acid has a positive effect on mitochondrial health (33), liver/kidney health, and inflammation (33). One of the most interesting characteristics about Alpha Lipoic Acid, which is the reason why *researchers refer to it as a "super-antioxidant", is its ability to regenerate both fat soluble Vitamin E (9,29) and water soluble Vitamin C (9,29)* after they have been used in free radical scavenging. So powerful are Alpha Lipoic Acid's antioxidant properties, that *it has been used in the treatment of the potentially fatal Amanita mushroom poisoning*.

One of the major problems with commercially available supplement form of Alpha Lipoic Acid is its bioavailability. Most of the benefits seen in studies on Alpha Lipoic Acid occur when the R-Stabilized form of Alpha Lipoic Acid was used (not the commercially available Alpha Lipoic Acid). The R-stabilized form is an unstable version of Alpha Lipoic Acid, which can lose its molecular integrity if not prepared or stored properly.

Vitamin E

Studies on vitamin E have shown this antioxidant to be one of the most abundant and efficient scavengers of free radicals (12). As a result, it plays a major role in decreasing the risk of degenerative diseases and cancer (37,38), while preserving cellular membrane health and cardiovascular health (23). A major benefit of this fat-soluble vitamin is the fact that after it has scavenged a free radical, *it can basically be recycled to be used again in the battle against free radical and oxidative stress*. Alpha Lipoic Acid and Vitamin C play a crucial role in this antioxidant recycling (23).

The key to Vitamin E is to find one that includes all members of the vitamin E family, 4 tocopherols and 4 tocotrienols (37). Many of the store bought brands contain only Alpha-dl-tocopherol, which, by itself, does not promote the health benefits of the entire Vitamin E family. Food sources of Vitamin E include vegetable and fish oils, seeds and nuts, whole grains, and fruits such as apricots.

Vitamin C

A 1985 double blind placebo controlled study found that individuals taking ascorbic acid (Vitamin C) had significantly greater weight loss than the control group.

Vitamin C is a very versatile vitamin with regards to its antioxidant abilities. Deficiencies in Vitamin C have been shown to be a risk factor in cardiovascular disease (8,18) and oxidative stress (8,18). Vitamin C supplementation may also reduce the inflammatory biomarker C-reactive protein after only two months of treatment (10).

A major benefit of Vitamin C is that it **has been shown to regenerate Vitamin E *(8,38)*,** as well as and has the ability to improve antioxidant capacity of the blood through its positive effects on red blood cell glutathione (8,18). When choosing a Vitamin C product, choose one that incorporates a full spectrum of bioflavonoids to ensure maximum vitamin activity. Good food sources of Vitamin C include citrus fruits and juices, green peppers, cabbage, spinach, broccoli, kale.

CoQ10

Coenzyme Q10 has long been studied and known for its positive effects on mitochondrial health and energy production (13,25,28). More recently studies have shown that CoQ10 plays a role in neurodegenerative diseases, cancer and diabetes complications (13,32). This antioxidant is similar to Alpha Lipoic Acid, in that it also has the ability to recycle Vitamin E (13,32).

CoQ10 has been shown to be an effective treatment in migraine attacks. A 2005 study out of the Headache and Pain unit of the University Hospital in Zurich, Switzerland, found nearly 50% of the migraine sufferers had superior results (with regard to frequency of headaches) when taking the CoQ10.

OTHER ANTIOXIDANTS

Outside the Antioxidant Network are many valuable antioxidants including Selenium, Beta-carotene, N-acetyl Cysteine, Polyphenols, carotenoids, flavonoids, phenolic acids, EGCG, along with others. Most recently a potent antioxidant with superior anti-aging effects found in red wine has made it into the media headlines: Resveratrol.

Resveratrol may have anti-carcinogenic properties (3, 26), anti-inflammatory properties (22), as well as positive effects on neurodegenerative diseases associated with oxidative stress

(69). This tremendous compound has also been shown to have anti-estrogenic properties, believed to promote cardiovascular health (26).

ORAC

The antioxidant capacity of foods can be measured through the use of a rating scale called ORAC (Oxygen Radical Absorbance Capacity). In other words, the ability of the compounds found in food to scavenge free radicals. The beauty of ORAC measurements is they take into account the synergistic bioactivity of all the antioxidant compounds in a certain food, not just single substances.

Regular everyday foods such as organic strawberries, prunes, raspberries, blackberries, cherries, and blueberries have considerably high ORAC values. Beware of superfoods as they may involve tricky marketing schemes trying to get consumers to buy grossly overpriced foods in hopes of resurrecting youthful vitality.

Below is a sampling of some of the published data on a few highly rated foods:

Food Source	Antioxidant Capacity
Cinnamon (ground)	61000
Red Beans	13727
Blueberries (wild)	13427
Red Kidney Beans	13259
Pinto Beans	11964
Blueberries (cultivated)	9019
Cranberries	8983
Artichokes	7904
Blackberries (Cultivated)	7701
Prunes	7701
Raspberry	6058
Strawberry	5938
Red Delicious Apple	5900
Granny Smith Apple	5381

Worth noting is the degradation of foods (particularly vegetables) during cooking. Steaming seems to allow for greater retention of ORAC, while conventional boiling can significantly reduce the value.

THE PARADOXICAL NATURE OF GEOMETRICAL SHAPES AND DIETING

If weight loss/body fat loss weren't such important topics, there probably wouldn't be so many diet books written on the topic, quick fix supplements to make it easier, and $10 monthly gym memberships to at least get you thinking in the right direction (even if you never use it).

> It has been estimated that the US fat loss and diet market may reach over $70 Billion a year by 2010.

The recommendations come from all sources, some in-the-know, others because it worked for them. From the nutritionist recommending what they learned from their years of institutional education to the dieter who neurotically watches their weight, telling you a calorie is a calorie is a calorie, and all you have to do is watch your points. The local personal trainer in her early 20's informs you that all you need to do is exercise and the bag of Doritos and margaritas from the night before just magically peel off your thighs and love handles.

The endurance athlete will tell you to eat more carbs and do more cardio. The former bodybuilding competitor will tell you what worked for them while they were competing. So, who is right? How about the USDA? After all, they created the food pyramid guidelines that we are recommended to follow in order to maintain or achieve proper health.

Speaking of the food pyramid, do we really need that many grains and starchy carbohydrates in our diet? Does the human machine require the amount of carbohydrates that are heavily promoted by the USDA guidelines (the food pyramid recommends 6-11 servings per day). Using a little common sense, we know there are essential amino acids (proteins), essential fatty acids (fats), but there are no essential carbohydrates? Understanding that our body can produce energy from proteins through gluconeogenesis, as well as through fats via lipolysis, do humans really require all those carbohydrates that fill the base of the USDA food pyramid?

In his groundbreaking book, In *Defense of Food*, author Michael Pollan talks of how we did change our diets according to the scientifically unproven recommendations of the USDA food pyramid. Pollan mentions how we cut fat out of our diets, yet became fatter. But thanks to the miracles of modern pharmaceutical medicines (tens of billions of dollars in statin sales over the last 5 years), it actually appears that our cholesterol levels have gone down.

Low fat this, low fat that, and yes, we became, fatter. Come to think of it, didn't a fat blocking chemical that "they" put into potato chips require a label on the bag cautioning that it actually could cause anal leakage. *WHAT??* Yes, the modern day trade-off for not getting fat. Your insides will leak out, but you can eat all the chips, cookies, and low fat snacks you want. Never mind self-control and personal accountability.

> A 1997 press release by Frito-Lay admitted that Olestra caused "anal oil leakage", according to a study commissioned by the company.

Would it be considered wise to eat the cereal box the cereal comes in, because the nutritional values may be close? Or perhaps blending up some Styrofoam, plastic wrap, and a non-stick Teflon like substance, then adding milk and strawberry flavoring and you have a milkshake with known carcinogens to chug at your own risk. Probably not wise when we look at it from this perspective.

> The popular TV show Mythbusters measured 1g of cereal vs 1g of the cardboard box the cereal came in. The cardboard box had 20% fewer calories, but the cereal had more fat, starch, sugar, and protein (the cardboard had hardly any real nutrients).

It is almost as if what is considered the norm has done a complete 180 degree turnaround. With the obese outnumbering the non-obese, roughly 60/40, is obesity the new norm? (Kind of reminds one of the passengers on board the spaceship in the movie Wall-E.) Every morning there is a traffic line at the local fast food donut shop or a commercial every 5 minutes for some new processed carbohydrate snack. And people wonder what could possibly be causing the current obesity epidemic. What has happened to the norm?

> A 2003 audit by the Australian Divisions of General Practice found that over a 6 week period, children watching roughly 2.5 hours of TV per day would be exposed to roughly 406 advertising messages for junk food.

Accepting mediocrity should never be the answer, especially with regards to health, fat loss, and obesity. In today's culture with obesity rates at an all time high, there has never been a better time to overcome inertia and start gaining momentum in the journey

As of 2010, when you type in the word "diet" in the books section of Amazon.com, **53, 323** result pop up.

toward optimal health. For those not willing to accept mediocrity, educating yourself and changing your habits is usually a good place to start. Any diet and exercise program may work for a period of time. The spark has been lit, but all too soon, the flame may die out.

As frustration kicks in because the results are not as rapid, many choose to throw in the towel and accept mediocrity or switch to the next great diet. After all, why else would there be so many books and diet centers if people did not have problems with adherence?

So, is it the diet itself that is not working, or is it the mindset of the individual? Or is it both? In many cases, these diets may only work for a short period of time because they do not take into account……..common sense?

Before digging into the next box of Pop Tarts or pre-wrapped, uncrusted, bleached white bread, peanut butter and jelly sandwich, ask yourself these 5 questions:

1. *Where are the calories coming from?*
2. *What are the hormonal effects of this food?*
3. *Are there chemical additives that may promote weight gain?*
4. *Will the timing of these nutrients affect my weight goals?*
5. *What is the status of my digestive system or gut health?*

Utilizing common sense rather than falling prey to heavy marketing, it becomes easier to understand the importance of the answers to these questions. In order to be effective and work for an extended period of time, any fat loss (note: fat loss not just weight loss) regimen must take into account the entire human organism.

It is not simply calories consumed or calories burned. Nor is it as simple as "they" would have us believe, that a calorie is just a calorie. Looking at nutrition and fat loss from an evolutionary perspective, one can draw conclusions that our ancestors were eating food they could hunt or gather, not chemically laden, synthetic substitutes used to trick our bodies into thinking we are ingesting nutrients.

The perfect storm for obesity is upon us. Our diets have never been higher in processed foods and sugar-laden drinks (thanks to the food pyramid guidelines). Estrogen levels are skyrocketing while testosterone levels are plummeting. There is a medication for almost every ailment one can imagine, and then some. If something is wrong, just take a pill to forever rid you of the symptoms, never mind figuring out the root cause of the problem in the first place. One has to wonder if there will soon be an obesity vaccine, as with the current obesity trends, it does not seem that our healthy eating guidelines are working.

> A 2006 study found that men 50 or older in 1988 had higher testosterone than men 50 or older in 1996. The study also found the men in 1996 had higher testosterone than their 50+ year old male counterparts in 2004. Basically, every 10 years, men's testosterone seems to be decreasing.

Our foodstuff is not only supersized, but lacking in so many vitamins and minerals that our grandparents probably would not even recognize it as food. It seems wherever you turn, soy and corn have crept into everything we eat. With all the low fat diets out there, it is amazing that our cholesterol and serum triglycerides levels are still so high.

SATURDAY MEALS WITH THE VERY HUNGRY CATERPILLAR

Is it truly the fat in our diets that is making us fat? Could it be, the high percentage of high glycemic carbohydrates we consume through such food items as soda, processed foods, bagels, white breads, cereals, milled grains, microwave meals, high sugar juices, etc.., etc.. etc?

The carbohydrate overload we currently face in our diets reminds me of one of my son's favorite books, The Very Hungry Caterpillar. No matter how many carbohydrates the caterpillar ate, he was "still hungry". Quite possibly due to the fact that the carbs he was eating provided an immediate insulin spike, but then led to an increase in serotonin production and eventual energy crash. To compensate for this energy crash, the caterpillar craved more carbohydrates and thus began the unhealthy eating cycle, until his Saturday meal, when he eventually got sick.

There is an easy do-it-yourself method to determine if it is carbs or fat that makes us fat. ***No carbs for 2 weeks vs. low fat for 2 weeks! Which had the greater weight/fat loss?*** Let's look at what the scientific literature says.

A 2003 research paper out of the Duke University Medical Center reviewed the efficacy of low carbohydrate ketogenic diets and how these diets affect weight and cardiovascular health. The researchers found that low carbohydrate ketogenic diets were very effective for weight and fat loss purposes. But what was truly significant was the effect the diet had on serum triglyceride levels and HDL cholesterol. Both demonstrated favorable changes when subjects took part in low carbohydrate ketogenic diets.

Another 2003 study, this one from the New England Journal of Medicine compared the effects of 3 and 6 months of low carbohydrate dieting vs. conventional dieting. Big surprise here: *The low carb groups lost nearly triple the amount over the first 3 months and nearly double the amount of weight over the entire 6 month period*. In a similar study directly comparing low carb vs. low fat diets as a treatment for obesity, the researcher found significantly greater weight and fat loss among obese children eating a low carb diet compared to those eating a low fat diet.

In what can be referred to as a politics of food backfire study, a research team set out to determine if the then recommended National Cholesterol Education Program Diet was all that it was cracked up to be. After all, this diet was based on the recommendations of our medical experts. *"THEY"* recommended we dramatically lower our cholesterol/fat intake and eat more grainy carbohydrates to create a more favorable cardiovascular profile and decrease our obesity rates. According to this comparison study, their recommendations may have been slightly off, as the low carb group had almost twice as much weight loss, when compared to the National Cholesterol Education program diet.

Last are two research papers by world renowned Harvard Professor/Doctor, Dr. Walter Willet. In a 2002 review from the American Journal of Medicine, Willet and Leibel found that dietary fat intakes of up to 40% of total macronutrient intake have little or no effect on the fat that accumulates on our bodies. The researchers found that it is not the fat in our diets that accounts for the current obesity epidemic facing our society. *So much for fat making us fat*.

In his second paper, Willet echoes the same findings as the previous paper, but this time goes on to tout the benefits healthy fats play in our diets. Of particular importance are the findings regarding the potential medical problems that can arise with a reduction in healthy dietary fats. That's right, decreasing healthy dietary fat intake to an extent, while increasing carbohydrate intake can actually lead to adverse health effects. Not only can the fat accumulate, but the potential for adverse health problems also increases.

That may be quite an earful, especially if you just finished a bag of Snackwell's fat free cookies (are they still on the market?) or some Olestra laden potato chips. If the latter, personal experience has taught that Depends undergarments are a cheap solution for the previously mentioned plumbing issues associated with these chips.

What is the next step? First recommendation might be to pick up some excellent books on healthy eating. I highly recommend reading in order:

1. *The Paleo Diet* by Dr. Loren Cordain: Dr. Cordain does an excellent job of educating the reader about how the human organism is meant to eat according to our genetic makeup. Most people seem to forget that we are omnivores, and Dr. Cordain provides significant scientific research reminding us in this excellent, easy to read book.

2. *In Defense of Food* by Michael Pollan: Pollan's books have become significantly popular over the past years. His works, alongside Eric Schossler's excellent book *Fast Food Nation*, have been the subject of a 4 star movie, and have been touted on the Oprah Winfrey Show. In this book, Pollan basically gives the reader insight as to where our food comes from (not as in-depth as the *Omnivores Dilemma* book) and how our food choices can affect our health.

3. *The 150 Healthiest Foods on Earth* by Dr. Jonny Bowden Generally regarded as one of, if not the best nutritionist on the planet, Dr. Bowden walks the walk and talks the talk. From his highly pragmatic approach to functional foods, to his never ending knowledge of the latest scientific research, Dr. Bowden's books are a must read for anybody interested in bettering their

health. I would highly recommend reading Bowden's other books, or adding his website www.jonnybowden.com to your priority list of favorites.

4. ***Good Calories, Bad Calories* by Gary Taubes**: Quite possibly the most comprehensive book ever written on the subject of food and our health. Taubes is a research mastermind with a knack for digging up every detail regarding this subject. You may have to read this one at least twice!!!

These books should give you a good start. Now, the question revolves around ketogenic/low carb diets and how do you put together a healthy version of this diet in order to get lean.

A ketogenic diet is basically a carbohydrate restricted diet that causes the body to produce ketone bodies. These ketone bodies are then used by the nervous system and brain as fuel. The rest of the body switches to the utilization of free fatty acids as its primary fuel source, as there are minimal carbohydrates available for energy. In other words you are burning fat for your primary fuel source. Studies comparing low carb ketogenic diets to low fat/high carb diets have shown significantly favorable decreases in weight loss and cardiovascular markers when utilizing ketogenic diets.

For some of the best books on the market about ketogenic dieting, fat loss, and body composition, it is highly recommended that you read ***Ultimate Diet 2.0* by Lyle McDonald, *The Anabolic Solution* by Dr. Maurio DiPasquale, and *BodyOpus* by Dan Duchaine**. These books are packed with extremely valuable information backed by tons of scientific research. Dr. DiPasquale and McDonald have become highly sought after experts in this field, while the late Dan Duchaine was a pioneer in the realm of fat loss, body-recomposition, bodybuilding/figure athlete contest preparation.

As this is intended not to be a diet book the best way to give you a brief overview of what a cyclical ketogenic diet looks like is to provide you with a 7-day food log reflecting a cyclical ketogenic diet guidelines utilizing Paleolithic nutritional standards. As you read through the diet, notice how the macronutrients are broken down into daily percentages. Pay particular attention to how high the fat intakes per day are and also how each day is adapted according to the daily training status of the individual.

MONDAY

Food Item	Servings	Calories	Fat (g)	Cholest (mg)	Sodium (mg)	CHO (g)	Sugars (g)	Fiber (g)	PRO (g)
Wegman's Organic grass fed Organic sirlion Steak	4	480	14	260	180	0	0	0	92
Whole Foods (365) Pine Nuts (Raws)	1.5	285	29	0	0	6	2	2	6
Anceint Harvest quinoa Garden pagodas gluten free	2	410	2	0	8	92	2	8	8
Plainville Farms Ground Turkey 94% fat Free	3	480	21	180	255	3	0	0	72
Organic Avocado	1	289	26	0	0	15	0	12	3
Whole Catch Wild Alaskan Cod Fillets	2	180	1	80	160	0	0	0	40
Whole Foods Organic Broccoli Florets	2	20	0	0	12	4	2	4	4
Challenge Organic Butter	1	100	11	30	90	0	0	0	0
ON casein Protein	1	120	1	10	250	4	1	1	23
Fage Total greek yogurt	1	300	23	40	65	7	7	0	15
King Oscar Sardines, Mediterranean style	1	150	10	110	320	0	0	0	13
Whole Foods Raw Macadamia Nuts	1	220	23	0	7	4	1	3	2
Tree of Life- Organic Goji	1	110	1	0	130	25	15	5	4
Blue Berries Raw	1	84	1	0	2	21	15	4	1
Cinnamon	1	0	0	0	0	0	0	0	0
Metagenics Omega-3 Fish Oil Soft Gels	7	140	14	28	0	0	0	0	0
Ito En sencha Shot	2	0	0	0	40	0	0	0	0
Vibrant Health Green	2	88	2	0	100	14	2	6	6
Totals	34.5	3456	179	738	1619	195	47	45	289

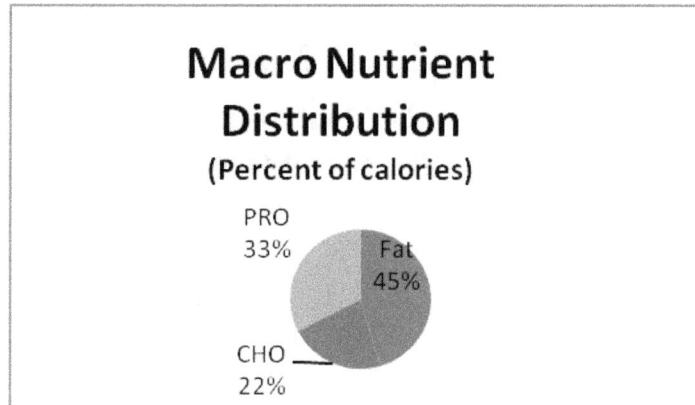

Macro Nutrient Distribution
(Percent of calories)

PRO 33%

Fat 45%

CHO 22%

17

TUESDAY

Food Item	Servings	Calories	Fat (g)	Cholest (mg)	Sodium (mg)	CHO (g)	Sugars (g)	Fiber (g)	PRO (g)
Whole Foods Market Alaskan Wild Caught Stockeye Salmon	4	240	12	96	72	0	0	0	30
Organic Avocado	1	289	26	0	0	15	0	12	3
Wild Harvest Organic Fresh Herb & Greens Salad	1.5	30	0	0	53	5	0	3	2
Whole Foods Market Organic Free Range/ No Antibiotics chicken Breast	3	375	4	195	218	0	0	0	78
Whole foods Raw Macadamia Nuts	1.5	330	35	0	11	6	2	5	3
Wegman's Organic Beef Strip Steak	4	520	18	180	160	0	0	0	92
Whole Foods Organics Broccoli Florets	2	20	0	0	12	4	2	4	4
Whole Foods Market roasted Brussel Sprouts	1	120	9	0	500	8	0	4	4
Challenge Organic Butter	1	100	11	30	90	0	0	0	0
Fage Total Greek Yogurt	1	300	23	40	65	7	7	0	15
ON Casein Protein	1	120	1	10	250	4	1	1	23
Cinnamon	1	0	0	0	0	0	0	0	0
Metagenic's Omega-3 Fish Oil Soft Gels	7	140	14	28	0	0	0	0	0
Ito En Sencha Shot	2	0	0	0	40	0	0	0	0
Vibrant Health Green Vibrance	1	44	1	0	50	7	1	3	3
Total	32	2628	154	579	1521	56	13	32	257

Macro Nutrient Distribution
(Percent of calories)

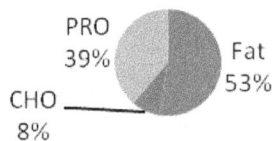

PRO 39%

CHO 8%

Fat 53%

WEDNESDAY

Food Item	Servings	Calories	Fat (g)	Cholest (mg)	Sodium (mg)	CHO (g)	Sugars (g)	Fiber (g)	PRO (g)
Organic Valley Organic Large Eggs	2	140	10	430	130	2	0	0	12
Great Range Bison Steak Medallions	1	180	3	65	75	0	0	0	37
King Oscar Sardines Mediterranean Style	1	150	10	110	320	0	0	0	13
365 Brand Roasted & Salted Fancy Mixed Nuts	1	180	16	0	65	6	1	2	4
Bob's Red Mills Steel-Cut Oatmeal	2	340	6	0	0	58	0	10	14
Trader Joe's Grassfed Angus Beef Ground Beef	2.5	675	53	175	188	0	0	0	50
365 Brand Roasted & Salted Fancy Mixed Nuts	1	180	16	0	65	6	1	2	4
Whole Foods Market Alaskan Wild Caught stockeye Salmon	4	240	12	96	72	0	0	0	30
Grilled Vegetables	1	350	0	0	0	0	0	0	0
Blue Berries Raw	0.5	42	0	0	1	11	7	2	1
Optimum Nutrition Nitrocore 24 Ultimate Chocolate	1.5	300	8	68	270	21	3	8	36
Tree of Life- Organic Goji Berries	0.5	55	1	0	65	13	8	3	2
Organic Avocado	1	289	26	0	0	15	0	12	3
Metagenics Omega-3 Fish Oil Soft Gels	1	20	2	4	0	0	0	0	0
Metagenics Omega-3 Fish Oil Soft Gels	5	100	10	20	0	0	0	0	0
Ultimate Nutrition Mct Gold	2	252	28	0	0	0	0	0	0
Vibrant Health Green Vibrance	1	44	1	0	50	7	1	3	3
Total	28	3537	202	968	1301	139	21	42	209

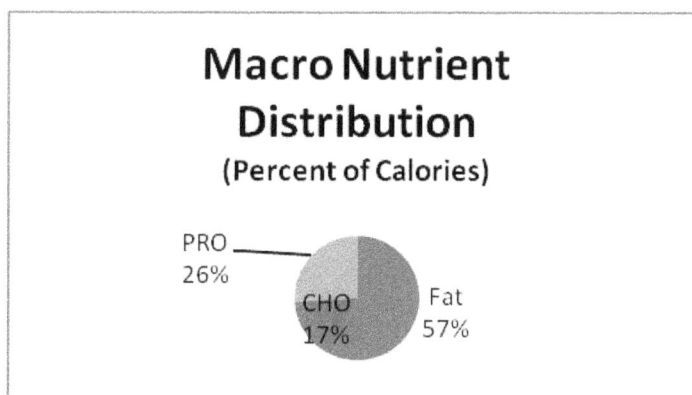

Macro Nutrient Distribution
(Percent of Calories)

PRO 26%

CHO 17%

Fat 57%

19

THURSDAY

Food Item	Servings	Calories	Fat (g)	Cholest (mg)	Sodium (mg)	CHO (g)	Sugars (g)	Fiber (g)	PRO (g)
365 Brand Roasted & Salted Fancy Mixed Nuts	2	360	32	0	130	12	2	4	8
Organic Valley Organic Large Eggs	6	420	30	1290	390	6	0	0	36
Nature's Promise Organic Olive Oil Cooking Spray	15	0	0	0	0	0	0	0	0
Olivia's Organics Spring Mix	1.5	15	0	0	90	5	0	3	3
King Oscar Sardines, Mediterranean Style	2	300	20	220	640	0	0	0	26
Member's Mark (Sam's) balsamic Viniagrette, Organic	1	70	6	0	360	4	4	0	0
365 Brand Roasted & Salted Fancy Mixed Nuts	1	180	16	0	65	6	1	2	4
Whole Foods Market Organic Free Range/no antibiotics Chicken Breast	3	375	4	195	218	0	0	0	78
Grilled Vegetables	1	350	0	0	0	0	0	0	0
Ultimate Nutrition Mct Gold	2	252	28	0	0	0		0	0
Metagenics Omega-3 Fish Oil Soft Gels	4	80	8	16	0	0	0	0	0
Coffee, Black	1	2	0	0	5	0	0	0	0
Cinnamon	1	0	0	0	0	0	0		0
Hood Heavy Cream	1	50	5	20	0	0	0	0	0
Wegman's Organic Grass Fed Organic Sirloin Steak	1	120	4	65	45	0	0	0	23
Vibrant Health Green Vibrance	1	44	1	0	50	7	1	3	3
Yerba Prima Physillium Whole Husk	1	15	0	0	4	5	0	5	0
Total	44.5	2633	154	1806	1997	45	8	17	181

Macro Nutrient Distribution...

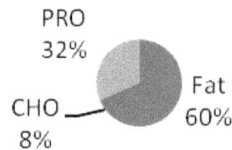

PRO 32%

CHO 8%

Fat 60%

20

FRIDAY

Food Item	Servings	Calories	Fat (g)	Cholest (mg)	Sodium (mg)	CHO (g)	Sugars (g)	Fiber (g)	PRO (g)
Great Range Bison Steak Medallions	2	360	5	130	150	0	0	0	74
Organic Avocado	1	289	26	0	0	15	0	12	3
Coffee, Black	1	2	0	0	5	0	0		0
Hood Heavy Cream	2	100	10	40	0	0	0	0	0
Ancient Harvest Quinoa Garden Pagodas Gluten free pasta	3	615	3	0	12	138	3	12	12
Plainville Farms Ground Turkey 94% Fat Free	2.5	400	18	150	213	3	0	0	60
Ito En Sencha Shot	1	0	0	0	20	0	0	0	0
Wild Oats Spicy salmon Sushi	2	820	28	50	1420	122	20	28	22
Bob's red Mills Steel-cut Oatmeal	3	510	9	0	0	87	0	15	21
Optimum Nutrition nitrocore 24 Ultimate Chocolate	2	400	10	90	360	28	4	10	48
Beach Cliff Sardines- in water	1	150	8	115	230	0	0	0	19
Bob's red Mills Steel-cut Oatmeal	3	510	9	0	0	87	0	15	21
Optimum Nutrition nitrocore 24 Ultimate Chocolate	2	400	10	90	360	28	4	10	48
Tree of Life- Organic Goji Berries	2	220	2	0	260	50	30	10	8
Ancient Harvest Quinoa Garden Pagodas Gluten free pasta	1	205	1	0	4	46	1	4	4
Cinnamon	1	0	0	0	0	0	0	0	0
Tree of Life- Organic Goji Berries	1	110	1	0	130	25	15	5	4
Vibrant Health Green Vibrance	2	88	2	0	100	14	2	6	6
Total	32.5	5179	142	665	3264	643	79	127	350

Macro Nutrient Distribution
(Percent of Calories)

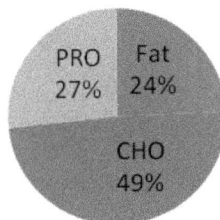

PRO 27%
Fat 24%
CHO 49%

SATURDAY

Food Item	Servings	Calories	Fat (g)	Cholest (mg)	Sodium (mg)	CHO (g)	Sugars (g)	Fiber (g)	PRO (g)
Bob's Red Mills Steel-cut Oatmeal	3	510	9	0	0	87	0	15	21
Optimum Nutrition Nitrocore 24 Ultimate Chocolate	1	200	5	45	180	14	2	5	24
Tree of Life- Organic Goji Berries	1	110	1	0	130	25	15	5	4
Organic Valley Organic Large eggs	2	140	10	430	130	2	0	0	12
Quinua	2	320	5	0	20	58	0	6	12
Brunswick Herring Seafood snacks	1	130	8	65	460	0	0	0	16
Great Range Bison Steak Medallions	2	360	5	130	150	0	0	0	74
WHFoods Sweet Potato	1	95	0	0	10	22	16	3	2
Purely Decadent w/ Coconut Milk Chocolate Peanut Butter Swirl	2	420	26	0	80	42	24	12	6
Whole Foods Market Wild Alaskan Halibut Steaks	1.5	293	7	102	135	0	0	0	52
Whole Foods- Locally grown Green beans	2	88	0	0	2	20	4	8	4
Frey Natural Red organic Wine Red Organic Wine	2	160	0	0	0	0	0	0	0
Brunswick Herring Fillets	1	140	8	65	270	0	0	0	15
Metagenics Omega-3 Fish Oil Softgels	5	100	10	20	0	0	0	0	0
Vibrant Health Green Vibrance	2	88	2	0	100	14	2	6	6
Total	28.5	3154	96	857	1667	284	63	60	248

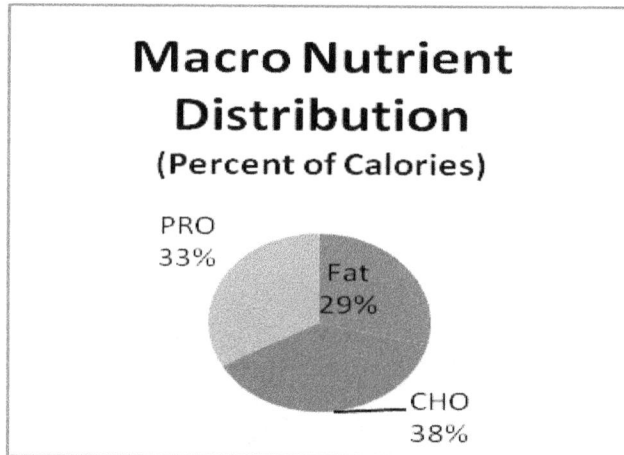

Macro Nutrient Distribution
(Percent of Calories)

PRO 33%

Fat 29%

CHO 38%

SUNDAY

Food Item	Servings	Calories	Fat (g)	Cholest (mg)	Sodium (mg)	CHO (g)	Sugars (g)	Fiber (g)	PRO (g)
Great Range Bison Steak Medallions	2	360	5	130	150	0	0	0	74
365 Brand Roasted & Salted Fancy Mixed Nuts	1.5	270	24	0	98	9	2	3	6
Coffee, Black	1	2	0	0	5	0	0	0	0
Hood Heavy Cream	1	50	5	20	0	0	0	0	0
365 Organic (Whole Foods) Chunk ight tongol tuna- No salt added	2	120	0	70	100	0	0	0	28
Driscoll's Rasberries	1	60	1	0	0	8	0	0	1
Blackberry, Raw	1	62	1	0	1	14	7	8	2
Whole Carrots	1	25	0	0	40	6	3	2	1
Horizon Organic Organic Cottage Cheese	1.5	180	8	30	585	6	5	0	20
Whole Foods Market Organic Free Range/ No antibiotics chicken breast	3	375	4	195	218	0	0	0	78
Whole foods Market Roasted Brussels Sprouts	2	240	18	0	1000	16	0	8	8
Vibrant Health Green Vibrance	2	88	2	0	100	14	2	6	6
Metagenics Omega-3 Fish Oil Soft gels	7	140	14	28	0	0	0	0	0
Total	26	1972	82	473	2297	73	19	27	224

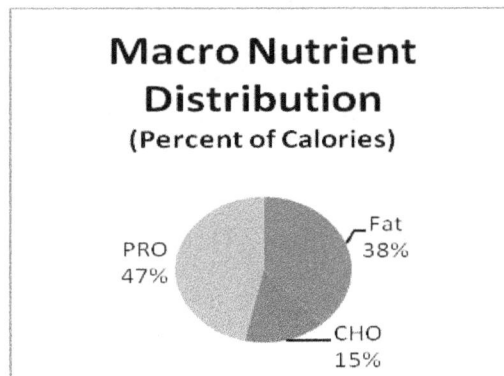

Macro Nutrient Distribution
(Percent of Calories)

PRO 47%
Fat 38%
CHO 15%

You are probably asking yourself; *"this is all great information, but does this type of dieting really work for individuals looking to get leaner"*. After all, there is quite a bit of fat in the diet???? *The proof is in the pictures*! →→→→→→→→→→→→→→

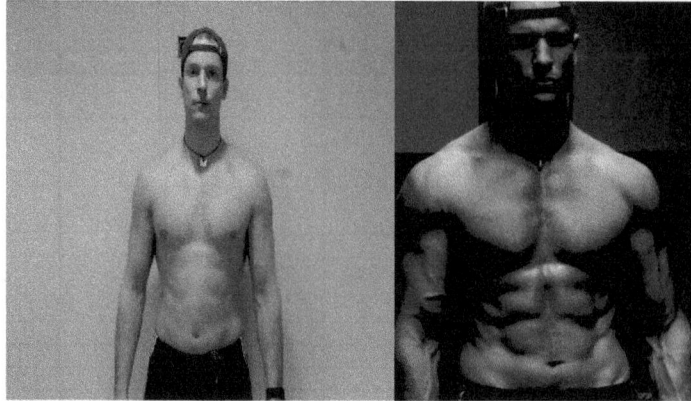

Age 37 BEFORE　　　　**Age 37 AFTER**

March 2012　　　　**July 2012**

If you still don't believe it is the carbs in your diet that may be the culprit for fat gain, weigh yourself. Perhaps cutting carbs and following Paleolithic nutritional strategies for two weeks, then re-weighing yourself may be worth a try.

Besides excessive dietary carbohydrate intake, lack of exercise and poor food choices (i.e. fast food, too many trips to the dessert tray) what other factors could be behind this obesity crisis we are now facing? According to the National Center for Health Statistics 2005-2006, 5% of Americans are "extremely" obese, 34% are obese, and 32.7% are overweight. Let's examine a few of the possible culprits.

CHAPTER II

LIGHTING THE FIRE AND MAINTAINING THE FLAME

The most obvious and probably the greatest determining factors in any success story are the motivation to succeed and the gumption to adhere. Many well-intentioned individuals never see the fruits of their labor, because they cannot see their goals through to the end. For a while, some people can burn as bright as the sun on a hot summer day; but once their motivation runs out, they simply turn into a piece of charcoal waiting for some type of spark to ignite them again.

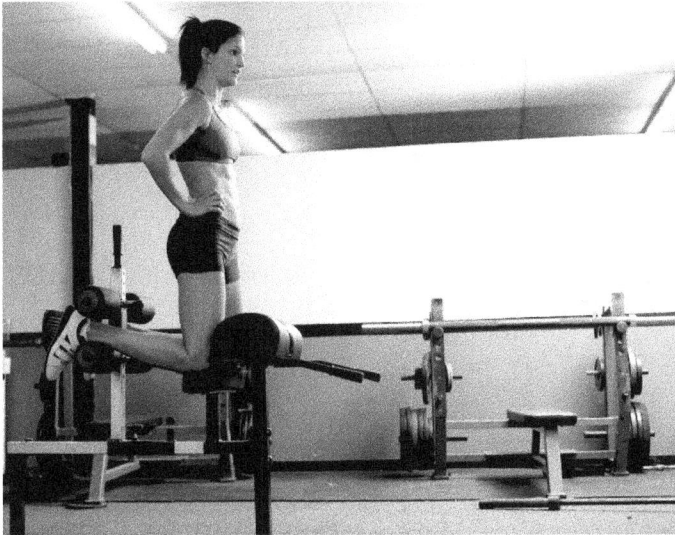

In the realm of fat/weight loss, the motivation to finally "get in shape" is usually the spark that ignites the flame. But therein lays the problem. Good intentions without a proper course of action may lead to a witch-hunt with nothing to gain and everything to lose. For example, how many times have you had somebody tell you that they need to lose a couple more pounds, with no plan of action of how they are going to do it? It is like going on a road-trip without a map.

After performing nutritional coaching and body fat modulation for a few hundred clients, I can honestly say that it is not only a motivational/adherence issue, but also a planning issue. As the old adage states, "failure to plan is planning to fail". Those who have succeeded in their body composition goals were the ones who were able to steer the course even though life provided some obstacles along the way. Their motivation to change is so great, that no matter what dietary roadblock lay in front of them, they somehow managed to find their way back on track. Those roadblocks are things like processed carbohydrates, foods high in trans fats, microwavable meals, and fast foods, just to name a few.

> According to an article in Time Magazine, 48% of Americans will make a New Year's Resolution, with 65% of those keeping it for a small part of the year, and the other 35% "falling off the wagon" much sooner.

Those that plan and make their meals in advance are less likely to reach for the high glycemic load snack when their blood sugar drops. This in contrast to those who fail to plan and in essence plan to fail. They seem to find comfort in the fact that cereal is just an arm's reach away and supposedly "healthy" soy bars stock their shelves (check out the website www.soyonline.com or read the book *The Whole Soy Story* by Dr. Kaayla Daniel for some terrific insight on soy).

If motivation and perseverance are issues in your life, sometimes stepping outside your comfort zone and looking at what others have done to accomplish their goals may provide some perspective. Sometimes, it is these inspirational stories and the people who have overcome unseemingly difficult obstacles to achieve success that allows us to truly appreciate the power of the human spirit. Take for instance, the story of Nando Parrado and his rugby teammates who were stranded in the Andes Mountains for 72 days.

For 72 days, the survivors of the plane crash had the entire deck stacked against them. With hardly enough food to feed a field mouse, broken bones, internal injuries, and crippling minus degree temperatures, their chances of survival were minimal, to say the least. After over two months in these conditions, Parrado and a team of 2 other Uruguayan rugby teammates decided to overcome these obstacles and trek out of the Andes Mountains to find help. Ahead of these courageous survivors was a 10-day trek through some of the most fierce and unrelenting terrain in the world. Never mind the fact that they didn't have any of the professional gear that many modern day mountaineers would need to make this trek.

The book, *Miracle in the Andes* by Parrado and the 1990's feature film, "Alive", document this tremendous example of human spirit, perseverance, and the will to survive. If these guys could survive and climb out of the Andes Mountains, then surely you could survive any temporary discomfort associated with your weight loss journey. It is about achieving your goals; as not only does your health depend on it, but, the quality of your life demands it.

Another truly inspirational story can be seen nearly every year on Patriot's day in Boston, roughly around noontime. In front of live onlookers and thousands of TV viewers nationwide, a message on two T-shirts appears, inspiring any and all who bear witness. The message reads, "Yes You Can", and is proudly displayed on the t-shirts worn by Rick Hoyt and his father Dick Hoyt.

The story began back in 1962 when Rick was born and due to oxygen deprivation to the brain during birth, he would become diagnosed as a quadriplegic with cerebral palsy. Confined to a wheel chair, but not to be denied a life filled with experiences and memories, Team Hoyt would soon become a national role model of inspiration.

As the story goes, roughly 30+ years ago, Rick approached his father about running a 5-mile road race to benefit an athlete who had also become paralyzed and confined to a wheelchair. The two ran their first race, with a physically exhausted father pushing wheelchair-bound son the entire five miles. The two finished near last, but the experience would change both for the rest of their lives.

According to their books and website, "later that same night, Rick told his father, *'Dad, when I'm running, it feels like I'm not handicapped'"*. In this author's opinion, those are the only words any parent would need to hear in that situation to find the gumption to sacrifice one's body to endless limits in order to make their child's dreams come true. (*I say that from my perspective, as a father to a 3 year old son.*)

And so, over one thousand races later, Team Hoyt is the model for success and perseverance. Their motto, "Yes You Can", can be heard and seen everywhere, from Ironman Triathlons to Fortune 500 speaking engagements. If these two can overcome the odds against them, there comes a time when you need to look at your reflection in the mirror and ask the same question. Hopefully the answer is "yes you can!" You can learn more about Rick and Dick Hoyt and their incredible story at their website www.teamhoyt.com.

In summary, if you cannot seem to overcome fat loss issues due to adherence issues and planning, remember, that "***it is easier to blame than take accountability.*** Understanding this concept, here a few effective strategies to keep the motivation alive until you achieve your goals.

I. **Take a Picture:** If body composition is your goal, then stop looking in the mirror from that same angle that makes you look good and have somebody take some pictures of how you really look. Ever notice when you think you are doing something right (body composition wise), then somebody takes some holiday pics, and when you see them you think to yourself "is that me", or "I didn't realize I had a double chin", or the old "wow, I thought the fact that because I was lifting more weight in the gym and the scale was going up meant I was putting on muscle (*Yes, speaking from experience here*)". The old adage goes "a picture is worth a thousand words" speaks volumes here. Without photo shoot staging, image document enhancement and photo doctoring, a quality picture will not lie, but will also provide you with an accurate image as to where your body composition needs work (if at all). Perhaps it may also stimulate you to get to the gym and start monitoring your diet.

II. **Find a Quality Workout Partner:** There is nothing like going through a gut - wrenching workout with somebody else sharing in your pain the entire time. Not only will a good workout partner keep your adherence high by committing to be there for the workout, but can also increase motivation as the competitive spirit begins to kick in. A top notch workout partner will be there to spot you, allowing for those extra reps, where without him/her you would have racked the bar a long time ago. They can monitor time under tension, correct technical breakdowns to avoid injury, and yell at you because "you look like a cross between Woody Harrelson and Jon from Garfield with a hairline that resembles an upside horseshoe rusting in the sun on a hot summer day". (*Once again, speaking from experience.*)

III. **Hire a "qualified" strength coach/personal:** This one is obvious. When you want legal work done, reading the latest edition of Legal and Witness Magazine may not be the best option. When you need dental work done, perhaps watching what the celebrity dentist on the dental version of "the biggest loser" may not be the best idea. So, why should your approach to body composition be any different?

Quite possibly, the best starting point for finding a quality strength coach is to find somebody who has been certified through renowned strength coach Charles Poliquin's PICP certification program (www.charlespoliquin.com). This program teaches a strength coach just about all the practical aspects they need to know to become a top quality professional in the industry. After all, just look at Poliquin's track record as the most successful strength coach in the world for the past 30 years (countries hire him when they need a Gold medal or World championship) and you will realize why the program is so good.

Other more heavily marketed certifications, which are generally recognized by the public, include the NASM-CPT (National Academy of Sports Medicine), NSCA (National Strength and Conditioning Association) CSCS or CPT, and ACSM (American College of Sports Medicine) CPT or health and fitness specialist. These provide a basic foundation of general anatomy and physiology, kinesiology, biomechanics, nutrition, and injury prevention among others. Many health clubs, gyms, and training centers require these as their minimum qualifications for employment.

IV: Keeping a Journal or Following a Program: If you don't know where you are going, then how do you expect to get there? A properly designed strength and conditioning program can provide you with a valuable tool for providing information on what you have done thus far, what else you need to do, what has worked and what has not.

V: Attend a seminar: The value of attending a seminar can be very under-appreciated, as the motivation one gains from learning new information can bring about a whole new approach and energy to one's workouts. The "I can't wait to try this when I get home" attitude takes over, igniting a fire to the already roasted charcoals that represent your motivation levels. With excellent presenters, seminars can represent a sort of battery recharger for those who are running on empty.

VI: Read an Inspirational Book: The stories of human willpower and perseverance can be a great way of providing perspective on just how difficult your challenges may be, especially when compared to those of others. Once put into "perspective", overcoming your obstacles and achieving your goals may be a little easier. Some great reads for some inspiration are:

1. *It's Only A Mountain: Dick and Rick Hoyt, Men of Iron* by Sam Nall. If you are lacking inspiration or motivation, or feeling bad about your physical limitations that may be preventing you from achieving your fat loss goals, this heart wrenching book is a must read.

2. *Miracle in the Andes* by Nando Parrado. Another story about human achievement, the will to survive, and the perseverance to succeed. This book is very compelling as it provides a first-hand account of the actions and emotions of a struggle for survival. Compared to hardships of the characters in this book, weight loss/fat loss should be a cinch.

3. *Awaken the Giant Within* by Tony Robbins. Tony Robbins has built a multimillion-dollar empire on his ability to inspire others to achieve more in their lives. For that reason, he must know a thing or two about motivation and perseverance. In this book he provides some useful "nuggets" to help one get off the couch and into the race.

4. ***The Last Lecture*** by Randy Pausch. This inspirational "lecture" entitled, "Really Achieving Your Childhood Dreams" is all about finding the motivation to follow your dreams and the perseverance to overcome any obstacle that comes in your way.

5. ***The Monk Who Sold His Ferrari*** by Robin Sharma. I know, I know, but this book is a personal favorite of mine. It may be difficult for any of us to quit our jobs, move to the Himalayas with Buddhist Monks, and come back looking 30 years younger with zero stress in our lives, but the story is highly inspirational and the guidance provided by Sharma allows us to aim for a higher quality of life.

VII: Compete in Something: There is nothing like having a goal with a deadline looming in the uncertain future. The deadline of a goal can be a critical element for successful adherence and motivation. Besides not wanting to be embarrassed, the will to succeed and the competitive spirit play excellent motivators in this strategy. I have seen many successful athletes push through workouts and adhere to nutritional protocols because they knew the curtains were going to go up for their performance in X amount of time.

VIII: Environment: Sometimes finding the right environment or just a change of scenery can bring energy back to your workout, not seen since you finally decided to toss out your last pair of Guess jeans (or those of us who have held onto our Z Cavaricci's long enough). Finding a gym with an upbeat and motivating environment can be difficult, as many commercial health clubs are now filled with plasma screen TV's, alarms that sound when you grunt or drop weights, and free lollipops at the front desk. Throw in a couple of 80's Gorilla wear outfits and some aerobics/group tendonitis classes dancing to techno Phil Collins' beats, and you have, well, the modern day health club experience.

Where have the days gone of going to the gym to……..get in shape. Now it seems to be more of a "get me out of the house" or "get a date" type environment.

Whatever happened to exercises such as deep squats and deadlifting, never mind Olympic lifts and pure strongman training. It seems as if most modern health clubs have 1 or 2 squat racks, accompanied by a myriad of machines that rotate, vibrate, and in some cases, constipate (at least it looks that way when people are exerting themselves on vibration training platforms).

Find a good environment, and you may find new levels of motivation to steer you past any fat loss obstacles that may be in your way. Stay motivated, and persevere.

Remember:

Believe, Work…………………………….Become!

CHAPTER III

TOXICITY

It may not be as simple as just eating less or exercising more. The human metabolism has the potential to be affected by a myriad of environmental toxic chemicals, ranging from those found in our food and water sources, to our everyday household cosmetics and cleaners [7]. Renowned human metabolism expert, Dr. Paula Ballie-Hamilton, draws similarities of the aforementioned chemicals to those used in fattening cattle. In other words, **we may be ingesting or absorbing those same chemicals used to fatten livestock**. So, if those chemicals are used to help animals gain weight, could they possibly have the same effect on humans? Perhaps one look at the current obesity trends and you may find your answer. How can these environmental chemicals have that type of effect on human metabolism?

> According to the CDC, obesity is defined as a BMI (body mass index) of 30 or greater. In 2008 only one state (Colorado) had an obesity rate of less than 20%, with six states having at least 30% of their population being obese. Compare this to just *25 years ago in which no state had more than 19% of its population that could be considered obese*

Dr. Baddie-Hamilton explains that these chemicals can have an impact on how the stomach communicates with the brain, otherwise known as our satiety mechanism. By damaging the "you have eaten enough" food mechanism, the result could cause us to eat much more than we should. Studies have shown a correlation between chemical impairment and the promotion of weight gain. They showed that environmental xenobiotic chemicals or chemical estrogen mimickers have the ability to damage the body's adipogenic mechanisms through disruption of the endocrine system [3,6].

> **Sample of just some of the Ingredients found in a fast food strawberry milkshake:**
>
> Milkfat, non-fat milk, sugar, sweet whey, high fructose corn syrup, guar gum, monoglycerides and diglycerides, cellulose gum, sodium phosphate, carageenan, citric acid, E129 and "artificial strawberry flavour": **What exactly is artificial strawberry flavour? Glad you asked, here are just a few of the possible ingredients:** amyl acetate, amyl butyrate, amyl valerate, anethol, anisyl formate, benzyl acetate, benzyle isobutyrate, butyric acid, cinnamyl isobutyrate, cinnamyl valerate, cognac essential oil, diacetyl, dipropyl ketone, ethyl butyrate, ethyl cinnamate, ethyl heptanoae, ethyl heptylate, ethyl lactate, ethyl methylphenylglycidate, ethyl nitrate, ethyl propionate, ethyl valerate, heliotropin, hydroxyphrenyl-e-butanone (10% solution in alcohol), ionone, isobutyl anthranilate, isobutyl butyrate, lemon essential oil, maltol, 4-methylacetophenone, methyl anthranilate, methyl benzoate, methyl cinnamate, methyl heptine carbonate, methyl napthyl ketone, methyl salicylate, mint essential oil, neroli essential oil, nerolin, neryl isobutyrate, orris butter, phenethyl alcohol, rose, rum ether, undecalactone, vanillin, and solvent.

Not only do synthetic chemicals have the potential to "trick" your body into eating more by inhibiting the satiety mechanism, but they may also damage the body's ability to burn off existing fat stores, which is where many of these chemicals are stored. Talk about a one-two punch. **Not only are you eating too much and you don't know it, but now your body is not**

letting go of the fat you are storing because it makes a nice storage spot for the xenobiotic chemicals you are absorbing or ingesting. It is kind of like going to the dentist and having a root canal, and on your way out, the receptionist decides to give you a swift kick in the nuts.

Entire books have been written on the topic of environmental toxins and their adverse effects on human health. Therefore it is well beyond the scope of this singular chapter to delve into more detail than an initial introduction on how these chemicals may be affecting your ability to lose both weight and body fat. If you are still not convinced that environmental toxins may be limiting your body's ability to burn excess fat stores and calories, a few books I highly recommend reading are Dr. Mark Schauss' *Achieving Victory Over a Toxic World*, Dr. Sherry Rogers' *Detoxify or Die*, and Dr. Paula Ballie-Hamilton's *Toxic Overload*.

Now that we understand that chemicals can have a significant impact on our health and weight management, what are some of these toxins and what can we do about them? A great website to start with is the Environmental Working Groups website www.ewg.org. Some of the chemicals affecting our health are found during our everyday routine. In his book, Achieving Victory Over a Toxic World, Dr. Mark Schauss goes on to demonstrate the minor toxic exposures before we even leave the door for work in the morning. From the flame retardants in the mattresses we sleep on, to the chemicals in our cosmetics, food supply, and water, the toxic exposures just seem to be unavoidable and add up, everyday, over a life time.

How do we combat this toxic overload? Certainly not by living in a bubble! Methods of detoxification are a good place to start.

When one mentions detoxification, what exactly are they talking about? Our body has several different mechanisms or filters that it uses to cleanse and rid itself of wastes and toxins. Some of these filters along with their processes include, the skin (sweating), the lungs (expelling CO_2/inhaling O_2), the colon, the kidneys, and last but certainly not least, the liver.

With regards to detoxification, the two filters we will be talking about are the kidneys and liver. Each day the kidneys process about 200 quarts of blood, filtering out approximately 2-3 quarts of toxic byproducts and water (depending on levels of toxic exposures and water retention). It also plays a critical role as an endocrine organ, affecting PH and blood pressure regulation, maintenance of calcium/potassium balance, etc.. What happens inside the kidneys is a chemical process by which byproducts from the blood are absorbed into the urinary system to be excreted later, while the filtered blood is then circulated back through the body.

The liver is regarded as the main detoxification organ of the human body. It breaks down all environmental pollutants/toxins which enter our body through our skin, food we eat, air we breathe, water we drink, etc... Detoxifying nearly two quarts of blood every minute, this efficient organ can clear nearly 99% of the toxins and bacteria from the blood during the first round of cleansing.

The liver is so important that every vein from our digestive system empties into it to filter out pollutants and toxic byproducts from our food and drink, (with today's modern westernized diet, many people suffer from overworked livers). No wonder there are so many diseases popping up each day, as doctors have found that diminished liver function is often a precursor to many diseases.

Not only identified as a primary detoxification organ, the liver also wears many other hats. It serves as a storage center for glucose in the form of glycogen, as well as storage of critical vitamins required by the body. It also manages thousands of enzymes, produces and regulates hormones, produces bile, and regulates tissue and blood clotting. Just by

> Did you know that the Tyrannasuarus Rex would always look to eat the liver of its fallen prey first, as it somehow sensed the greatest supply of vitamins (possibly the B vitamins) in this organ?

listing only a few of the functions, it is evident that the liver can easily become overworked, especially with an excessive toxic burden compromising its effectiveness.

The two processes of liver detoxification are known as Phase I detoxification and Phase 2 detoxification. The liver's primary method of detoxification is similar to that of a processing plant. Toxins are shuttled to the liver through the bloodstream or digestive system for chemical processing in which the compounds of the toxin are chemically changed and packaged up for excretion at a later time.

Phase I is where the toxins are chemically altered and packaged up for secretion. This occurs through an enzyme system known as the P-450 enzyme system. An individual's sensitivity to certain chemicals can provide insight into the efficiency/effectiveness of one's P-450 system.

A simple way of determining the health of one's P-450 activity is to measure the sensitivity toward caffeine. If a person is very sensitive to caffeine, their P-450 system may not be efficient at transforming it to a water-soluble form, in which the body can easily excrete it through the kidneys.

Without proper detoxification ability, a myriad of health issues can occur. Basically an internal system breakdown can occur, as other organs will become overworked due to the lack of efficient functioning of the liver as a detoxification filter.

Phase 2 detoxification utilizes the production and secretion of bile. This system is actually six different pathways through which toxin excretion can occur. The six pathways are:

- **Amino Acid Conjugation**
- **Glutathione Conjugation**
- **Methylation**
- **Acetylation**
- **Sulfation**
- **Glucuronidation**

Each of these pathways involves different enzymatic processes requiring various vitamins, minerals, and amino acids (and their metabolites) to function properly. Working collectively to properly detoxify the body, each pathway is also responsible for the detoxification of certain chemicals and toxins, as their constituents have affinities toward certain chemicals and toxins. Feel free to pick up any number of books available on the dangers of impaired detoxification or functional human anatomy for further detail on these processes.

To sum it up, if your detoxification process is failing you, all the environmental toxins from the food you eat, the deodorant you rub under your arm each morning, and the fumes you inhale during your morning commute are absorbed directly into your system. With no place to go, these environmental toxins can be absorbed by fat cells or left to linger somewhere in one, if not all, of your body's systems.

Depending on whom you ask, methods of detoxification can vary greatly with regards to effectiveness. For each method there seems to be the die-hard advocates and their rally-cry opponents. Let's take a quick peek at a few of the options:

a. **Sweat:** Whether from Hot Yoga, Far Infrared Sauna Therapy, Indian Sweat Lodges, and even high sweat inducing workouts, sweating is one of the body's natural mechanisms for ridding itself of toxins.

b. **Paleolithic Nutrition:** This method is an effective way to ensure your body is ingesting minimal amounts of toxins found in our food supplies. Organic berries and vegetables, wild caught fish, grass fed meat and dairy, etc, etc. Studies have shown Paleolithic Nutrition, or eating the foods one is genetically programmed to eat, to be very effective in lowering cardiovascular risk markers, lowering C-reactive protein, increasing insulin sensitivity, decreasing bodyweight, and decreasing blood pressure.

Studies have actually taken place in which the researchers have followed Australian aborigines out of their natural environment and into a westernized culture [8,9,10,11]. Here they consumed a westernized diet consisting of processed foods, cereal grain carbohydrates, food additives, low levels of saturated fats (egg whites instead of whole eggs for example), and sugary drinks. After making the transition from their traditional lifestyle to a westernized lifestyle, many of these aborigines developed symptoms of metabolic syndrome or diabetes, including elevated cholesterol levels, insulin resistance, body fat accumulation, and increased blood pressure [8,9,10,11,12,13].

One of the most remarkable outcomes of these studies occurred when the researchers returned some of these aborigines back to their traditional hunter/gatherer lifestyle for a 7-week period. Amazingly, but not surprisingly, almost all the subjects realized significant improvements in carbohydrate and lipid metabolism, leading to decreased blood pressure, cholesterol, body fat/obesity, increased insulin sensitivity, as well as improvements in other symptoms of metabolic syndrome and diabetes (8,9,10,11,12,13). These studies have shown that just by altering one's lifestyle for a period of 7 weeks, one can reverse a negative health and wellness profile without the use of modern day pharmaceuticals or medical procedures. Even more interesting is how there wasn't and still isn't more publicity based on these studies.

So, what does a Paleolithic Nutrition look like? If one can hunt, fish, catch, or gather it, they can eat it (poisonous plants/berries/mushrooms aside). *Read Dr. Loren Cordain's excellent book "The Paleo Diet" for an in-depth analysis of this type of nutrition, as well as a menu of meals and weekly food planning. This book is highly recommended.*

c. **Massage**: By improving circulation, one can improve the function of the internal organs. Basically with improved circulation, there is an increased oxygen supply and blood cleansing that occurs. Healthy blood is then circulated throughout the body, while toxic blood is shuttled to the liver for cleansing. Along with this increased circulation, enhanced digestive function and lymph flow becomes evident. Besides, what better way to detoxify your body than to lay there and get a relaxing total body massage.

d. **Neutraceutical Detoxification:** Today's diet consists of a recommended daily allowance of certain nutrients, vitamins, and minerals. Unfortunately, these recommendations can be drastically deficient due to the fact that the RDA is the minimum amount that is required not to get sick. But when you are talking about people dealing with increased stressors, toxic exposures, lack of digestive acids/enzymes, leaky gut syndrome, diets consisting of high levels of processed carbohydrates, etc, the RDA is just not going to cut it!

Never mind the fact that even natural organic food today has much less vitamins and mineral content than its counterparts just 30 years ago. This is the result of excessive soil stripping, synthetic crops *(Read Michael Pollan's Omnivores Dilemma to learn all about synthetic corn and how it rotates with soy)*, and increased pesticide use.

Chinese medicinal herbal remedies have also been used for centuries to strengthen the liver and increase the body's ability to detox. Below are a just a few of the more common neutraceutical supplements used for detoxification purposes:

1. **Wheatgrass and Greens:** Chlorophyll, found in high quantities in both wheatgrass and greens powders, is known for its ability to pull toxins from the body, cleanse blood supply, and improve oxygen supply to the circulatory system. Wheatgrass (along with certain seaweeds) has been found to be very high in this detoxifying agent. The health benefits of wheatgrass are so effective that many positive research studies are echoing these findings. For instance, wheatgrass was found to be beneficial to patients undergoing chemotherapy. While having zero negative effect on the chemo results, the wheatgrass was found to minimize the usage of blood building meds, resulting in positive effects on blood cell counts. Wheatgrass has also been used in the treatment of gastrointestinal issues and chelation of heavy metals.

   Wheatgrass has become such an important element in the detoxification process, that it is one of the prime "ingredients" in the detoxification programs at the world renowned Hippocrates Health Institute in Florida.

2. **Fiber:** Fiber comes in many forms and from many foods. Vegetables, legumes, nuts, beans, and some "unprocessed grains" are all strong sources of fiber. Some of the best supplemental sources of fiber with regards to detoxification are citrus

pectin fiber and psyllium husk. Basically acting as a broom, fiber expands once inside the digestive tract, pushing toxic particles down through the intestines and colon until eventually excreted. Fiber is an important part in the detoxification process. Certain types of fiber have also been associated with decreased risk of cancer, diabetes, estrogen dominance, and cardiovascular disease.

3. **B-Vitamin Complex**: In particular, vitamin B6, B9 (often referred to as folic acid), and B12 (preferably methylated) are regarded as the lipotropic B-vitamins. They promote the production and flow of bile. Regarded as one of the six types of Phase II detoxification, methylation is the metabolism of B-vitamins. Basically a methyl group is donated to a toxin, forming SAM (S-adenosylmethionine). SAM, which is synthesized from methionine, acts to then neutralize estrogens as well as promote and restore bile flow. So, without adequate methylated B-vitamins available, these processes may lose their efficiency and quickly be rendered ineffective.

4. **Vitamin C:** As a major vitamin responsible for the body's ability to eliminate sulfur and other antibiotic based drugs, inadequate levels of vitamin C may cause a dysfunction in the human detoxification processes. Along with its potent antioxidant properties, Vitamin C has been shown to promote the increase in red blood cell glutathione, which in turn allows for more efficient Phase II detoxification.

5. **Phosphatidylcholine:** The most abundant phospholipid of the cellular membrane, phosphatidylcholine protects the liver from invading toxins and other bacteria. Basically without this protective "shield", the overburdened liver can no longer function properly, leaving the body susceptible to greater toxic buildup and eventual sickness.

6. **Glycine**: This amino acid is critically important in the detoxification systems of the human body. Being one of the amino acids (along with cysteine and glutamic

acid) that makes up the human antioxidant, Glutathione, when levels of glycine are down, so are levels of Glutathione. Playing a major role in the detoxification of xenobiotics such as benzene, xylene, and toluene, glycine is also the most commonly used amino acid in Phase II detoxification. All the more reason to eat a diet high in proteins. Check your stomach HCL levels for adequate production of pepsin to breakdown those proteins, and try supplementing with Glycine if there is concern. By the way, both Glycine and Taurine are very reasonably priced supplements, even for quality products.

7. **Taurine:** Taurine is an amino acid that is commonly deficient in individuals with increased sensitivity to chemical (weakened P-450 detoxification system). Being made from cysteine, which is another important component of glutathione, tuarine levels will rapidly decrease in individuals with overburdened detoxification systems and daily exposures to environmental toxins.

8. **Calcium D-Glucarate**: Calcium D Glucarate is the bioavailable form of glucaric acid. When trying to learn why diets high in certain fruits and vegetables had positive effects on degenerative diseases and cancer, researchers found one of the major common links to be, you guessed it, Calcium D Glucarate. As a primary agent in Phase II detoxification (Glucoronidation), glucoronic acid not only has potent effects on detoxifying estrogens, food additives, and chemicals from the body, but it can also increase testosterone levels by correcting estrogen/androgen ratios.

9. **N-Acetylcysteine** (NAC): A metabolite formed from the amino acid cysteine, NAC has been shown to increase glutathione synthesis. For this reason, NAC is a highly important antioxidant in the Phase II detoxification process. N-acetylcysteine has been shown to reduce the risk of certain types of cancer, enhance immune cell function, and the scavenging of heavy metals in the body. This inexpensive supplement works well with Vitamin C.

Herbs and Adaptogens

Holy Basil (Ocimum Sanctum or sometimes referred to as Tulsi): This Indian herb is not only known for its neurorprotective and hepoprotective properties, but it has also been shown to induce calmness, reduce cortisol levels, regulate thyroid functioning, and enhance cognitive functioning. Of significance is this adaptogen's ability to regulate blood sugar levels and reduce brain fog. Back in ancient times, this herb was even used to treat people bitten by desert scorpions and snakes.

Licorice Root: The "Sweet Root" is known as a remedy for liver damage and cirrhosis. This ancient herb has been effective in treating chemical, pesticide, lead, and arsenic poisoning. Through its anti-inflammatory properties, Licorice root has been used in the battle against autoimmune diseases and intestinal permeability issues (aka: leaky gut syndrome). Another important use has been in the regulation of the adrenal function. By aiding in the restoration of the adrenals, many individuals taking licorice have found elevated morning energy and awareness, as well as stress alleviation. This may be due to its modulatory effects on the stress hormone, cortisol.

Reishi Mushroom (Ganoderma Lucidum): Known in Chinese medicine as the "spirit plant", this potent family of mushrooms is a treasured adaptogen in Chinese medicine. These mushrooms have been known to strengthen the immune system, enhance vision, relax and strengthen connective tissues, strengthen the endocrine system, improve cardiovascular function, improve cognitive function, assist with kidney function, alleviate insomnia, and, of course, aid in the detoxification processes of the human body by protecting the liver.

Shisandra: This berry has been used for the treatment of everything from night sweats to diarrhea. Whether it be reducing stress or enhancing the immune system, this versatile adaptogen is a highly regarded element of Chinese

Medicine. It has been shown to have liver cell regenerative properties, but of even greater significance Shisandra is known to have beneficial effects on increasing hepatic glutathione levels.

GoldenSeal: Known for its antimicrobial effects, the "Orange Root" has been used in the battle against intestinal pathogens and many other disorders of the GI tract. Through its anti-inflammatory and astringent properties, Goldenseal has been used in the treatment of liver disease, colitis, and ulcers.

Turmeric rhizome: Not just a popular tea or spice for food, turmeric also has many Ayurveda properties. From its well-documented anti-inflammatory properties to its ability to remedy digestive and gastrointestinal issues, turmeric is a widely used and is an easily obtainable herb. Other benefits include antiseptic and antibacterial properties, as well as potential benefits for those suffering from arthritis.

Lycium: Better known as the Goji Berry, Lycium is believed to be one of nature's most potent antioxidants. Due to its relative closeness to the sun (typically found in extremely high altitudes), this berry must develop "thick skin" to withstand the potentially damaging rays. With this "thick skin" comes it's incredible antioxidant properties.

Understanding Chinese Medicine saying, *"The liver opens the eyes"*, one can understand why people have claimed enhanced vision and eyesight when taking this potent antioxidant on a regular basis (possibly due to the large amount of flavonoids and carotenoids). Goji berries can regenerate liver cells, as well as protect the liver from damage from hepatotoxic chemicals. Lycium has also been used for its cardiovascular, blood sugar, and immune benefits. As a matter of fact, some individuals have even used Lycium as a supplement to cancer treatment.

Uva Ursi Leaf: Otherwise known as bearberry, this evergreen shrub leaf is widely accepted for its antiseptic and diuretic properties. Typically used for urinary tract function and health, Uva Ursi has been recommended for kidney stones and bladder infections. It is also beneficial in promoting liver, spleen, pancreas, lung, and heart health, as well as regulating blood sugar levels.

Juniper Berry: These berries have quite an array of uses. From stomach and indigestion issues, to kidney and bladder health, the juniper berry has many non-medicinal uses as well, including beer (found in Sweden).

Peppermint Leaf: Peppermint has been used as an effective liver and gallbladder -stimulating herb. By improving bile flow it helps rid the body of toxins, and promotes healthy kidney functioning and digestion. Peppermint has also been used for respiratory issues, circulation, cramping, and stomach issues.

Yellow dock root: Yellow dock has been used in the treatment of skin, liver, and digestive problems. It may be one of the most powerful herbs in repairing poor liver function and ridding the body of toxins. Along with the stimulation of bile and digestive enzymes, yellow dock can be used as an astringent for rashes, bites, burns, hemorrhoids, and various other skin problems. Yellow dock root also has anti-inflammatory and laxative properties. It can even be used as mouthwash.

Milk Thistle Seed: Widely known and recognized as a liver specific herb, Silybum marianum contains silymarin, which is known for its protective properties on the specialized cells of the liver that are responsible for the removal of bacteria and toxins. Individuals have been prescribed Milk thistle to fight long-term poison/toxin exposure, as well as to repair the liver from damage caused by medications and drugs. Milk thistle basically has the ability to enhance the body's detoxification processes by binding to, neutralizing, and eliminating toxins.

Dandelion Root: The dandelion is well established as an important herb in the human body's detoxification processes. With high amounts of beta-carotene and potassium, dandelion has been used to treat liver, kidney, and digestive disorders. From the regulation of blood sugar, to the scavenging of free radicals, this electrolyte-balancing herb may be a potent ally in the regulation of human health.

NOTE*When shopping for detoxification herbs, it may be wise to learn the differences between the potential effects of these herbs. For instance, some herbs will have laxative effects, which can stimulate the intestines to flush out various toxins. On the other hand, other herbs may bring about diuretic effects, eliminating toxins through the excretion of fluids from the urinary tract.*

e. **Detoxification Centers**: Check out the website for the Hippocrates Health Institute in Florida www.hippocratesinst.org. From daily exercise and macrobiotic eating, to sauna and massage therapy, this facility is known world-wide for promoting positive healing effects and life altering wisdom. One of their main ingredients: Wheatgrass.

For further education on toxic exposure and detoxification, the following books are highly recommended:

1. ***Achieving Victory over a Toxic World*** by Dr. Mark Schauss: Not only does this book hit on some very emotional and personal notes in Dr. Schauss' life (his daughter's battle against grand maul epileptic seizures), but it is also packed with very useful information on toxic exposures, where these toxins can be found, and possible methods of neutralizing their effects on the body.

2. ***The Hundred Year Lie*** by Randall Fitzgerald: To be honest, this eye - opening book is very hard to put down. Once you finish it not only do you want to tell everybody you know to read it, but you will also find yourself re-reading it. Packed with information, Fitzgerald's timeline

section on toxic exposures and the health of our society is worth the price of the book alone. A must read!!

3. *The Body Restoration Plan* by Dr. Paula Ballie-Hamilton: Along with Dr. Sherry Rogers, Dr. Ballie-Hamilton has to be regarded as one of the best environmental health doctors on the planet. In this book, not only does she provide a valuable introduction as to why you may be toxic, but she also provides a plan (complete with diet) for what to do about it.

4. *Detoxify or Die* by Dr. Sherry Rogers: This book is quite possibly the most eye-opening and important book on toxic exposure and how it affects our health. If you have never read one of Dr. Rogers' books, *Detoxify or Die* is a pretty good place to start. From her tireless research, to her ability to translate complex scientific information into easy to read and understand writing, Dr. Rogers is truly a genius in the health and wellness community.

5. *The Anti-Estrogenic Diet* by Ori Hofmekler: Easy to read and to the point, the author of *The Warrior Diet* now tackles a problem facing much of our society today: excess estrogen. Hofmekler describes where these excess estrogens come from, what they do to the human body, and what to do about it. Good book, easy to read, and straight to the point.

CHAPTER IV

DIGESTIVE PROBLEMS

Did you know that roughly 70-80% of your body's immune system is located in your gut (3,5).? Knowing this, then why do so many people fail to take care of it? Perhaps like most, they have never heard about this through the popular media outlets. Their doctor has never educated them on this subject, and, it certainly has not been discussed by the experts on any major television networks. Damage to the "tight junctions" of the epithelial cells of the intestinal lining has been associated with poor dietary habits (26), NSAIDs (26), antibiotics (29), stress (24), inadequate kidney function (1), low levels of healthy gut flora (including lactobacilli and bifido bacterium), and exposures to environmental toxins (18).

Just as important as gut health, so is the ability of the digestive system to properly break down food, absorb the constituents, and excrete waste products. If you cannot digest and break down your foods properly, how can you expect to absorb enough nutrients, vitamins, and minerals to maintain optimal health? Combined with an overburdened liver, digestive problems such as "leaky gut syndrome" (intestinal hyper permeability) cause your body to battle with itself. This creates an autoimmune response to the large food particles and unfiltered waste products that have leaked through the intestinal fissures and into your bloodstream (9). Because of the increased permeability, the body is then susceptible to bacteria and environmental toxins also seeping into the bloodstream (18).

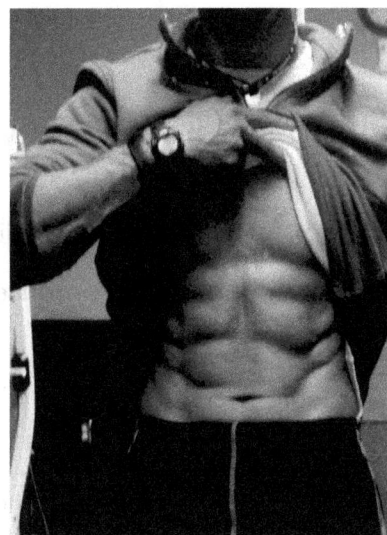

Your body sees these particles as dangerous invaders, sending out the firefighters (cytokines →lymphocytes) to put out the fire. The net result of the body's battle to extinguish the flames is the production of oxidants/free radicals. These can lead to systemic inflammation and some of the previously discussed symptoms in other parts of the body.

What can we do to fix our digestive problems so we begin to absorb the vitamins, minerals, and nutrients from our food properly while avoiding the potentially dangerous symptoms associated with compromised digestive function? Fixing your diet may be a good place to start. A healthy diet can lead to many positive outcomes, the least of which is repairing your gut. Secondly, repairing the intestinal lining and increasing digestive tract functioning should be an obvious choice.

In the realm of functional medicine, practitioners and doctors utilize specific methods of screening the body for deficiencies and intestinal permeability. Outside of your general doctor ordering a gastric analysis or Heidelberg capsule test, a reasonable mineral absorption test may be a hair mineral analysis or Zinc Tally test. These tests can be used to help determine if a client is producing enough stomach acid to effectively breakdown their food so they can properly absorb zinc. In addition they may provide valuable insight into hydrochloric acid levels in the stomach and absorption of other nutrients, vitamins, and minerals.

Oh, that burning in my stomach

Any discussion about digestion is not complete without an evaluation of one of the most important substances produced by our body during the digestive process: Hydrochloric Acid (stomach acid).

Contradictory to what is pushed on us through heavy marketing campaigns paid for by patent and profit driven pharmaceutical companies and doctors who receive much of their continuing education through these same pharmaceutical company sponsored events, *in many cases high stomach acid levels are not the cause for acid reflux (GERD)* (13,15). In fact, it may be the exact opposite. Low stomach acid levels combined with a dysfunctional LES (Lower Esophageal Sphincter) and fermenting sugar (from those poor dietary habits) in the stomach are frequently the causes of acid reflux (13).

So the answer is yes, it is stomach acid (HCL) that causes the heartburn pain and irritation. But too much? Unlikely. When chronically poor nutrition, excessive drinking, smoking, food allergies and sensitivities, environmental toxin exposures, or elevated levels of stress are present, the lining of the stomach can become irritated and inflamed (23). As a result, certain cells that make up the lining of the small intestine (parietal cells) can no longer function properly and begin to die off. These cells are responsible for the production of HCL (hydrochloric acid), otherwise known as "stomach acid".

With this decrease in the number of parietal cells comes a decrease in the production of HCL, along with another important digestive compound secreted in these cells called intrinsic factor (12,27). With this lack of digestive ability, LES (lower esophageal sphincter) functioning can become compromised, leading to improper valve functioning, allowing the stomach acid you do have to reflux back up into the esophagus. This refluxing can then cause the burning and irritation that is symptomatic of heartburn.

It is interesting to note that the term heartburn refers to pain and inflammation of the esophagus and not pain and irritation of the stomach. But yet, if we do complain of heartburn, a gastro scope or esophageal X-ray may be recommended. Even further yet, the pharmaceuticals we may be prescribed are typically used to "knock out" stomach acid, even though we have never had our actual *STOMACH* acid levels checked? Understanding that the refluxing acid in our esophagus is a symptom of what is actually going on in our stomach, wouldn't it be wise to check our stomach acid levels first prior to prescribing acid blocking medications? (*Hair Mineral analysis and tubeless gastric analysis are two very non-invasive methods of measuring stomach acid levels.*)

Have you noticed that the ads for certain acid reflux medications and drugs no longer mention "elevated or high stomach acid levels" in their commercials? Perhaps they can't, because it may not true.

As of 2008, an estimated 100 million Americans get heartburn, generating **over $10 billion in sales.**

It is interesting to note that people are taking a drug that they assume is for high stomach acid levels, while the culprit may be the opposite, low stomach acid levels (as well as the previously mentioned dysfunctional LES). Studies have shown that when stomach acid levels, not esophageal acid levels, are tested, oftentimes those suffering from GERD (acid reflux) have insufficient levels of HCL (11). Rather than taking a pharmaceutical, why not try to correct the actual deficiency by bringing the HCL levels back to normal?

The best way to think about digestion and stomach acid is: ***how can we expect the food we eat to be efficiently broken down into the nutrient constituents without the presence of proper amounts of stomach acid?*** If you do not have enough stomach acid present, you may not be able to properly break down your food thereby creating a malabsorption of minerals, vitamins, and nutrients (31).

If your stomach acid levels are low, chances are you are not absorbing many crucial minerals such as magnesium, zinc, or iron. Combine this with a decreased absorption of certain B-vitamins and you may be heading toward some negative health consequences. Lastly, if you are not breaking down your proteins into their amino acid constituents your bodily reparation, hormonal functioning, and neurotransmitter functioning may be compromised (7,16).

When food is eaten, it passes down the esophagus through the LES and into the stomach. As food enters the stomach, the lining is then stretched. The stretching triggers specialized cells known as G Cells, to release gastrin (as well as Histamine), a hormone that regulates the release of HCL from the parietal cells. As the parietal cells secrete more stomach acid to break down the food, they also begin to secrete intrinsic factor to help with B12 absorption.

To bring more complexity to this process, the gastrin also stimulates the release of pepsin (well actually pepsinogens, which are then converted into pepsin when they come in contact with stomach acid). Once this process takes place, proteins can be broken down into amino acids for absorption. Hormones such as secretin, cholecystokinin (CCK) and other pancreatic and digestive enzymes are secreted to aid in furthering the digestive processes.

As you can see, digestion from mouth to end product is quite a complex process. If there is a deficiency in any step of this process, complications in the breakdown and absorption of food may occur. Normally, stomach acid levels rise gastrin begins to level off. But, if your stomach acid levels are low to begin with, gastrin may be secreted in excess leading to peptic ulcers, atrophic gastritis, or even the H. pylori infection.

Another example is the domino effect that may occur with a decrease in the release of pepsin due to low levels of HCL. Pepsin is the enzyme required for the breakdown of proteins. Stomach acid (HCL) and pepsin go hand in hand. If HCL levels are low, pepsin levels follow suit. And with low pepsin levels comes a decreased ability to breakdown proteins into amino acid.

If proteins are not properly broken down, a deficiency in certain amino acids can result. Some of these amino acids are essential for the production of hormones in the body. For example the hormones thyroxine and catecholamines are synthesized from the amino acids tyrosine and tryptophan. A deficiency in these amino acids has been shown to affect behavior patterns in both men and women [16]. Depression, anxiety, irritability and insomnia may result from the change in brain chemical composition because the lack of building blocks needed to make many important hormones.

Other health issues that may arise from having low levels of stomach acid include the manifestation of bacteria, including H. pylori, as well as deficiencies in key vitamins and minerals including B12, B6, Zinc, iron, magnesium, copper, and others. From asthma to cancer, the body becomes susceptible to multiple forms of disease and dysfunction when lacking these vital compounds.

With regards to bacterial overgrowth, there is a symbiotic relationship with these houseguests. They help to maintain our health through various functions. In fact, the gut flora is the first line of defense against infection and disease. Gut flora may play a key role in diabetes and obesity, as well as autoimmune diseases. Eating a proper diet and supplementing with probiotics may increase healthy gut flora [4]. These healthy bacteria also play a prominent role in the absorption of minerals and the manufacturing of important B vitamins.

With too little stomach acid, the bad bacteria are allowed to multiply by creeping their way up the intestinal track from the small intestine, eventually settling in the stomach. Here they can colonize, wreaking havoc on the digestive processes. Without proper stomach acid levels, this bacterial overgrowth can lead to a myriad of health issues [23].

Leaky Gut Syndrome

Another interesting phenomenon that occurs with low stomach acids levels is "Leaky Gut Syndrome". When the food particles are not broken down properly, they can compromise the lining of the small intestine.

When the small intestine is functioning properly, the lined walls act as a semi-permeable barrier between the intestinal tract and our bloodstream. This keeps bacteria and particles that are too large from passing through the wall and into our bloodstream, yet still allowing those that are properly digested into it [8]. Under healthy circumstances, nutrients, electrolytes, and water are selectively absorbed through the intestinal barrier, while other particles manage to pass between the cells through adhesions of the junctions [19]. It is these gaps between the cells that we need to worry about.

Increased intestinal permeability is otherwise known as leaky gut syndrome. It is not a disease, but studies have shown intestinal permeability can lead to a variety of symptoms that can manifest into more serious complications including fatigue [20], asthma [2], depression [20], IBS [9], Crohn's disease [22,25], cystic acne [9], rheumatoid arthritis [28], migraines [30], and various other autoimmune dysfunctions. Amazingly, it has also been associated with diabetes [18], kidney disease [24], and autism [10].

An interesting side note, many professionals in the medical community still view "leaky gut syndrome" as one of those holistic healthcare diseases. If you tell your doctor you think you may have this condition, he will probably look at you like you have two

> Polycephaly is a condition in which an animal has more than one head.

heads and think you are crazy. It is only a matter of time before this becomes a legitimate health issue in the eyes of doctors. Pharmaceutical companies are now targeting the proteins of the epithelial lining for a new line of drugs [14].

I can see the commercial now: Do you find yourself going to the bathroom often? Do you have symptoms of arthritis, migraines, fibromyalgia, depression, or Crohn's disease? Do you suffer from fatigue? If so, the new wonder drug, "Leakitor" may be appropriate. Talk to your doctor if you are experiencing any of these symptoms, because in clinical studies, "Leakitor" was found to alleviate symptoms by 50% (when combined with proper diet and other lifestyle changes, of course). Leakitor may not be for everybody, as those with heart disease, high blood pressure, elevated oxidized LDL, liver problems, kidney problems, are pregnant or nursing, or a heartbeat may experience serious side effects including Alzheimer's, cancer, depression, and elevated liver enzymes. Ouch…….. Ah yes, the next billion dollar pharmaceutical blockbuster.

In summary, if stomach acid levels are not up to par, you may not be getting the most out of your food (vitamins, minerals, proteins), especially if what you are eating has remarkably low if any nutritional value to begin with. When taking heartburn medications and antacids, without a proper gastric analysis, you may be pushing your stomach acid levels even lower, which in turn leaves the body susceptible to multiple forms of disease and sickness over the long haul (58 Koop).

Restoring stomach acid levels may be an effective method of increasing vitamin and mineral absorption, increasing protein digestion, and decreasing the side effects of improper digestion and heartburn. If stomach acid levels are tested low, combining proper nutrition intervention with supplementary digestive enzymes and HCL+Pepsin is a good place to start when trying to enhance overall quality of health. Consulting with a qualified functional medicine doctor is recommended to determine if these are necessary.

Other nutraceutical supplement interventions that may be effective in digestive repair include zinc, glutamine, Aloe, probiotics, vitamin C, vitamin A, and methylated B-vitamin complex.

CHAPTER V

YOUR HORMONES ARE OUT OF BALANCE

A Brief overview.

Through the course of a single day, your body goes through a significant amount of hormonal variations to maintain homeostasis or hormonal balance. Let's scratch the surface and look at how our hormones may be affected by the normal actions of daily life.

It's 6 a.m. and the alarm clock is chiming a classic childhood song on one of the oldies stations that saturate the radio waves. Our body wakes up and thus begins the day. Early morning cortisol levels provide us with energy needed to awaken from a restful night's sleep. As you continue to energize throughout the morning, you may also reach for a cup of coffee for the extra stimulant effect.

The caffeine in the coffee can trigger a fight or flight response from the catecholamines, inducing an increase in heart rate, blood pressure, and heightened energy. From here you may decide to have breakfast. Certain breakfast food choices will elicit specific hormonal and neurotransmitter responses. For instance, a bagel will dramatically spike up insulin secretion while ramping up the production of the neurotransmitter serotonin. On the healthier side, a steak and macadamia nuts will elicit a more favorable insulin response while increasing the production of the neurotransmitters acetylcholine and dopamine.

Once you finish breakfast, you brush your teeth and throw on some hair gel and deodorant. Unknowingly, you are smearing chemical estrogens known as xenoestrogens onto your scalp and under your armpits. These estrogen mimicking chemicals can be found in any number of personal care products, raising your body's toxic burden while increasing environmental estrogen stored throughout your bodily tissue, specifically in the fat cells.

Out the door, you hop into your car and off to fight the morning commute on your way to work. For the first 45 minutes it's a smooth ride until another driver decides to cut you off. A fight/stress response is accompanied by a release of more cortisol. A beep of the horn and the obligatory hand gesture and you are now stressed and in a bad mood for the rest of your commute.

Upon arrival at work, you learn from your boss that your presentation to one of the company's largest clients was a hit and they have agreed to utilize your product for another year. Your luck has changed and so has your mood. With success comes the secretion of the anabolic hormones. Now, your mood is positive, while your mental clarity is up and stress levels down.

Throughout the rest of the morning, you work on the finishing points of the deal and perhaps indulge in a little celebratory offering from the vending machine down the hall. Once again, there is a hefty spike in your insulin levels triggering a similar secretion of serotonin. About a half hour later you feel the energy crash from the high glycemic snack, and a mid-afternoon nap may be in order during your lunch break.

During this nap your body and brain are in recovery and repair mode thanks to the actions of certain hormones. The nap may help to reduce your body's levels of stress hormones while aiding in the production of anabolic hormones.

Upon waking up from your mid-day siesta, you decide to have some green tea and get back to work. Around 3p.m. you are feeling the hunger cravings again and reach for a supposedly healthy granola bar for some energy. Little did you know, this processed granola bar would spike your insulin up again followed by an energy crash later.

It is now an hour later and time to put an order in for the mid-afternoon pick-me-up, better known as coffee. This coffee may have the same effect as the morning version, giving you an energy jolt while stimulating your catecholamines and slightly elevating your stress hormones.

It is now 5p.m. and time to leave work and head to the gym for a workout. Arriving at the gym after a 60 minute commute, you are ready to burn some energy, at least what little energy you still have. After getting changed, you try to decide: Cardio or weights. Well, your endurance athlete friend says cardio is better at burning calories, while weights may get you big and bulky. Which to choose? With that you opt for 55 minutes on the elliptical machine followed by 10 minutes of abs. Little did you know, with that decision, you opted for the exercise modality that elicits the greatest stress hormone response, whereas the weight training would have elicited the greatest anabolic hormone response (depending on how you train).

About 20 minutes into the cardio you begin to hit your groove, feeling the resultant rush or runner's high from the release of endorphins and other neurotransmitters. Unbeknownst to you, at about the 50 minute mark, your stress hormones are peaking. After completing the cardio, you work the abs for an additional 10 minutes and head home.

Once home, you grab dinner, specifically a carb laden dinner. Once again, you ingest more carbs and just a little protein, so the insulin rollercoaster can continue. With dinner you decide that since you worked out, you deserve to kick a couple of cold ones back. One thing is for certain, from the looks of the spare tire above your waist, you were unaware that beer not only has some powerful effects on your insulin and cortisol, but it also contains estrogen.

After a few beers, it's on to the couch to catch up on TV. Sitting there, you feel yourself beginning to crash. The energy crash from the combination of depleted adrenals, low blood sugar, and overall fatigue has you zombie walking to bed for a well-deserved night's sleep.

Thanks to your body's natural regulation mechanisms, at about 3a.m., while in deep sleep, you begin to secrete growth hormone pulses to aid in healing and recovery from the previous day. A few hours later, your body begins to awaken you with the production and secretion of cortisol. And thus the hormonal cycle begins again.

Enter Stress

We encounter various forms of stress throughout our lives. In some cases, it becomes constant in our daily lives and can be responsible for many degenerative health issues. With this stress comes the increased production of our body's stress fighting hormones. These hormones can put an excessive burden on the body's adrenal system and forces other organs of the endocrine system to take up the slack. Decreases in androgen hormone production, increases in catabolic hormone production, decreased insulin sensitivity, and compromised thyroid function can all result.

Along with these negative hormonal effects, stress creates the oxidative by-products known as free radicals. With increased free radical production and endocrine disruption other bodily systems become compromised. From ineffective detoxification function of the liver, kidneys, and lymphatic system, to increased risk of cardiovascular episodes and cancer, your hormones play a major role in regulating your health. When overburdened by stress, an abundance of disruptive events occur and challenge your body's ability to maintain homeostasis.

Hormones are not as simple as the earlier story would illustrate. There is an endless feedback loop of mechanisms and complex enzymatic reactions that must occur to regulate the release of these hormones. Your body tries to maintain balance between hormones, as a fluctuation in one may throw off homeostasis. Whether it's fat loss or fat gain, feelings of elation or feelings of depression, feats of incredible strength or incredible weakness, hormones play a key role.

> Did you know sunlight is highly important in the normal physiological functioning of the human body. Sunlight enters the eyes and travels along the optic nerve until it reaches the pituitary gland where it triggers the release/production of various hormones.

Hormonal Balance and Regional Fat Distribution

From metabolic control and regulation of fat storage, to mood and energy levels, hormones play a major role in human functioning and health. Each hormone plays a role in this delicate balance to maintain optimal health. When one part of this hormonal cascade is dysfunctional, a domino effect is likely to occur, affecting any number of systems throughout the human body.

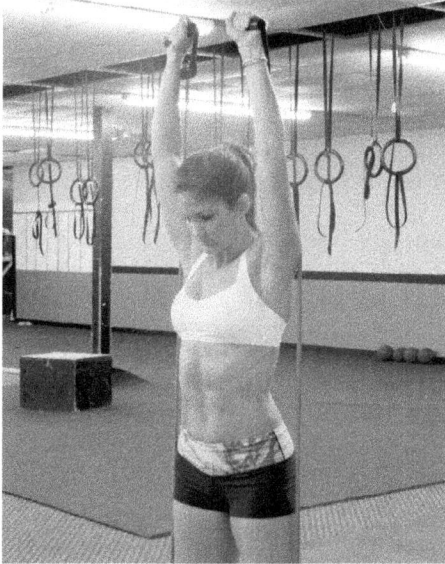

Of particular importance is the role hormones play in regional fat storage. The late research scientist, Per Bjorntorp, is quite possibly the most significant contributor to the science of hormonal control and regulation of body fat storage. Much of his research has not reached the widespread audiences of the mass media for reasons unbeknownst to this author.

In some of his earlier works, Bjorntorp was already beginning to correlate fat distribution patterns and their hormonal regulation. Noticing deficiencies in certain anabolic hormones or excess secretion of storage and/or catabolic hormones led to fat distribution patterns in men and women. From his early research on serum androgen levels and fat distribution in women to his magnificent studies on testosterone replacement in men with excess belly fat, Bjorntorp's work has played a critical role in the science of hormones and fat distribution.

Truly a pioneer in this field, Bjorntorp began seeing similarities in fat distribution patterning and hormonal profiles of his subjects as early as the late 80's early 90's. In 1991, the International Journal of Obesity printed his research paper *"Adipose Tissue Distribution and Function"*, in which Bjorntorp provided some magnificent insight into the hormonal regulation of fat storage. Excesses or deficiencies in certain hormones could lead to fat accumulation in different areas of the human body.

Many of Bjorntorp's other works were published in the pages of other highly respected journals, echoing similar findings. His aptly named *"Hormonal Control of Regional Fat Distribution* (1997)" can be found in the pages of the Human Reproduction publication, Hormonal Research and the International Journal of Obesity also published several of his studies including *"Endocrine-Metabolic Pattern and Adipose Tissue Distribution* (1993)", *"Adipose Tissue Distribution and Function* (1991)", and *"The Regulation of Adipose Tissue Distribution in Humans* (1996)".

Much of Per Bjorntorp's research is still ahead of its time (almost 25 years later). Many professionals in the health and nutrition field are still either unaware or unconvinced of the importance of the works of this medical pioneer. One functional medicine expert, Charles Poliquin, has taken the work of Bjorntorp and others one step further with the creation of his extraordinary Biosignature Modulation. Poliquin's cutting edge method is the culmination of decades of meticulous research, experience, and statistical evaluation of his extremely precise record keeping and thorough measurement techniques. Biosignature Modulation has been called "the blueprint to fat loss/storage".

On his website www.charlespoliquin.com, Coach Poliquin refers to Biosignature Modulation as the culmination of 20+ years of skinfold data collection compared against blood, urine, and salivary hormone testing over that same period of time.

How does Biosignature Modulation work? A skilled biosignature practitioner, with a pair highly calibrated calipers, records skinfold measurements from 12 major body fat sites (Chin, Cheek, Pectoral, Triceps, Umbilical, Supralliac, Subscapular, Mid Axillary, Knee, Calf, Hamstrings, and Quadriceps). The ratio between the triceps and each of the other 11 sites provides the practitioner with an accurate depiction of their client's hormonal balance and possible problem areas.

Hormonal Dominos

How do some of your major hormones affect weight gain? If you are eating poorly with highly insulogenic chemical laden processed foods making up the majority of your diet, the sensitivity to the hormone insulin may be compromised. More than a change in diet may be required to increase efficiency and sensitivity. If you are stressed, whether physically (poor nutrition is stressful on the body) or emotionally, your body may have consistently elevated levels of the stress hormone Cortisol, which signals the body to go into storage mode. Storage of calories and eventually fat accumulation is the result.

If your thyroid is not functioning optimally, your metabolism may slow down, which in turn may lead to weight gain. If your testosterone levels are low, you may see a dramatic increase in body fat accumulation due to the decreases in lean muscle tissue. With a decrease in testosterone, you may also see an increase in the female hormone estrogen, which is conveniently stored in fat cells. Thus with more estrogen, you will need more and larger fat cells to accommodate.

Growth hormone has an effect on fat loss through its actions on lipolysis. GH can stimulate the receptors on fat cells to increase mobilization, so they can be used as fuel (47,65).

Through stimulatory hormones, the pituitary gland is responsible for the regulation of the production of many of the major hormones including growth hormone, androgens, thyroid, estrogen, and cortisol. For instance, the pituitary gland produces luteinizing hormone and follicle stimulating hormone, which in turn stimulate the production of testosterone in the testes.

Adrenocorticotrophic hormone is another hormone produced in the pituitary. ACTH stimulates the adrenal gland to produce cortisol and DHEA. The same goes for the pituitary's role in thyroid hormone production, with thyroid stimulating hormone being produced in this "master gland".

Other hormones such as insulin, the catecholamines, glucagon, serotonin, and neuropeptide Y are under the regulation of other glands such as the adrenals and brain. Fat cells have even been shown to be endocrine tissues themselves, with the production of hormones such as leptin and ghrelin (5,36).

Not only do many of the hormones stimulate the release and regulation of other hormones and the accompanying bodily processes, but they are also a part of a negative feedback loop, which in turn inhibits the release of other hormones. In essence, the hormonal system is one large feedback loop which a stimulating hormone triggers the release of another hormone. The release of the hormone will cause the desired/undesired physical response. Once the response has been accomplished, an inhibitory hormone may then be released to counteract the actions of the stimulatory hormones.

As you can see, the entire endocrine system is quite complex and well beyond the scope of one chapter in a fat loss and body composition book. Entire medical school textbooks are written on this topic. Hopefully, this chapter will serve as an introductory primer to the delicate balance between hormones. Let's take a closer peek at each of the major hormones and some of the "minor" ones.

Quite possibly the most comprehensive textbook available on the topic of hormones is Hormones by Norman and Litwack. You may be able to pick up a copy of this for a good price on Amazon used books.

Alcohol and Hormones:

- Research has shown a decrease in testosterone was observed in healthy male subjects for up to 24 hours post alcohol consumption (despite increased levels of Lutenizing Hormone and Follicle Stimulating Hormone), with 12 hours being the lowest. This probably due to the increased breakdown of testosterone in the liver by reductase enzymes (76). In a separate study, after 4 weeks of alcohol consumption, it was found that men's testosterone decreased after 5 days and kept dropping during the duration of one study (31).
- Elevated cortisol levels mirrored the duration of testosterone decreases (76).
- Alcohol has been shown to increase the aromatization of testosterone into estradiol (32).
- Alcohol induced liver damage has been associated with thyroid dysfunction. Studies have shown that chronic alcohol abuse can lead to thyroid problems, including conversion of T4 to T3 thyroid hormone.
- Studies have shown the hormonal response to low blood sugar levels can be affected by acute alcohol consumption (42).
- Alchohol has even been shown to have negative effects on growth hormone levels in animals (79).

Insulin

Insulin may be the mother of all hormones. After you eat a meal, the levels of circulating blood glucose increase. To normalize the blood sugar levels (balance between insulin and glucagon), insulin is released from the pancreas. The presence of insulin signals activation of proteins inside the muscle and liver cells. These proteins then stimulate receptors on the liver and muscles to absorb the glucose into the tissues, which is then stored as glycogen.

Under normal healthy conditions, the peaks and valleys of insulin release are moderate. When insulin resistance is an issue, the receptor site sensitivity is diminished leaving excess glucose in the bloodstream. This glucose is

Average blood sugar levels:
Normal fasting before meal: 70-100mg/dl (though some doctors suggest >90mg/dl can be a predictor of pre-diabetic
1 to 2 hours post meal: Under 120mg/dl, with <100mg/dl considered normal 2 hours after eating

taken up by the liver where it is then converted to fat. From here it is shuttled back to the bloodstream where the cycle of obesity is allowed to continue.

When blood sugar levels get too low, the hormone glucagon is released from the pancreas stimulating the liver to release glucose into the bloodstream. Glucagon has a counter-regulatory relationship with insulin in that it regulates the amount of glucose released into the bloodstream. Blood sugar balance is similar to a seesaw with insulin on one side and glucagon on the other. As insulin goes up, glucagon goes down and vice versa.

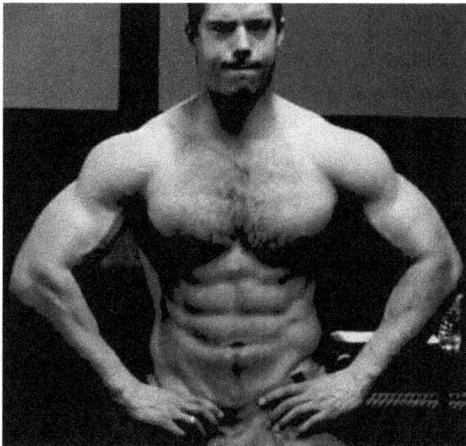

Monitoring the hormonal effects of food, in particular the Glycemic load, and the timing of those nutrients is important. With either an increase in the amount of insulin needed to decrease blood sugar levels or an abrupt saturation of the muscle and liver tissue, the excess glucose has to go somewhere. If you have had poor dietary habits for an extensive period of time, are synthetic exogenous anabolic hormone free, or are not a complete genetic freak, the answer may be between just above your belt line and below your chest. It could also be pasted to your upper thighs/buttocks area, making shopping for clothes less than pleasurable. The triceps is another area fat likes to accumulate, making it look like you are waving twice when bidding adieu. Yes that is right, the fat cell recruiters are more than welcoming to any new recruits you want to send their way.

The fat cells open their loving arms to more recruits, and many come from high sugar drinks and processed foods, not to mention the problems with hydrogenated fats. Unfortunately, these fat cells increase in both number and size. With this increase in size and number of fat cells, more storage for additional fat cells is created, providing a platform for phytoestrogens and environmental toxins to set up home base. The addition of these toxins makes the fat in these cells less apt to be released. With the release of these fatty acids leads comes the release of the stored toxins, which may cause your body to become ill.

Besides the storage of excess glucose and stimulating cells to use carbohydrates as preferential fuel source, insulin has also been shown to affect fat utilization and mobilization in other ways. It can also decrease the activity of the catecholamines and their ability to bind to receptors, leading to a decreased ability to mobilize fat cells. In other words, if insulin is present, then the catecholamines will not bind with their receptor sites, decreasing the body's ability to utilize fat as a fuel source.

When the amount of insulin required to normalize blood sugar levels is not adequate, more is needed to signal the insulin sensitive receptors on the muscles, liver, and fat cells to absorb glucose in order to bring the circulating blood glucose levels back to normal. If enough insulin is not released from the pancreas, the blood sugar levels stay elevated.

> The herb Fenugreek has been shown to have positive effects on insulin sensitivity. In a 2001 double blind placebo controlled study the researchers found significant improvements in blood sugar, insulin sensitivity, serum triglycerides and HDL cholesterol after only 2 months of fenugreek usage in type 2 diabetics (34).

With consistently elevated blood glucose levels, the doors for negative metabolic effects are wide open. Increased risk of body fat, hypertension, diabetes mellitus, metabolic syndrome, elevated triglycerides, decreased HDL, as well as many other symptomatic diseases can quickly arise with insulin resistance.

The relationship between insulin and other hormones can also have a vast effect on the physiology of the human body. The balance between insulin, cortisol, and testosterone is an often overlooked factor with regards to human health and fat loss. A disruption in the delicate balance between these hormones can lead to a cascade of negative effects ranging from increased inflammation to metabolic syndrome, as the body is no longer in an optimal state to fight infection and disease.

In simple terms, when you have increased resistance to insulin, a disruption in the balance between catabolic and anabolic hormones can result. The increased insulin resistance (seen as a stress on the body) elevates the secretion of the stress hormone, cortisol. Or in some cases, the increased stress levels signal an increase in cortisol, which then signals the body into storage mode in order to survive the stress. This storage mode leads to an increase in insulin release.

Testosterone

Have you ever noticed how many commercials there are on TV for low T or decreased levels of testosterone in men? Yes, it is sad to say, testosterone levels are slowly dropping, and in some cases becoming extinct (see hermaphroditic lake frogs).

How important is testosterone to your health? Well, a drop in testosterone has been linked to everything from bone health and low back pain to chronic inflammation and cancer. Testosterone plays a role in keeping energy levels up and inflammation levels down. With receptor sites from head to toe, testosterone deficiency can be a real "downer".

> **Testosterone and fat loss:**
>
> - Testosterone has been shown to increase lipolysis by increasing fat cell receptor activity (83).
> - Testosterone blocks the fat storage effects of the lipoprotein lipase enzyme.

Beginning in the hypothalamus of the brain, testosterone production is stimulated through a series of hormonal actions. Gonadotropin releasing hormone is secreted from the hypothalamus, which then signals the pituitary gland to secrete Luteinizing hormone. The luteinizing hormone is a signal for the synthesis and release of testosterone.

The trouble with testosterone is that its production is not an easy one or two step process. Testosterone is actually a prohormone because it can be converted into DHT (dihydrotestosterone) or aromatize to estrogen.

> Did you know that in the average man, roughly 53% of testosterone is bound to albumin, 45% bound to Sex Hormone Binding Globulin (SHBG), and 2% is free. The more free testosterone, the more active the hormone.

DHT or dihydrotestosterone is a potent metabolite of testosterone that is particularly important to the functioning of the central nervous system. Studies have shown DHT to have similar effects to testosterone on the growth in number of neural cells. Besides its potency, another important characteristic of DHT is the fact that it cannot aromatize to estrogen, unlike testosterone and androstenedione. With all its anabolic properties, the problem with DHT is that it is theorized to be produced because of estrogen.

> **DHT (Dihydrotestosterone) Facts:**
>
> - Most androgenic hormone found in the human body, approximately 3-4X stronger than testosterone.
> - The 5-alpha reductase enzyme removes at double bond (C4-5) from testosterone to for DHT.
> - DHT may play a role in balding and acne.

How important is testosterone? In studies on muscular hypertrophy and strength adaptations, researchers have found significant increases in bench press and squat, as well as muscle fiber hypertrophy, in the group who took the testosterone.

> Nettle root has been shown to have the ability to decrease the actions of Sex Hormone Binding Globulin's (SHBG) ability to bind with free testosterone. Research has shown the compounds found in "stinging nettle" may have an affinity for the sites in which SHBG binds to.

Balance must be maintained between testosterone and other hormones because a cascade of negative health events may result if testosterone levels are allowed to drop too low. With enough testosterone present, the catabolic effects of cortisol may be mitigated. Low testosterone levels have been associated with decreased insulin sensitivity and type II diabetes.

Testosterone has even been associated with the hormone leptin. Research has shown a rise in testosterone to be accompanied by a rise in leptin, and the same occurrence with a drop in each [72].

When looking at the steroid hormone pathways, it becomes clear just how complex the process of synthesizing testosterone can actually be. It is evident there are many opportunities for something to go awry, leading to aromatization to estrogen, cortisol production, or conversion to DHT. With any of these situations the full benefits of testosterone may not be realized. On a similar note, notice how easy it is for testosterone to aromatize (convert) to estrogen: just one step.

Cortisol

"You mean all that long distance running and spinning classes are the reason I can't lose any bodyfat or gain any muscle? *That doesn't make sense because the famous female celebrity trainer on the popular weight loss show keeps saying, 'It comes down to two very simple things: calories in vs calories out.'"* Perhaps with regards to initial weight loss only, this can be effective. In the realm of lean muscle tissue accumulation and body fat loss, the situation may not be quite as simple.

When partaking in excessive endurance training without strength training, you may actually be getting fatter as they lose weight. *Enter Cortisol.*

Cortisol is the stress hormone that stimulates our body to go into protection mode during times of crisis. Picture a caveman who realizes there will be minimal food in the upcoming winter. His body somehow knows he is going to need to store more and more calories to prevent starvation during the cold months ahead. With this perceived stress, his body goes into protection mode by increasing storage of macronutrients in the cells and body tissue. With this increase of macronutrients, more energy is stored and thus weight gain occurs.

An extremely lean caveman would have had a difficult time surviving the winter months with little fat storage to draw upon when the opportunity to hunt and gather presented itself. Turn the clock forward thousands of years. The body still works the same, but the availability of food is much different. The problem is that stressors are ever-present, whereas back then it may have been intermittent.

How does cortisol cause weight gain? After its secretion from the adrenal gland, cortisol can decrease the action of specialized receptors on cells, called GLUT-4 receptors. These are responsible for signaling the shuttling of circulating glucose into muscle and fat cells. With the decrease of glucose absorption in the cells, there is more glucose floating around the bloodstream, which may lead to various metabolic conditions.

The excessive levels of cortisol can then create a vicous cycle. People can become more stressed as they begin to gain weight, so they eat more unhealthy food to make themselves feel better. With more unhealthy food choices comes more insulin resistance, and of course….more weight gain, particularly around the stomach area. Numerous studies have found excessive belly fat storage to be strongly correlated to elevated cortisol levels [25,26].

As can be seen, individuals under high stress with poor dietary habits may have cortisol and insulin working against them. Understanding that hormones are dependent upon each other, when cortisol or insulin levels are elevated/resistant, testosterone levels may be compromised, thus creating a recipe for even greater difficulties in fat loss.

Another negative effect of cortisol is the loss of muscle tissue. Excessive cortisol can lead to the breakdown of muscle proteins into their amino acid constituents to be converted into usable fuel by the liver. With less muscle comes a metabolic slowdown, and with this metabolic slowdown comes stress. With greater levels of chronic stress comes elevated cortisol levels, and the cycle begins again.

Too much cortisol can be responsible for many psychological problems including anxiety, insomnia, and depression. It can also cause physiological ailments including: cancer, cardiovascular risk factors, obesity, Cushings Syndrome, and many other adverse health effects.

Do not be mistaken as cortisol is not all bad. In fact, cortisol is the hormone that helps the immune system to fight off inflammation. Strange how when found in excess levels, cortisol can cause inflammation, but when found in normal levels is actually one of the body's primary defenses against inflammation. Normal cortisol levels typically peak early in the morning around 7 or 8 am, and drop to a daily low sometime mid afternoon, roughly around 4pm.

Growth Hormone

Over the past few years growth hormone has received a bad rap from its excessive usage by professional athletes and bodybuilders. Too bad for all the negative conjecture and accompanying media surrounding growth hormone because when produced naturally or taken in the correct doctor prescribed dosages, it has often been referred to as "a fountain of youth".

Known as a peptide hormone, growth hormone is synthesized from amino acids. It may be capable of increasing muscle mass and decreasing body fat, healing structural tissue, decreasing inflammation, improving cardiovascular function, and basically, fending off the physical symptoms of aging. In excess, too much growth hormone has been linked to cancer, cardiovascular risks, and diabetes.

Secreted from the anterior pituitary gland, growth hormone production is stimulated by Growth Hormone Releasing Hormone (GHRH) produced in the hypothalamus. Somatostatin is the hormone released from the hypothalamus that inhibits growth hormone production.

Once growth hormone has been released, it then travels to the liver, stimulating the liver to secrete a hormone called Insulin like Growth Factor-1 (IGF-1 or somatomedin), which has a similar chemical structure to insulin.

The IGF-1 is then responsible for numerous bodily functions as well as maintenance of physical health. Growth hormone can also affect the mobilization of fat cells as IGf-1 receptors are found on the fat cells in your body. When these receptors are activated, they in turn send a signal to begin breakdown of fat so it can be used as fuel.

Specialized receptors on the cells known as adrenergic receptors are responsible for regulation of lipolysis (fat cell mobilization). They are triggered into action by the catecholamines, epinephrine, and norepinephrine. The alpha-receptors inhibit fat cell mobilization and the beta-receptors stimulate it. Growth hormone stimulates the beta-receptors to increase their responsiveness to the catecholamines.

With regards to fat accumulation, many studies have shown that a decrease in growth hormone can lead to an increase in body fat and obesity (29, 33, 54, 61). When obese subjects are treated with growth hormone their body fat decreases. Understanding the existence of a negative feedback loop between hormones and physical functioning, when a person becomes obese, the fat cells can actually lower growth hormone levels; thus, creating another vicious cycle for weight gain.

Typically peaking in levels around 3 or 4 a.m., growth hormone is also released in large amounts after a large meal. Counter to the effects of insulin, growth hormone is released to help in the suppression of a large insulin spike after you eat one too many chocolate cupcakes and washed them down with a super sized sugar laden beverage.

Growth hormone production is also stimulated by exercise. Studies have shown that higher intensities and lactic acid production are associated with higher growth hormone output (43). Similar effects have also been found in changes in exercise prescription. It is theorized that when workouts become stale, growth hormone production levels off, whereas individuals who changed up their workouts kept seeing positive effects with regards to growth hormone production.

Estrogen

Did you know that estrogen levels are rising in both humans and animals at alarming rates? Have you ever heard of so many men getting surgery for gynomastasia or breast cancer? Did you ever think we would see the day when manziers, mirdles, and mantyhose would be more a plotline for a sit-com episode? How about the fact that beer bellies are beginning to outnumber flat stomachs or that hermaphroditic mutant frogs outnumber single sex frogs in certain lakes?

> As of 2009, the American Cancer Society estimated that nearly 1,910 new cases of invasive breast cancer would be diagnosed *among males.*

One of the major culprits is the family of estrogen mimicking environmental toxins and chemicals known as xenoestrogens. Estrogen is known as the female sex hormone. Formed from the synthesis of androstendione from cholesterol, estrogen is formed primarily in the ovaries of women by the stimulating actions of luteinizing hormone (LH) and follicle stimulating hormone (FSH). Estrogen is produced in two forms. First is the form of estrogen known as estradiol, which is formed from testosterone by the enzyme aromatase. The second form of estrogen is known as estrone, which is formed from androstenedione.

> **Aromatazation of testosterone can lead to unwanted side effects including:**
> - Body fat accumulation
> - Development of gynecomastia (female breast tissue)
> - Water retention
> - Undeniable urges to comparison shop dishware at Crate and Barrel and Williams Sonoma.

Androstenedione is one of the precursors to actual testosterone. A male who does not convert his androgens properly to testosterone may have excessive aromatase activity. This elevated aromatase activity can lead estrogen conversion either via the precursor androstenedione or actual testosterone.

Is Estrogen really that bad? If you are male, a resounding yes. For females to an extent, well, yes. Xenoestrogens (environmental estrogen mimickers) have been linked to breast cancer [19], prostate cancer [80], growth of tumors [84], obesity and cardiovascular risk [24], and many other physiological dysfunctions.

Below is a non-exhaustive list of Xenoestrogens and where they can be found:

- Bisphenol A: plastic bottles, inks, the inner lining of food cans, plastic containers, etc..
- Organchlorines: plastics, pesticides
- Butylated hydroxyanisole (BHS): common food preservative found in processed foods.
- Pthalates: found in baby lotions, skin creams, perfumes, scented items, and cosmetics.
- Parabens: cosmetics, shampoo, hair styling, sunblock, soaps, and skin creams
- Benzones (benzophenone-3, 4-methyl-benzylidene): Sunscreen
- Bovine Growth Hormone: found in non-organic meats, dairy, poultry, and eggs.
- Stearal Chloride: found in cosmetics, body lotion, and face creams.
- And many more........

Tips to avoid Xenoestrogen exposure:

- Eat certified organic foods

- Use BpA free water bottles or aluminum water bottles.

- Avoid processed foods

- Use paraben free, chemical free health and beauty products

- Do not heat food in plastic bags or containers. Use glass instead.

- Avoid processed soy and flax products.

Major problems with estrogen include how and where it is stored, its accessibility to the cell membranes, and how easily it can be produced from its androgen precursors. Surprisingly, estrogen in the form of estradiol can be created in just one chemical step from testosterone; meanwhile it can take five chemical steps to synthesize testosterone from cholesterol. It is almost as if the body would rather produce estrogen with its ease of conversion.

Thyroid Hormone

According to the textbook, *Endocrinology*, the authors state "Thyroid hormones are extremely important and have diverse actions. They act on virtually every cell in the body to alter gene transcription: under- or over-production of these hormones has potent effects [59]". In fact, thyroid hormone is the only hormone *(it depends if you consider vitamin D a hormone)* that has receptor sites on every cell of the body. For that reason, maintaining proper thyroid levels should be paramount as it has profound effects on many areas of the body.

The thyroid hormones, thyroxine (T4) and triiodothyronine (T3) are produced in a small gland at the base of the throat called the thyroid gland. These hormones are synthesized from the amino acid tyrosine and also responsible for synthesizing the catecholamines, epinephrine and norepinephrine. Thyroxine (T4) is known as the inactive form of thyroid hormone, and triiodothryonine (T3) is the active form. In large concentrations, these hormones can increase the fat burning effects of the catecholamines, as they can increase the number and sensitivity of the adrenergic receptors [77].

From controlling your appetite, to maintaining body temperature and energy levels, the thyroid gland is a major player in both your overall physical and emotional wellbeing. It can affect your sleep patterns as well as sex drive. Of particular importance to this book are the effects thyroid hormones have on metabolism and protein synthesis. Thyroid hormones have such profound effects on human metabolism that bodybuilders and figure athletes have used injectible T3 (Cytomel) to increase their metabolic rate, and in turn, burn more body fat.

> Guggulsterones have been shown to be effective modulators of thyroid hormone activity [74,75]. As a side benefit, these Ayurvedic herbs may also increase cardiovascular health and decrease inflammation [20].

In healthy individuals, roughly 80% of the thyroid hormone produced is the inactive form T4, while the other 20% is T3. To become active, T4 is stripped of one of its outer ring iodine molecules through a process known as deiodination, thus converting to the more active form, T3. Incidentally, the antioxidant/mineral Selenium plays a critical role in this conversion, as the enzyme selenodeiodinase is responsible for stripping the iodine molecule from the outer ring of T4. Without proper selenium levels, this process may become quite inefficient, leading to a cascade of negative events, the least of which is a drop in your metabolic rate. A deficiency in iodine may have similar effects, as this is also an important component in the synthesis of thyroid hormones.

Speaking of slowing down metabolic rate, the stress hormone cortisol can effect thyroid production in two ways:

1. Cortisol has receptors on the pituitary gland that can actually shut down the production of TSH, thyroid-stimulating hormone [67].

2. Cortisol can affect the conversion of inactive T4 to active T3 by impairing the enzyme (5-deiodinase) from stripping an iodine molecule from the outer ring [22].

Estrogen can affect thyroid hormone as it can increase the amount of TBG, Thyroxine Binding Globulin [81]. When a hormone is bound to one of these blood proteins known as binding globulins, it may become unavailable for uptake into its receptor cells. This can lead to a ripple effect in the production feedback loop. Certain foods, especially certain vegetables when eaten uncooked, can have negative effects on one's thyroid functioning.

Soy, stress, and lack of minerals such as zinc and magnesium are believed to dramatically affect thyroid functioning. Studies have shown that diets high in improperly fermented soy can alter thyroid function [21]. Likewise, diets low in zinc and selenium have been shown to have similar effects. As for stress, it may be safe to say that too much stress in one's life can lead to alterations in almost all hormones. Regarding the effect of stress on thyroid hormone production, it has been theorized that stress can signal the brain to alter the production of TSH, allowing the body to become hypothyroid.

The Catecholamines

The Catecholamines (epinephrine/adrenaline, norepinephrine/noradrenaline, and dopamine) are similar to growth hormone in that they are also formed from amino acids, specifically Tyrosine and its derivatives. However, unlike growth hormone, the catecholamines are catabolic in nature, because they trigger the breakdown of tissue/cells to be used as fuel.

Derived from the amino acid phenylalanine, tyrosine (from the greek word "tyros" for cheese as it is found in casein protein) is responsible for the synthesis of the catecholamines, as well as other hormones including thyroid and adrenal hormones.

Dopamine is the precursor to norepinephrine. Norepinephrine is the precursor to epinephrine. Tyrosine is responsible for the synthesis of dopamine, so without the amino acid tyrosine, catecholamine production may be halted.

Dopamine, the "feel good" neurotransmitter or neurohormone, plays a key role in several functions of human health including movement, mood, nervous system activation, pain perception, and especially brain function with regards to the reward and motivation systems.

Parkinson's disease and the neurological symptoms associated with it are linked to depressed dopamine levels. Addiction is another dopamine related health consequence. Certain drugs can increase dopamine levels, putting the user in a euphoric state. Then comes the crash, and the only way to fend off the rebound effects is to raise dopamine levels again by taking more drugs.

Without optimal dopamine biosynthesis and processing, basic human functioning may be severely altered. With regards to this book and fat loss and fat cell mobilization, we are concerned with the function of dopamine as a precursor to the other catecholamines, norepinephrine and enpinephrine (as well as its role in motivation).

Noepineprhine is secreted by the sympathetic nervous system. Secreted from specialized cells in the adrenal medulla, epinephrine is part of the endocrine system. The sympathetic nervous system, which is responsible for the fight or flight stimulatory response is where the catecholamine norepinephrine exerts its effects. In contrast, the endocrine (hormonal) system is the major stomping ground for epinephrine.

From increased blood flow to the working muscles to decreased blood flow to the digestive system, we have all felt the effects of the catecholamines. Increases in heart rate, body temperature, and even that "adrenaline" rush are all responses to the physiological efforts of the catecholamines.

It is through the adrenergic receptors that the catecholamines exert their fat loss effects, specifically the beta -eceptors for fat cell mobilization. The beta adrenoreceptors are broken down into beta-1, beta-2, and beta-3, with beta-2 being found in muscle tissue and all three being found in adipose tissue. The alpha-receptors, on the other hand, inhibit fat cell mobilization when bound to by the catecholamines. This reason causes many supplement companies to target ingredients that can both "turn on" beta-adrenergic receptors and "turn off" alpha adrenergic receptors.

For more in-depth information on this topic, it his highly recommended to read the writings of body re-composition expert Lyle Mcdonald. His books The Ultimate Diet 2.0 and the Stubborn Fat Solution are packed with thoroughly researched and referenced information**.

Norepinephrine (NorAdrenaline)	Epinephrine (Adrenaline)
Activation of cAMP	Activation of cAMP
Binds to Alpha receptor, activates G Protein	Increases vasodilation
Increases blood flow to skeletal muscle	Increases lipolysis
Increases Vasoconstriction	Increases oxygen supply
Increases blood pressure	Increases heart rate
Acts on Alpha receptors	Suppresses digestion
	Increases glycogenolysis
	Increases gluconeogenesis

General actions of Alpha and Beta adrenoreceptors:

Alpha Adrenoreceptor	Beta Adrenoreceptor
Inhibitory	Stimulatory
Inhibit lipolysis	Stimulate lipolysis
Increase Vasoconstriction	Increase Vasodilation
Inhibit adenylate cyclase (A-2)	Stimulates adenylate cyclase (B-2)
Decreases cAMP	Increases cAMP production
	Increase glycogenolysis

High circulating levels of the catecholamines can lead to some serious health consequences. These high levels can be caused by toxicity, tumors, or even prescription medication usage. What do doctors typically do to suppress the side effects associated with elevated catecholamine levels (ie: blood pressure)? You have probably heard the term "beta-blocker" in a commercial or at your doctor's office at some point. There are also "alpha-blockers". Simply put, these medications block the alpha adrenoreceptors from being stimulated by the catecholamines.

As can be seen, the catecholamines play a critical role in many bodily functions, with fat cell mobilization and storage being examples of just some of their vast physiologic effects.

Leptin

What would a modern day fat loss book (post 1995) be without at least a small description of the hormone leptin? Lesser known than the previously discussed hormones, leptin may play a lead role in the battle of the bulge.

Produced in the White Adipose Tissue (WAT), along with another hormone called resistin, leptin plays a critical role in appetite, hunger, and satiety control. In

> Did you know the word Leptin is derived from the greek word "leptos", which means "thin"?

essence, leptin lets you know when you are full. It is similar to other hormones because it circulates through the bloodstream and binds to receptor sites. But it is distinctly different because it is synthesized in the fat cells. Proof that fat cells are actually endocrine organs.

When measured, the majority of obese individuals actually had elevated leptin levels. These obese individuals develop a resistance to the leptin, similar to insulin resistance. The sensitivity of the leptin receptors decreases, and more leptin is then needed to do the job. Eventually the effectiveness of the high concentrations of leptin is not enough and the system begins to break down. Obesity can lead to leptin resistance, thus creating a vicous cycle for weigh gain and fat accumulation.

> Leptin was discovered in 1994, when researchers tried to identify the appetite controlling mechanism in the ob/ob mouse. The ob/ob mouse is known for its abilty to become excessively obese due to an unregulated appetite.

Think about it this way: leptin is produced in the fat cells. The more obese you become the more fat cells you have. The more fat cells you have, the more leptin you are capable of producing. The more leptin you can produce, the more leptin resistant your leptin receptors can become. Therefore, the more hunger signaling hormone levels are able to elevate, and the more you eat, etc, etc, etc...

Ghrelin

The hormone Ghrelin signals the body when it is hungry, increasing prior to a meal and dropping after a meal.

Resistin

The more obese you are, the more resistin you make (4,46). Similar to leptin, resistin is also produced in the White Adipose Tissue (WAT). The more obese you are, the more fat cells you have, the more resistin you are capable of producing, and so the viscous cycles begins again. The name describes this hormone appropriately because resistin causes insulin resistance (44), or "Resist-Insulin".

Glucagon

Glucagon is a digestive hormone, released when food, particularly protein, leaves the stomach and enters the small intestine. It slows the exit of food from the stomach making you feel full. Glucagon acts to raise blood sugar and signal the liver to pump out glucose. It is one of a number of counter-insulin hormones, including cortisol, GH, and epinephrine.

Somatostatin

Also known as Growth Hormone Inhibiting Hormone (GHIH), it inhibits the release of growth hormone and thyroid stimulating hormone. Somatostatin can also shut down the b-cells responsible for insulin secretion.

Hormonal Summary

Between all hormones of the human body exists a delicate balance. Each hormone has regulatory and counter-regulatory effects due to the negative feedback loop that is the human endocrine system. If one hormone is left unchecked or out of balance, the widespread ripple effect can be seen in various forms of illness and negative health implications. Keeping your hormones balanced can be one of the most critical factors in achieving optimal health.

Hormones and human physiology can be a difficult subject to grasp, especially the complex interactions between each. Understanding that this chapter has only been a brief introduction to these hormones and their interactions, it would be recommended to read the following books for much greater detail on many of these hormones:

1. *The Cortisol Connection* by Shawn Talbott: This highly recommended book provides the reader with a complex topic and breaks it down into layman's terms so it is easy to understand. From the nuts and bolts of the physiology behind cortisol and its interactions with other hormones to a highly practical education on how to regulate cortisol levels, *The Cortisol Connection* is a must have for any and all interested in the stress hormone and its effects on human health and fat loss.

2. ***Why Zebras Don't Get Ulcers* by Robert Sapolsky:** This highly acclaimed book by MacArthur Foundation "genius" Grant recipient, Robert Sapolsky is quite possibly the most definitive book out there on stress and stress related disorders. His manner of providing truly useful information with some great humor makes this book a must read. Another book by Sapolsky that is a quicker read packed with great information is ***The Trouble With Testosterone.*** Check that one out as well.

3. ***The Testosterone Syndrome* by Dr. Eugene Shippen:** This quick and easy to read book on testosterone and testosterone replacement provides some valuable information on what testosterone does for us, how it interacts with other hormones, and the health consequences that accompany a drop in this anabolic hormone. Not only does Shippen go into great detail about some of the culprits that may be causing lowered testosterone, but he also provides information on the good and bad of multiple types of replacement therapy.

4. ***Mastering Leptin* by Byron Richards and Mary Richards:** Packed with a lot of scientific research/information, this is a great book providing valuable information on leptin and its wide spread effects throughout the human body. From the valuable tips to the explanation of the effects leptin has on other hormones, this is a great read for anybody wanting to know more about the science of this "obesity" hormone.

5. ***The Schwarzbein Principle (I and II)* by Diana Schwarzbein:** These books are a must have for anybody interested in learning why and how their hormones affect every aspect of their health from weight gain to aging. Both books are easy to read but provide valuable information on hormones, nutrition, exercise, and lifestyle. As one of the best endocrinologists in the world, Schwarzbein also provides various case studies of how hormonal regulation helped these patients renew their vigor and health.

6. ***Hormonal Balance* by Dr. Scott Isaacs:** This comprehensive book provides excellent information on all the hormones and their interactions with each other. Dr. Isaacs makes a great case for how imbalances in these hormones can lead to various health

disorders. I highly recommend this book as you may find yourself reading it more than once.

7. ***Your Thyroid and How to Keep it Healthy* by Barry Durant-Peatfield**: Debunking the myths surrounding thyroid dysfunction, Dr. Durant-Peatfield goes into great detail regarding the possible causes of thyroid dysfunction, the myriad of symptoms associated with this health issue, and the proper testing needed to determine if a thyroid issue is at the source of your physical ailments.

CHAPTER VI

PH BALANCE

Looking at nutrition from an evolutionary perspective can be one of the most effective strategies for maintaining vibrant health. Eating a diet completely defunct of the foods similar to those consumed by our Paleolithic ancestors may lead to a cascade of health problems. One of the most often overlooked, but most important, is the development of chronic metabolic acidosis (2) otherwise known as an acidic PH.

Foods like processed carbohydrates, highly processed protein/fat foods, cheeses and many others found in the common westernized diet, can have a dramatic effect on the human body's PH balance. This pattern, combined with the fact that much of the alkalizing foods are absent from our current modern diet (6), leads to an acidic environment in which many health problems may occur. Type II Diabetes, metabolic syndrome, high blood pressure, advanced gaining, high oxidized cholesterol, inflammation and of course weight gain are just a few.

When a highly processed carbohydrate is broken down in the body, the glucose is quickly shuttled into the bloodstream, causing the bloodstream to become slightly acidic. With proper kidney function, a buffer known as bicarbonate will be secreted to neutralize the hydrochloric acid and bring the body back to a neutral PH of 7.365. In the case of too much acidity, calcium may also be excreted from the bones to help in re-alkalization of the body.

This excretion of calcium can be problematic, as it can open up the door for further health complications including case osteoporosis and kidney stones. To further exacerbate the issue, an acidic internal environment can actually deplete the body's ability to absorb and utilize minerals. This leads to an endless cycle of mineral depletion and the health issues that accompany these deficiencies.

Similar to calcium, the body also depletes its stores of the amino acid glutamine to help in restoring PH levels. Through a process known as nitrogen fixation, glutamine is bound by hydrogen ions to form ammonium, which acts as a natural buffer for acidity.

Another negative effect of excessive acidity is a decrease in oxygen levels. With a state of deprived oxygen, cells become sick, germs and bacteria are allowed to thrive, and PH levels are further thrown off. As can be seen, the effects of excessive acidity can be far ranging.

From reduction in enzyme activity to the possible damage and strain on the kidneys, allowing the diet to become acidic through poor nutritional choices can open the body up to many negative health consequences. One consequence of particular interest to this book is weight gain and the accumulation of body fat. Without optimal levels of oxygen, the body can slow down. With a slowing metabolism comes weight gain and decreased energy.

> How important is the lymphatic system? Did you know that there is 3 times more lymph fluid than blood in the body? One study showed that 80% of overweight women have sluggish lymphatic systems.

Is there a way we can keep our body in a balanced PH state even if we are eating healthy foods containing protein such as meat and eggs, which have been shown to acidify the bloodstream? Two research papers out of the Research Institute of Child Nutrition in Germany have shown that with the addition of alkaline foods (ie: greens, vegetables, and berries) leads to a balanced PH (12). This may serve as evidence for the potential dangers of a purely fat/protein diet lacking proper alkalizing food like vegetables.

Of interest is the fact that high quality protein intake has been shown to improve your capacity to excrete excess acids (12). Rather than hanging around in your body, excess organic acids are excreted through your urine when you go to the bathroom.

A 2000 study found several factors to affect the acid-base determination of food. The factors to consider include the nutrient/vitamin/mineral composition of the food, the body's ability to break down these nutrients, the ratio of particular minerals, and the metabolic generation of sulfate from the breakdown of certain amino acids found in the food (13).

Is there any scientific validity showing that the human organism needs to be concerned about the acidifying effects of our daily food intake? A study in 2002 performed by researchers from the University of California at San Francisco found that the processed diets ingested by today's society may have caused a shift toward "diet induced metabolic acidosis". By eating a diet that does not live up to our genetically determined nutritional standards/requirements to maintain positive PH balance (16), we may see a negative change in the body's PH levels. Other studies on the evolutionary perspective of human nutritional requirements have shown similar results (8,16).

A recent 2009 study set out to study the physiologic effects of an optimal acid/base diet over a ten-day period. When they compared the subject's baseline physiologic state from their normal to the optimal acid/base diet, they found significant reductions in total and LDL cholesterol, and blood pressure as well as an increase in insulin sensitivity.

In a separate study involving subjects with type II diabetes, researchers found a Paleolithic nutrition type of diet to be more beneficial to cardiovascular health markers and insulin regulation than a diet known as the Diabetic Diet. In other words, *a diet created for the sole purpose of helping type II diabetics with insulin management was less effective in Glycemic control/insulin regulation than a diet named after our ancestral eating patterns.* The researchers concluded that a diet that may help to alleviate chronic metabolic acidosis (2,7) resulted in greater decreases in cholesterol, blood pressure, inflammation, bodyweight, waist circumference and an increase in insulin sensitivity.

And what happens as we age? Is there any decline in the body's ability to alkalize itself as we age and can we help to reverse this? A 2008 study out of Tufts University looked at the effects of increased dietary potassium intake over a 3 year period in adults aged 65 and older. *They found that, of the 384 subjects, those with the highest potassium intake (from potassium rich fruits and vegetables) were better able to preserve lean (muscle) body mass than their counterparts on acidic cereal grain and protein diets* (3).

Comparison studies between young adulthood and elderly subjects have found a decrease in the body's ability to maintain optimal PH balance due to a decrease in renal function, leading to a decrease in the body's ability to excrete excess organic acids. This compromised excretion of organic acids can in turn lead to a decreased ability to maintain optimal muscle mass (1,9,15).

Bottom line: make sure to eat your fruits and veggies (organic preferred, and be sure to include highly alkalizing greens such as wheatgrass, spinach, arugula, garden herbs, berries, etc...), and minimize acidifying food/beverage intake. Below are some helpful tips to help your body to restore balance to your PH.

Tips:

- Purchase some PH strips from your local health food store. Test your urine Ph level first thing in the morning on an empty stomach to ensure the most accurate reading. This test will give you a baseline of what your Ph level is. If you are acidic, the following tips can be quite helpful in restoring Ph balance.

- Stay away from sodas and other colas, as most contain phosphoric acid as their main ingredient. Phosphoric acid is highly acidic with a PH of roughly 2.8. Phosphoric acid has been linked to the depletion of calcium and other minerals from the bones, as well as a potent blocker in mineral absorption.

- You may want to stay away from dairy products as these can be highly acid forming, especially non-organic products. With antibiotic treatments, hormones, and a diet consisting of genetically modified corn or soy, animals on the non-organic dairy farms may not be healthy. If you are concerned about calcium intake and osteoporosis, read the above box.

> Did you know that the countries with the greatest consumption of dairy have the highest incidence of osteoporosis? The countries with the lowest consumption have the lowest incidence.

- Stay away from most processed foods, especially sodium, sugar, and high fructose corn syrup laden snacks as these can be especially acidifying.

- Eat an avocado a day to balance your bodies PH. Avocados are a great source of monounsaturated fat and protein. They are also high in lutein and minerals. Avocados actually have the highest vitamin E levels of any fruit and have more potassium than a banana. The fats from the avocado can help bring your body's PH up, as they are known to bind to excess acids preparing them to be eliminated from the body.

- Drink plenty of alkaline water. Most tap and bottled water is acidic, so try adding either PH drops or alkalizing electrolytes to your water to make it more alkaline.

- Add a lime or lemon to your water. Though these test acidic, in the body they have an alkalizing effect. A functional medicine trick is to add Celtic sea salt and a lime to water the night before and drink it first thing in the morning.

- Drink beverages made from multiple greens drinks throughout the day. A high quality greens drink is important, as many of the lower quality drinks have been tested for excess heavy metals. Make sure to drink the greens drink on an empty stomach and away from meals as it can interfere with digestion. In this author's opinion, the best tasting high quality greens drink on the market is Poliquin's Primal Greens. This high quality greens drink has a light minty taste making it perhaps the best product on the market.

- Eat a coconut or have some coconut water or oil. The luaric acid, a saturated fat, found in coconut oil is very similar to the fatty constituents of human breast milk.

- Take fish oil. DHA and EPA are quality fats that aid in the battle against excessive acidity. CLA and GLA are other good oils to promote fat metabolism and decrease fat storage.

- Invest in far infrared sauna therapy. Sweating can rid the body of not only toxins, but also excess acids.

- Decrease your stress and enjoy life...

1 Day Sample protocol to restore PH levels:

Wake up: 20+oz glass PH balanced water, Celtic Sea Salt, and 1 whole lime

Breakfast: Organic protein source with 1 whole avocado and/or blueberries, blackberries, or raspberries. Include fish oil supplement and 700-1400mg Acetyl L Carnitine. Eat protein first. After eating half of the protein, take HCL + Pepsin digestive supplement, then eat second half of protein, then eat the rest of the meal.

30-45 minutes after Breakfast: Greens drink in 20+oz PH balanced water.

Mid Morning Snack: Coldwater fish (ie; sardines or mackerel in olive oil), 1 Tbsp of Organic Coconut oil, fish oil supplement, and 700-1400mg Acetyl L Carnitine. Drink 20+ oz. of PH balanced water.

Lunch: Organic protein source with Quinoa and large organic salad. Include fish oil supplement. Eat protein first. After eating half of the protein, take HCL + Pepsin digestive supplement, then eat second half of protein, then eat the rest of the meal.

30-45 minutes after Lunch: Greens drink in 20+oz PH balanced water.

Mid Afternoon Snack: Avocado, raw organic almonds, and berries. Include fish oil supplement. Drink 20+oz of PH balanced water.

Dinner: Protein source and large helping of organic Brussels sprouts. Include fish oil supplement and high quality magnesium chelate supplement. After eating half of the protein, take HCL + Pepsin digestive supplement, then eat second half of protein, then eat the rest of the meal.

30-45 minutes after Dinner: Greens drink in 20+ oz. PH balanced water.

CHAPTER VII

VITAMIN/MINERAL DEFICIENCIES

Did you know that a deficiency in something as simple as magnesium can lead to a plateau in weight loss through its actions on multiple enzymatic reactions as well as other aspects of human functioning? Or, how about a deficiency in vitamin D? Did you know that deficiencies in vitamin D have been linked cancer, endocrine dysfunction, and cardiovascular health? Every vitamin and mineral from A to Zinc plays a crucial role in achieving optimal health. These can be considered "Nature's" medicine, as deficiencies in many of these can lead to adverse health effects and human dysfunction.

Avitaminosis is the term used to describe symptoms or disease caused by a vitamin deficiency or by a malfunction in the body's ability to synthesize, or convert the metabolic compounds. In modern Western medicine, a deficiency in one or many vitamins may be a common health problem that goes undiagnosed as the symptoms of the problem are treated rather than the cause of the problem. In this case, if the vitamin deficiency was recognized, more invasive measures would not have been necessary simply by adding the vitamin back into the diet may have been the solution.

In North America many people are now deficient in many vitamins and minerals due to a decreased availability of those compounds in our foods. When compared to the diets of our ancestors, the diets of today are distinctly deficient in many vitamins and minerals. Let's take a look at the possible negative health consequences that can arise from a deficiency in certain vitamins or minerals.

Vitamin A

In 1913 researchers at Yale and the University of Wisconsin isolated a compound consisting of retinoids from the actual retina of the eye. They then went on to name it the fat-soluble compound, Vitamin A. Of interest is how they isolated from the retina, and how vitamin A is known to have profound effects on vision.

The three forms of vitamin A are Beta Carotenes, Retinols, and Carotenoids. Beta-Carotene is responsible for most vitamin A production, while Retinol is the most abundant form found in food.

Vitamin A has been linked to:

- Vision (especially night vision) and eye health

- Production and repair of epithelial cells

- The cellular linings of the intestinal and urinary tracts

- Immune Function

- Cardiovascular health

- Gene expression

- Reproductive health

- And more……

Research has shown a deficiency in Vitamin A has been linked to:

- Vision dysfunction

- Blood disorders and anemia ***Note***If there is a pre-existing iron deficiency, supplementing with vitamin A may not correct a deficiency.

- Stomach disorders

- Liver problems

- Infection

- Cancer has been linked to deficiencies in vitamin A

- Heart disease and associated cardiovascular risk factors have been associated with a deficiency in vitamin A

- Fetal health has been associated with deficiencies in vitamin A

- Endocrine problems have been linked to deficiencies in vitamin A

- And more............

Vitamin B-12 (Cobalamin)

Cobalamin (vitamin B-12) is mostly found in animal proteins, eggs, and in some fish (yes, the superfood in a can sardines contain vitamin B-12). Most of it (or at least more than half) is stored in the liver. The absorption of B-12 is linked to the amount of hydrochloric acid is present in the stomach (more on this in the next chapter).

With a lack of HCL, something called intrinsic factor is not secreted in proper amounts. Intrinsic factor binds to the cobalamin and allows for proper absorption and transport of the vitamin. So, if there is a lack of HCL, there is a lack of intrinsic factor and leads to a decreased rate of absorption of B-12. It is for this reason that many individuals with achlorhydic stomachs need vitamin B-12 injections. No, not the B-12 certain famous major league baseball players were taking in the early part of the decade to "enhance" their on-field performances. B-12 deficiencies have been known to manifest in the upper extremities.

Vitamin B-12 has been linked to:

- Maintaining proper homocysteine levels

- Methionine synthesis

- Phase I and Phase II Liver Detoxification

- Maintaining bone marrow health

- Liver health

- Neurologic health

- Immune health

.

Deficiencies (**note** with lack of animal proteins in their diet, vegetarians can be susceptible to B-12 deficiencies) in vitamin B-12 have been linked to:

- Alzheimer's and other neurodegenerative diseases

- Autoimmune diseases

- Elevations in homocysteine

- Cancer

- Cardiovascular diseases

- Neuropsychiatric disorders

- Gastrointestinal disorders

- And more….. In fact, entire books could be written on this one vitamin alone.

Vitamin B9 (Folate, Folic Acid)

Vitamin B9 is otherwise known as folic acid (or folate). How fitting that a major vitamin in the fight against cancer is called B9. The importance of this vitamin can be seen in the fact that foods are/were required to be fortified with B9 to decrease the risk of associated ailments and negative health consequences. Strongly linked to the development of cancer and cardiovascular diseases, B9 is widely known for its role in keeping homocysteine levels at bay.

Found in fruits, green vegetables, and some animal foods, folic acid must be taken in through the diet since the body does not readily synthesize this important vitamin. The average healthy person needs to absorb about 50-100mcg of B9 per day to replenish the supplies used up throughout the day.

Folic Acid has been linked to:

- Cardiovascular function

- Maintaining healthy homocysteine levels

- Detoxification and liver health

- Anti-carcinogenic, especially in those whom consume moderate to high amounts of alcohol

- Cognitive functioning

A deficiency in vitamin B9 (Folate) has been linked to:

- Cancer

- Cardiovascular risk factors

- Increased homocysteine levels

- Compromised liver function

- Cognitive and neurodegenerative disorders

Vitamin B6 (Pyridoxine)

Vitamin B6 or Pyridoxine is found in liver, animal meats, vegetables, and yes,....whole grains. It is a highly important vitamin involved in many physical processes including synthesis of neurotransmitters, amino acids, and many other physiological components of metabolism, detoxification, immune health and human functioning. Pyridoxine is also critical in the metabolism of homocysteine. Of particular importance to this book is the role B6 plays in the production of serotonin, dopamine, glcyine, and the catecholamines, as these play critical roles in liver detoxification and fat cell mobilization and metabolism.

Vitamin B6 has been linked to:

- Metabolism of homocysteine

- Metabolism of glycine, serotonin, tryptophan, dopamine, and glutamate

- Production of catecholamines and GABA

- Liver health and detoxification processes

- Cardiovascular health

- And much more.........

A deficiency in vitamin B6 (Folate) has been linked to:

- Certain types of cancer

- Peripheral neuropathy has been linked to excessive B6

- High levels of homocysteine have been linked to a deficiency in pyridoxine

- Cardiovascular risk factors

- Inflammation

- Impaired liver function

- Cognitive dysfunction and depression

- Seizures have been associated with low levels of B6

Vitamin B1 (Thiamine)

Thiamine is the B vitamin that can be found in seeds, nuts, vegetables, and wheat germ. A water soluble vitamin mainly stored in the skeletal muscle tissue of animals is a highly important B vitamin which is responsible for glucose metabolism. Thiamine is also stored in the heart, liver, kidneys and brain, giving it a storage capacity of about 1 month, where problematic health consequences may take approximately one week to develop without appropriate thiamine intake. Prolonged diarrhea can actually decrease the body's ability to absorb thiamine.

This B vitamin plays a highly important role in energy production and glucose metabolism. In particular, many enzymatic processes require thiamin, as the enzymes used in these reactions depend on thiamine for production/function. Nervous system function is also dependent on this B vitamin. (****NOTE*** *If folic acid is deficient, a thiamine deficiency may indirectly result****)*

Vitamin B1 (Thiamine) has been linked to:

- Heart health

- Protection against neurodegeneration

- Glucose metabolism

- Nervous system function and health

A deficiency in Vitamin B1/Thiamine (otherwise known as beriberi) is linked to:

- Peripheral neuropathy, which is a primary symptom of dry beriberi. Go figure, *dry beriberi is associated with HIGH CARBOHYDRATE INTAKE.*

- Heart failure and cardiovascular risk factors are associated with wet beriberi

- Nervous system dysfunction

- Cognitive dysfunction

- Burning sensation in the hands and feet

- Disruption of gait patterns

Vitamin B5 (Pantothenic Acid)

Pantothenic acid is relatively overlooked, but important vitamin for human functioning. The body is capable of synthesizing its own "B5" through bacteria in the in the large intestine, but if enough is produced to be utilized for healthy function has been the subject of scientific investigation. For that reason, we need to eat foods such as shellfish, fish, sweet potatoes, eggs, broccoli, mushrooms and liver for ingestible sources of pantothenic acid. Pantothenic acid, a coenzyme in many enzymatic processes including hormone and neurotransmitter synthesis, has been shown (at least its derivative Pantethine) to have lipid lowering effects as well as an effect on your adrenal health.

Pantothenic acid has been linked to:

- Maintaining healthy cholesterol and triglyceride levels

- Synthesis of hormones

- Synthesis of neurotransmitters

A deficiency in pantothenic acid has been linked to:

- Tingling in the extremities

- Insomnia

- Compromised adrenal function

- Blood glucose disorders

Vitamin B3 (Niacin)

Niacin is the B vitamin usually found in animal proteins including white meats such as chicken and pork, as well as beef. Niacin is very interesting in that besides actual ingestion, it can also be synthesized from the essential amino acid tryptophan. With regards to cholesterol levels, not only has niacin been found to lower LDL (bad cholesterol) but it has also been shown to raise healthy HDL cholesterol levels, as well as its many other important functions in human health.

Niacin has been linked to:

- Detoxification system health

- Lipid biosynthesis

- Anti-carcinogenic

- Cognitive functioning

- Reducing inflammation

- Cardiovascular health and function

Vitamin B3 deficiency (otherwise known as Pellegra) has been linked to:

- Elevated blood lipid levels
- Niacin (vitamin B_3) deficiency is typically characterized by dementia, dermatitis, and diarrhea
- Gastrointestinal problems
- Skin disorders
- And more.........

*****Note**** Fad diets have been linked to decreases in niacin levels.

Vitamin E

Known as one of the most important fat-soluble antioxidants, Vitamin E is one of the most abundant and efficient scavengers of free radicals. It plays a major role in decreasing risk of degenerative diseases and cancer, while preserving cellular membrane health and cardiovascular health. One of this fat-soluble vitamin/antioxidant's major benefits is the fact that after it has scavenged a free radical, *it can be recycled to be used again in the battle against free radical and oxidative stress*. Alpha Lipoic Acid and vitamin C play a crucial role in this antioxidant recycling.

The key to vitamin E is to find one that includes all members of the vitamin E family, 4 tocopherols and 4 tocotrienols. Many of the store bought brands contain only Alpha-dl-tocopherol which, by itself, has not shown to promote the health benefits of the entire Vitamin E family. Food sources of Vitamin E include nuts, seeds, fish oils, and whole grains.

Vitamin E has been linked to:

- Cardiovascular health

- Heart health

- Scavenging free radicals and combating oxidative stress

- Prevents oxidation of LDL cholesterol which has been linked to atherosclerosis

- Immune function

- Cancer prevention

Deficiencies in Vitamin E have been linked to:

- Cardiovascular risk factors

- Cancer

- Cystic Fibrosis

- Dementia

- Blindness

Vitamin D

Sometimes referred to as a hormone, Vitamin D may be one of the most important vitamins in the human body. Think about it, it has receptor sites on every tissue of the human body. What else besides thyroid hormone can claim this? It must be for a reason. Once thought of primarily as a bone

> Did you know that nearly 50% of breast cancers and nearly 80% of colon cancers have been linked to low levels of vitamin D?

modeling/remodeling vitamin, important in calcium regulation, D3 is now regarded as a major player in overall health and physical functioning.

Vitamin D actually has 2 forms, D3 (cholecalciferol) and D2 (ergocalciferol). D3 is the vitamin made by the skin or obtained through ingestion.

Vitamin D has been linked to:

- Prevention of cancers
- Physical performance
- Calcium absorption
- Glucose metabolism and insulin response
- Muscle function

A deficiency in vitamin D has been linked to:

- Growth of cancers
- Bone fractures
- Type I and II diabetes
- Rickets
- Muscular aches and pains
- And so much more…. ***As of this writing, the research on Vitamin D and the effects D3 has on human health is astounding. Literally, type in a physical ailment/disease and there may be some research linking inadequate vitamin D levels.***

Vitamin C

When lemon juice was listed as the cure for scurvy occurring in sailors, a "miracle" ingredient in those citrus fruits was brought to the world's attention. As the only animals (beside guinea pigs) that are unable to produce their own L-ascorbic acid, humans are then required to ingest Vitamin C through their diets for proper health and immune function.

Vitamin C has been shown to be a very versatile vitamin with regards to its antioxidant abilities. Deficiencies in vitamin C are known risk factors for cardiovascular disease and oxidative stress. Vitamin C supplementation has been shown to reduce the inflammatory biomarker C-reactive protein after only 2 months of treatment.

Of major benefit is the fact that ***vitamin C is known to regenerate Vitamin E,*** as well as the ability to improve antioxidant capacity of the blood through its positive effects on red blood cell glutathione. When choosing a vitamin C product, be sure to find one that incorporates a full spectrum of bioflavonoids to ensure maximum vitamin activity. Food sources of Vitamin C include citrus fruits and juices, green peppers, cabbage, spinach, broccoli, kale, cantaloupe, kiwi, and strawberries.

Vitamin C has been linked to:

- Scavenging free radicals and battling oxidative stress
- Collagen production
- Cardiovascular health
- Proper absorption of iron
- Immune health and function
- Liver health and detoxification
- Metabolism and synthesis of hormones
- Wound healing

- Carnitine production

A deficiency in vitamin C has been linked to:

- Scurvy

- Cardiovascular disease

- Free radical damage

- Poor wound healing

- Skin abnormalities

- General symptoms of sickness

- Bleeding gums and compromised dental health.

Vitamin K

One of the fat soluble vitamins, Vitamin K is known for its role in blood coagulation. Found in oils and leafy green vegetables, vitamin K can also be produced in the intestinal flora.

Vitamin K has been linked to:

- Proper coagulation

- Bone formation

A deficiency in Vitamin K has been linked to:

- Osteoporosis

- Hemorrhagic disease and excessive bleeding

ZINC

Did you know that zinc is required for quite possibly up to 300 enzymatic reactions occurring in the human body? From the common commercial uses like fighting colds, sunburn and diaper rash to lesser-known roles in testosterone production, immune function, and gastrointestinal tract health. Zinc is so important that it plays a role in the synthesis of cysteine histidine proteins. The highest concentrations can be found in the prostate and eye, while smaller concentrations can be found in the liver, brain, muscle, bones, and kidneys.

Found in seeds, beans, nuts, sardines, fish, eggs, liver, meat and whole grains, zinc levels found in farmed/planted/grown foods are usually dependent on the health of the soil they are cultivated in.

Zinc has been linked to:

- Up to 300 enzymatic processes
- DNA and RNA gene expression and signal transduction
- Binding to proteins
- Proper brain functioning
- Liver health and detoxification processes
- Normal growth and development
- Wound healing
- Cancer preventive
- Testosterone production
- And much more........

A deficiency in zinc has been linked to:

- Improper immune function
- Skin disorders

- Hair loss

- Decreased testosterone

- Weakened immune function

- Inflammation Digestive disorders and gastrointestinal disorders

- And much, much more...........Basically without zinc your health and physiological functioning may be impaired.

*** Note*** *When purchasing a zinc supplement, you should be concerned with the quality of the zinc used in the supplement as some forms are more absorbable than others. For instance, zinc carbonate and zinc oxide are some of the least absorbable forms of zinc while zinc oretate may be more bioavailable.*

MAGNESIUM

Before getting started on Magnesium, it is highly recommended that you read the book *The Magnesium Miracle* by Dr. Carolyn Dean. This incredible book is packed with information and provided in an easy to read manner. Upon reading this book, you will get a more in-depth picture of just how important magnesium is to human functioning.

Similar to zinc, did you know that magnesium is required in over 300 enzymatic reactions in the human body? Without magnesium "things" just don't happen, and "stuff" just doesn't get done. It is just behind potassium as the second most abundant cation found inside the cells. Everything from DNA and RNA synthesis to ATP production, magnesium is magnificently important to human functioning. Magnesium can be found in leafy green vegetables, nuts, unrefined whole cereals, spices, and other vegetables.

Magnesium has been linked to:

- DNA and RNA synthesis

- ATP production

- Hormone synthesis

- Hormone receptor binding

- Immune function

- And so much more…………

A deficiency in magnesium has been linked to:

- Heart problems

- High blood pressure

- Cardiovascular risk factors

- Circulatory problems

- Osteoporosis

- Psychological disorders

- Neuromuscular disorders

- Inflammation

- Asthma and bronchial problems

- And so much more...........

IRON

Found in food sources including meats, fish, poultry, beans, peas, and leafy green vegetables, iron is an essential mineral in hemoglobin and blood oxygen transport. The iron found in animal meats is more absorbable than that found in vegetable and other sources. Iron is mainly responsible for the transport of oxygen through the blood, as well as DNA synthesis and electron transport.

Iron has been linked to:

- Blood oxygen transport

- Electron transport

- DNA synthesis

- And much more……………

A deficiency in iron has been linked to:

- Anemia

- Abnormal platelet counts

- Cardiovascular disorders

- Gastrointestinal disorders

- Leg cramps and ice chewing are associated with iron deficiency

- Weakness

IODINE

Who knew iodine was so important. Just how important you ask? Well, there are receptors on every cell in the human body for thyroid hormone. So, if there are receptors everywhere for this one hormone then it must be pretty important. So where does iodine come into the picture? Well, iodine has one known primary function: to synthesize thyroid hormones. Besides salt, iodine can be found in eggs and milk. Does there seem to be a greater prevalence of people walking around taking thyroid medications with the current recommendations of decreased salt and eggs in our diets?

Iodine has been linked to:

- Synthesis of thyroid hormones

- Immune function

- Anti-carcinogenic

A deficiency in iodine has been linked to:

- Decreased synthesis of thyroid hormones

- Goiter (otherwise known as thyroid enlargement)

- Cretinism

- Mental retardation

- Compromised reflexive response

Selenium

Selenium, a mineral with high antioxidant capacity, is known to have many functions throughout the human body. From its antioxidant capabilities in battling free radicals to its function in the conversion of T4 thyroid hormone to T3, selenium is a highly important mineral antioxidant in human functioning. Selenium is found in food sources such as eggs, meats, fish, and nuts. Selenium levels can vary greatly in produce depending on the quality of the soil.

Selenium has been linked to:

- Anti-carcinogenic
- Synthesis of various enzymes
- Mitochondrial health
- Synthesis of selenoproteins
- Scavenging of free radicals and combating oxidative stress

A deficiency in selenium has been linked to:

- Heart Problems
- Decreased mitochondrial health
- Endocrine disruption
- Inflammation
- Infection
- Thyroid dysfunction
- Cancer

Manganese

Manganese is a highly underrated, but very important element of human function. Found in nuts, whole grains, leafy green vegetables, and fruits. As a critical component in the metabolism of glucose, amino acids, and cholesterol, manganese may play an even more critical role in human health as it is found in Superoxide Dismutase, the super-antioxidant of the mitochondria. With this role, manganese plays a critical role in the body's free radical scavenging capacity. Along with these functions, manganese is also important in many enzymatic reactions as well as skeletal growth and wound healing.

Manganese has been linked to:

- The synthesis of Superoxide Dismutase

- Metabolism of glucose

- Synthesis of hormones

- And much more…………

An imbalance in homeostatic Manganese has been linked to:
- Oxidative Stress and reduced free radical scavenging capacity

- Endocrine disruption

- Birth Defects

- Inflammation

- Joint problems

- Parkinson's Disease

- Diabetes

- Cardiovascular risk factors

- Seizures

Omega 3 Fatty Acids

How important are omega 3's? Well, they have been linked to everything from cardiovascular health to the development of autoimmune disorders. Whether it be fat loss or detoxification, omega 3's have been linked to numerous health factors. In fact, recently a deficiency in Omega 3's has been rated as the sixth largest risk factor for deaths among US citizens behind smoking, high blood pressure, obesity, physical inactivity, blood glucose disorders, and high LDL cholesterol (*and marriage.. Just kidding on the last one. I hope my wife doesn't hit me over the head again with a rolling pin*). In fact, some research has guesstimated that a lack of omega 3's to be responsible for roughly 72K to 96k deaths per year!!!

Let's look at the research regarding fish oil and health factors:

- Cardiovascular health

- Mitochondrial health

- Cancer
- Inflammation
- Autoimmune diseases
- Alzheimer's
- Cognition
- Neurodevelopmental disorders
- ADHD
- Obesity

- Diabetes
- Fat Cell Mobilization
- Leptin Production
- Joint pain and arthritis
- High Blood Pressure

The popularity of fish oil seems to be on the rise. Never before have there been television commercials expressing the performance enhancement and health benefits of fish oil as can be currently seen during the prime-time hours on major networks. This supplement gem seems to be greatly misunderstood though. The debate rages on from what type one should take, to which brands are better (lower in mercury, purity, twice processed, etc.) to even something as simple as dosages and best time of day to take fish oil.

CHAPTER VIII

POOR EXERCISE SELECTION

Understanding the fact that the more lean muscle you have the more efficient your metabolism becomes, then why is it on any given day at the local health club between the hours of 5 and 7pm, most if not all the treadmills and ellipticals are occupied by those looking to lose weight or burn fat? The problem lies in the fact that neither of these exercise modalities are really known as muscle builders. Rather, if used in excess, endurance training has been shown to stress the body, driving up cortisol levels [28], decreasing testosterone [30,35], and potentially leading to chronic overuse injuries [5,7,8,,18,19,20,25,27].

Endurance exercise and high intensity interval training [14] at different intensities have different effects on bodyfat and weight loss [1]. When performed in excess, the results can actually be detrimental to your weight loss goals, hormonal balance, and overall health [28,30].

Perhaps ensuring your endocrine system is in balance prior to partaking in this form of exercise may be a wise choice. After all, even world-renowned endocrinologist Dr. Diane Swarzbein usually does not allow her morbidly obese clients to take part in endurance training prior to correcting their hormonal balance. Instead, she prescribes resistance training.

The Benefits of Weight Training

The benefits of weight training are numerous. When done properly, resistance training can add lean muscle tissue to one's body, which will turn increase your metabolic rate while decreasing body fat levels.

Studies have shown that resistance training can increase resting metabolism to a significant degree and have a greater effect on fat loss than endurance training [21]. Studies have also shown resistance training has a positive effect on hormonal profile [15,16,17] without the negative endocrine effects seen in excessive cardiovascular exercise [12,34,35].

"I Don't Want To Get Big and Bulky, I Just Want To Tone!"

Many women tend to be scared of weight training, or at least increased intensity weight training. They are under the impression that only high reps and endurance training are the only way to increase muscle tone, while low repetition weight training builds too much muscle bulk. Many commonly express they "don't want to become big and bulky".

Muscle tone is defined as the continuous or passive contraction of muscles. **To acquire muscle tone, performing resistance exercises at a resistance that will lead to increases in muscle contractile element and sarcoplasmic hypertrophy is needed**. High repetition muscle endurance training, on the other hand, leads to an increase in the oxygen carrying capacity of the muscle, and to some extent very minor increases in sarcoplasmic and contractile element hypertrophy.

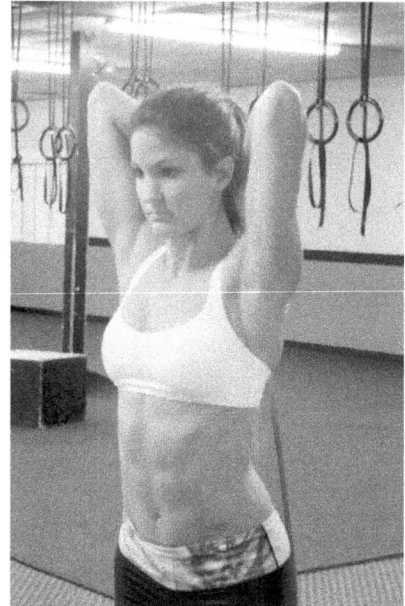

Hormones also play a major role in lean muscle accumulation. For instance, testosterone is regarded as the muscle-building hormone in humans. In theory the more testosterone you produce, the more muscle you are able to build. The fact that men and women produce different amounts of testosterone should shed some light on why most men are able to build more muscle than their female counterparts (*though nowadays with the increased risk of breast cancer in men, things may be changing*).

Men produce more testosterone. In fact, 10-20 times more on average. ***With 10-20X more testosterone, a male could be standing on a BOSU trainer, holding a medicine ball in one hand and a dumbbell in another, performing squats, shoulder presses, and curls while watching the hallmark network and still build more muscle than his female counterpart.***

Estrogen Rising

As mentioned in chapter 5, decreased testosterone levels and increased estrogen levels in men is slowly becoming an epidemic in today's society. Xenoestrogens and phytoestrogens are creeping into our everyday life. Estrogen mimickers can lead to a disruption of the endocrine system resulting in serious health problems. These deadly substances can be found in foods such as improperly fermented soy products (5,40). They are leached into our food through microwavable plastic bags and containers (*wouldn't recommend microwaving those vegetables in the bag they came in*). They are also seeping into our water supply through environmental chemicals, birth control pharmaceuticals, and plastic water bottles. Lastly, xenoestrogens have been found in our everyday cosmetics and household products (See www.ewg.org). Even certain alcoholic beverages are more estrogenic than others with the "MAN'S" drink, otherwise known as beer, being at the top of that list (33).

Let's take a break from the science and indulge in a little humor. So, if you are male and find yourself running to the mailbox to see if the new Bed, Bath and Beyond coupon has come in, you may want to consider having your serum testosterone levels checked. If you're a male and you find yourself spending more time talking about Grey's Anatomy with the staff at Payless Shoes, you may want to think about limiting the processed soy protein bars in your diet. If you're a male and you find yourself turning off Monday night football in exchange for your TIVO'd viewing of the Ellen Degeneres show, cutting out one of your 10 spinning classes may be a viable option. Lastly, if you are a male and you find that capri pants and muffin top half shirts outnumber jeans and t-shirts in your closet, you may want to partake in some strength training workouts a couple of times per week.

Exercise Order

Believe it or not, the order of your exercise may be just as important as the type of exercise you choose with regards to fat loss (11). Different exercise intensities have been shown to elicit different fat utilization responses (1,2,26). The order of strength training, interval training, and submaximal endurance exercise can also alter the fat burning effect of the exercises (11). *Studies have shown significant increases in total energy expenditure when high intensity work was followed by low intensity steady state work (11)*. As little as 45 minutes of high intensity followed by 15 minutes of low intensity can be effective.

Quality First

Let's examine the exercise order of a leg workout. In order to get the most out of a leg workout, it may not be wise to participate in a 1 hour spinning class, then go and test your 1 rep max in the squat. Probably would not want to go for the PR in the 100m after finishing a marathon either. The quality of the strength or power workout will be diminished by the fatigue induced from the prior long duration activity.

When it comes to cardiovascular training or metabolic conditioning, performing your high intensity work first has been shown to have a positive effect on fat cell mobilization (14). **The combination of high intensity intervals followed by longer duration, steady state fat burning cardio may be more effective for fat burning than long duration steady state training by itself**. For an even greater fat utilization, **cardio in the cold weather has been shown to expend 13% more energy, while utilizing 35% more fat during 1 hour of cardio (32)**.

Another effective method of ramping up fat utilization during a workout is to minimize carbohydrate ingestion in the hours prior to exercise. **Carbohydrate ingestion prior to a workout can significantly reduce the rate of fat oxidation (2)**.

Hypertrophy

To keep the adrenals healthy, while losing bodyfat and gaining lean muscle tissue, a combination of healthy diet (*individual tolerance to carbs must be determined*), proper cardiovascular/HIT training, and weight training may be required. With regards to weight

Studies as early as 1976 have been performed on rats to determine the different physiological outcomes induced by different methods of training. In one of the early studies the two types of hypertrophy were then referred to as compensatory hypertrophy and work-induced hypertrophy. Through the use of tenetomy and forced swimming, the researcher found differences in the way the hypertrophy actually occurred with the different training strategies. The compensatory hypertrophy strategy brought about increases in mitochondrial volume density, with a decrease in the myofibrillar volume and no changes in the sarcotubular (sarcoplasmic) density.

The work-induced hypertrophy strategy brought about an increase in the sarcotubular (sarcoplasmic) volume with no change in the myofibrillar or mitochondrial volume density. While this is technically not the same as relative strength/heavy weight training vs hypertrophy specific "bodybuilding" training, this study did show that different methods of training can technically lead to different forms of hypertrophy.

training, phases of heavy resistance and hypertrophy specific training can ensure both contractile protein (myofibrillar) and sarcoplasmic hypertrophy.

Contractile protein (myofibrillar) hypertrophy is the increase in the contractile elements involved in the generation of force and muscle tension. With heavy relative strength based weight training (1-5 reps), an increase in the density of the myofibrils (bundles of the contractile proteins actin and myosin) leads to an increase in the size of the actual muscle fiber. With minimal time under tension, the protein synthesis required for structural repair is less than that of sarcoplasmic hypertrophy (bodybuilding) training. Myofibrillar hypertrophy also requires a significant neurological contribution allowing for gains in strength with minimal gains in muscle hypertrophy (9,10).

Sarcoplasmic hypertrophy is an increase in the volume of the sarcoplasm, the cytoplasmic fluid that surrounds the myofibrils and its non-contractile elements. Unlike myofibrillar hypertrophy, the density of the contractile proteins does not change, but there is an increase in muscular size due to the increased volume of the surrounding sarcoplasm and the non-contractile elements (23,33).

With hypertrophy specific "bodybuilding" training, there is less protein degradation than heavy/relative strength training, but much greater time under tension. This time under tension combined with a greater volume of work leads to an increase in protein synthesis requirements and allows for greater structural repair demands.

A combination of both heavy strength training phases alternated with bodybuilding protocols may be one of the most effective training methods for developing lean muscle tissue. Below are sample templates of these training methods.

3 week Sample "bodybuilding" hypertrophy template:

Day I: Torso

Exercise	Rep Range	Sets	Tempo	Rest Interval
A1: Flat Dumbbell Bench Press	10-12	4	4020	60s
A2: Chin Ups	10-12	4	4020	60s
B1: Parallel Bar Dips	8-10	3	5010	60s
B2: Seated Cable Rows	10-12	3	4011	60s
C1: Supine Cable Flyes	12-15	3	3010	45s
C2: Kneeling Scarecrows	12-15	3	3010	45s

Day 2: Legs

Exercise	Rep Range	Sets	Tempo	Rest Interval
A1: Split Squats	10-12	4	4020	60s
A2: Kneeling Hamstring Curls	6-8	4	5020	60s
B1: Box Step Ups	10-12	3	1010	60s
B2: Stiff Legged Deadlifts	10-12	3	5010	60s
C1: Back Extensions	10-12	3	3030	45s
C2: Standing Calf Raises	10-12	3	3112	45s

Day 3: Biceps and Triceps

Exercise	Rep Range	Sets	Tempo	Rest Interval
A1: Supine Dumbbell Nosebreakers	10-12	4	4020	60s
A2: EZ bar Scott Curls	10-12	4	4020	60s
B1: Cable Tricep Pressdown	8-10	3	5010	60s
B2: Seated Dumbbell Curls	10-12	3	4011	60s
C1: Seated Dumbbell Ext Rotator	10-12	4	4020	60s
C2: Seated Cable Scap Retractions	10-12	4	4020	60s

3 week Sample strength template:

Day 1: Torso

Exercise	Rep Range	Sets	Tempo	Rest Interval
A1: Incline Barbell Bench Press	3-5	6	3010	120s
A2: Neutral Grip Chin Ups	3-5	6	3010	120s
B1: V Bar Dips	4-5	6	2011	120s
B2: Bent over Barbell Rows	4-5	6	3010	120s
C1: Standing Cable Ext Rot	4-6	3	2010	90s
C2: Dumbell 45deg trap 3 lift	4-6	3	2010	90s

Day 2: Legs

Exercise	Rep Range	Sets	Tempo	Rest Interval
A: Deadlift	3-5	10	2010	120s
B1: Lunges	4-5	5	2010	90s
B2: Prone Hamstring Curls	3-5	5	2010	120s
C1: Reverse Hyperextensions	4-6	3	2010	90s
C2: Seated Calf Raises	4-6	3	2010	90s

Day 3: Biceps and Triceps

Exercise	Rep Range	Sets	Tempo	Rest Interval
A1: Seated EZ Bar French Press	3-5	6	3010	90s
A2: Standing Barbell Curls	3-5	6	3010	120s
B1: Close Grip Bench Press	3-5	5	2110	90s
B2: Cable Preacher Curls	3-5	5	3010	120s

- Higher repetition ranges combined with fewer sets for the "bodybuilding" hypertrophy template vs longer rest, lower reps, and more sets for strength.

Training for Body Composition

Six pack abs. Toned arms and legs. Tight butt. We have seen all the slogans on the cover of virtually every fitness magazine. All of them with the same goal in mind: Improved body composition. Though diet probably plays the biggest part in achieving body composition improvements, proper training also plays a critical role. One type of training in particular, weight training, has been shown to be most effective in improving your body composition.

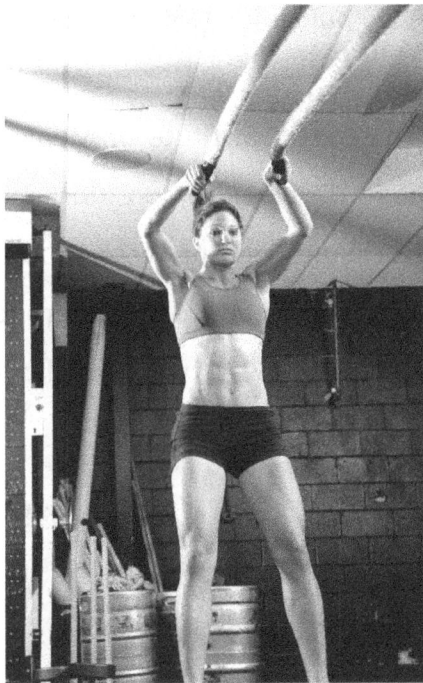

As we discussed earlier, the more lean muscle you add to your frame, the more efficient your metabolism becomes. As we showed, the most effective method for adding lean muscle is hypertrophy specific weight training. Hypertrophy based repetition counts with minimal rest periods are quite possibly the most effective fat burning tool you can add to your arsenal.

The basis for this type of training is to increase blood lactate levels while maintaining maximal time under tension. The increased blood lactate levels will lead to an increased secretion of growth hormone. Studies have shown that the greater the blood lactate levels the greater the growth hormone response (3,13,22).

Why does this matter? Growth hormone is the hormone that has been linked to positive body composition changes. Studies on the effects of growth hormone have shown that increased growth hormone levels leads to a subsequent positive alteration in body composition (6).

Through proper sarcoplasmic hypertrophy specific weight training, there is an increase in strength caused by the time under tension at a given resistance. With this increase in strength, hypertrophy gains, or gains in cross sectional area of contractile proteins are realized. The process of physically repairing the contractile proteins has been linked to a release of anabolic hormones, including growth hormone. Therefore, the greater the time under tension at a given resistance, the greater the blood lactate accumulation, the greater the potential for growth hormone secretion. This combined with minimal rest periods, to prevent the body from clearing high levels of blood lactate, and you have a one two punch for growth hormone secretion.

A fairly recent placebo controlled blind study out of the Garvin Institute of Medical Research in Australia measured the effects of growth hormone on body composition and physical performance of recreational athletes. Of the 96 participants, groups were broken down into the placebo group, the growth hormone group, and the combined treatment group (growth hormone and testosterone). After 8 weeks of treatment and a 6 week washout period, **the researchers found significant reductions in fat mass in the growth hormone treatment group**, while finding significant improvements in both fat mass reduction and muscle mass increases in the combined treatment group (24).

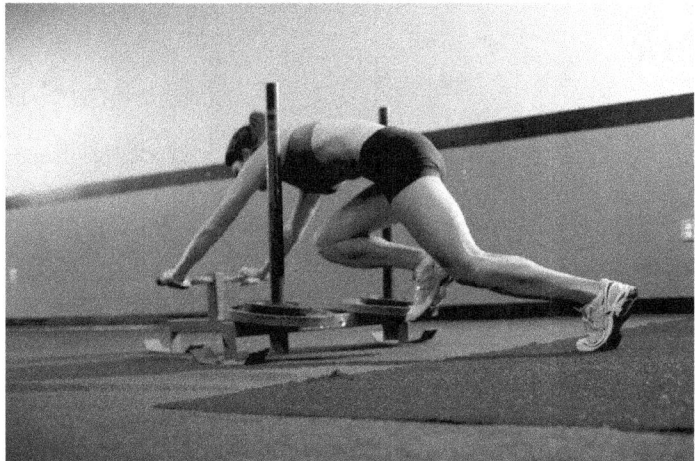

Keeping the lactate levels high while engaging in resistance-based training is the basis for many cross-training and boot camp style workouts. The combination of various forms of sprint intervals combined with either resistance training or calisthenics can be an effective method for increasing lactate levels, and therefore, enjoying the benefits of increased GH production.

Below are sample workouts of both weight training based body composition workouts and cross-training based workouts.

Weight Training Body Composition Workout

Exercise	Rep Range	Sets	Tempo	Rest Interval
A1: Dumbbell Split Squats	10-12	4	4020	45s
A2: Neutral Grip Chin Ups	10-12	4	4020	45s
B1: Parallel Bar Dips	8-10	4	5010	45s
B2: Walking Lunges	10-12	4	2010	45s
C1: Barbell Overhead Press	10-12	3	3010	45s
C2: Standing Dumbbell Curls	10-12	3	3010	45s
C3: Tricep Pressdowns	10-12	3	3010	45s

Compound Exercise Body Composition Sample Workout

Exercise	Rep Range	Sets	Tempo	Rest Interval
A1: Deadlifts	10-12	5	4020	10s
A2: Dumbbell Bench Press	10-12	5	4020	10s
A3: Back Squats	10-12	5	5010	10s
A4: Chin Ups	10-12	5	2010	120s

Total Body Weight training with Metabolic Sprints

Exercise	Rep Range	Sets	Tempo	Rest Interval
A1: Back Squats	10-12	4	4020	30s
A2: Incline Dumbbell Bench Press	10-12	4	4020	30s
A3: Versaclimber Sprint Interval	30s	3		45s
B1: Leg Press	25-30	4	1010	30s
B2: Pull ups	10-12	4	4010	30s
B3: Versaclimber Sprint Interval	30s	3		45s
C1: Back Extensions	10-12	3	3030	15s
C2: Kneeling Cable Crunches	10-12	3	3112	20s
C3: VersaClimber Sprint Intervals	30s	3		45s

Upper Body Body Composition Workout

Exercise	Rep Range	Sets	Tempo	Rest Interval
A1: Incline Barbell Bench Press	10-12	4	3010	10s
A2: Flat Dumbbell Bench Press	10-12	4	2010	10s
A3: Decline Barbell Bench Press	10-12	4	1010	10s
A4: Flat Dumbbell Flys	12-15	4	1010	90s
A5: Chin Ups	10-12	4	4010	10s
A6: Pronated grip Lat Pulldowns	10-12	3	2010	10s
A7: Seated Cable Rows	45-60s	3	1010	10s
A8: Reverse Cable Flyes (Scarecrows)	10-12	3	1010	120s

Cross-Training Workout Sample 1

Exercise	Rep Range	Sets	Tempo	Rest Interval
A1: Ring Chin Ups	10-15	5		0s
A2: Dumbbell Bench Press	25	5		0s
A3: Farmer Carry	40yds	5		0s
A4: Backward Sled Drag	40yds	5		120s

Cross-Training Workout Sample (go through this as many times as you can in 16 minutes)

Exercise	Rep Range	Sets	Tempo	Rest Interval
A1: Tire Flips	5	16m		0s
A2: Overhead Log Press	8	16m		0s
A3: 40yd Prowler Push	40yds	16m		0s

Millenium

Exercise	Rep Range	Sets	Tempo	Rest Interval
A1: Back Squats	10	10		0s
A2: Flat Dumbbell Bench Press	10	10		0s
A3: Chin Ups	10	10		0s
A4: Standing Overhead Press	10	10		0s
A5: Standing Dumbbell Curl	10	10		0s
A6: Tricep Pressdown	10	10		0s
A7: Dumbbell Squats	10	10		0s
A8: Pushups	10	10		0s
A9: Inverted Ring Rows	10	10		0s
A10: Plank Crunches	10	10		0s

Calisthenic Based Workout (Goal is to complete 4 rounds in 12 minutes or less)

Exercise	Rep Range	Sets	Tempo	Rest Interval
A1: Body Squats	50	4		0s
A2: Pushups	30	4		0s
A3: Floor Crunches	30	4		0s
A4: Chin Ups	10	4		0s

Calisthenic/Kettlebell Based Workout

Exercise	Rep Range	Sets	Rest Interval
A1: Kettlebell Swings	25,20,15,10,5,10,15,20,25	9	0s
A2: Super Murphy's	5,4,3,2,1,2,3,4,5	9	0s

One super Murphy is 5 pushup and 20 mountain climbers then jump to your feet

Functional Strength Workout

Exercise	Rep Range	Sets	Tempo	Rest Interval
A1: Hand over hand rope pull	30yds	5		0s
A2: Prowler Press	30yds	5		60s
A3: Atlas Stone Carry	30yds	5		0s
A4: Backward Sled Drag	30yds	5		60s

Cross Training Workout (5 rounds as fast as you can: timed)

Exercise	Rep Range	Sets	Rest Interval
A1: Burpees	10	5	0s
A2: Med Ball Slams	20	5	0s
A3: 120yd Sprint	120yds	5	0s
A4: Chin ups	10	5	0s
A5: 30yd fwd/30yd bckwd bear crawl	60yd	5	N

Team Builders

"Field Trip"

Exercise	Rep Range	Sets	Rest Interval
A: Farmer Carry	5280 feet	N	0s

Teams of 4. Each person carries as far as they can. Once one person fatigues the next one hops in. Keep alternating until you have completed the pre-determined distance.

"Field Trip"

Exercise	Rep Range	Sets	Rest Interval
A1: Prowler Push	300yds	N	0s
A2: Bckwd Sled Drag	300yds	N	0s

**Teams of 4. Each person pushes the prowler or drags the sled as far as they can. Once one person fatigues the

As you probably noticed, each of these workouts contains multiple exercise modalities combined with short rest intervals to ensure greater lactate levels and maximal growth hormone secretion. For more information on strength training for body composition the following books are highly recommended:

- *German Body Composition* **by Charles Poliquin**: Written by one of the most successful and respected strength coaches in the world, this is quite possibly the best body composition book available today.

- *Lose Fat Forever* **by Derek and Don Alessi**: Easy to read, yet filled with an abundance of practical information, this book provides the science and the application of effective body composition methodologies.

Supplements

Depending on how hard you are training and how well you are eating, a supplement regimen may also help in optimizing your health and fat loss goals. Too many individuals misperceive the term "supplement" with the latest and greatest powders, pills, or drinks found in the pages of monthly muscle magazines.

The term dietary supplement, as found on the Webster's dictionary webpage is defined as *a product taken orally that contains one or more ingredients that are intended to supplement one's diet and are not considered food.*

11 supplements that may help to optimize your health

1. **HCL/Digestive Enzymes:** With the decreases in stomach acid levels associated with poor dieting, age, stress, and other environmental factors, the ability to properly absorb the macro and micronutrients found in our food sources can be severely compromised.

As could be seen in chapter 4, GERD may be caused by a dysfunctional LES (lower esophageal sphincter) or *low stomach acid levels*. Understanding that these levels may be too low, wouldn't it be common sense to test the actual stomach acid levels rather than esophageal acid levels, and then correct the actual problem.

Some of the benefits of proper stomach acid levels include proper breakdown of macronutrients, stimulation of pepsin release for breakdown of proteins, overall immune health, and protection against various bacteria and microorganisms.

If you are not breaking down your food properly in your stomach, how can you expect to maximally absorb your vitamins, minerals, and macronutrients?

Some quality digestive enzyme/HCL products include Metagenics line of gastrointestinal support products (www.metagenics.com), Solaray HCL + Pepsin, and Poliquin's Digestive Enzymes or HCL 4.0.

2. **Fish oil (or other high quality Omega 3 fatty acids):** Enough cannot be said about the benefits of fish oils and Omega 3 fatty acids. From their function in fat loss to their cardiovascular benefits, fish oil and other Omega 3 fatty acids are a critical component in human health. So important that roughly 96,000 deaths per year in the US have been associated with a lack of Omega 3 fatty acids. Fish oils have been shown to protect the body from inflammation and cognitive dysfunction, as well as have positive benefits on everything from aging, Alzheimer's, and anxiety to blood pressure and immune functioning. If you are not currently taking a quality fish oil or Omega 3 supplement, you may want to consider one as the health benefits are numerous.

3. **Vitamin D3:** As mentioned in the vitamin and mineral chapter, besides Thyroid hormone, the body has receptor sites on every tissue/cell for only one compound, Vitamin D. That must mean that vitamin D is pretty important to human health. In the supplemental form of D3 (calciferol), vitamin D has been shown to have dramatic benefits on human health, as well as deficiencies in this critical vitamin being linked to everything from cancer and diabetes to thyroid and heart problems. With regards to fat

loss, the role vitamin D has in insulin regulation, thyroid function, and testosterone production may be of utmost importance.

I remember hearing a highly respected functional medicine doctor once say, "If you don't want to get sick this winter, make sure you take your vitamin D." With that said, if you are sick you cannot train. If you cannot train, it may be difficult to pack on fat metabolizing lean muscle tissue.

4. **Quality Multivitamin:** Much of the food we eat today lacks the vitamin and mineral content of our food sources just 30 years ago. And that goes for those who are trying to eat healthy foods. Never mind those who are known by their first name and asked if they want the "usual" at your local fast food restaurants.

A quality multivitamin should contain quality, highly absorbable forms of vitamins and minerals, rather than the cheap counterparts typically used in most of the more "popular" brands sold at the local convenience store. Look for one that has no fillers or artificial ingredients.

5. **Adaptogenic Herbs:** Termed by a Russian Scientist back in the 1960's the word adaptogen refers to any plant based herb that can bring the body back to balance by "adapting" to the physiological and psychological demands of the body. For instance if you have low energy, adaptogens may rejuvenate your energy stores. If you are stressed, adaptogens can have an anti-stress activity. These amazing herbs have been known to produce positive effects on everything from immune health and mental clarity, to decreasing inflammation and increasing cardiovascular health.

Through their hormonal adaptations (thought to modulate the HPA (hypothalamus-pituitary-adrenal) Axis, adaptogenic herbs can often restore homeostasis to the human system. In essence adaptogens enhance the body's ability to resist and adapt to physical and psychological stress.

6. **Antioxidants:** In case you have not seen the movie, there is a battle scene in The Lord of the Rings part 2: The Twin Towers. The heroes and their small gang of less than 500 humans and elves must protect the fortress Helms Deep from the evil army consisting of over 10,000 trolls, goblins, and Uruk-hai, created to wipeout mankind. Resveratrol, CoQ10, Alpha Lipoic Acid, Vitamin E (all tocopherols and tocotrienols), Vitamin C, Selenium, Pycnogenol, and various flavonoids, carotenes and various other antioxidants are the protective good guys. Too much oxidative stress, overburdened immune and detoxification systems, toxins, chemicals, and stress are the bad guys. The human body is the battlefield. Oxidative stress, overburdened detoxification processes and compromised immune function have been linked to almost every human health ailment. Antioxidants have been shown to be some of the primary defenses against these adverse health triggers.

7. **B Complex:** After reading the chapter on vitamins and minerals, you should realize the importance of the B-vitamins and the role they play in human health. Everything from cognitive functioning and cancer prevention, to energy production and immune function, B vitamins must be at optimum levels for the body to realize these and the many other benefits.

8. **Probiotics:** Increasing your healthy gut bacteria can have profound effects on your health. Roughly 70-80% of your immune system is found in the gut. Autoimmune disorders as well as various other negative health effects may stem from compromised healthy bacteria levels in the human gut.

9. **Carnitine:** So important is this nutrient substance, the late world-renowned functional nutrition expert Robert Crayhon wrote an entire book on it. Synthesized mainly in the liver and kidneys carnitine plays a highly important role in human energy production, transporting fatty acids to the mitochondria. Fat metabolism, serum testosterone levels and cardiac function are highly dependent on Carnitine levels.

Besides its role in fat metabolism and energy production, Carnitine has been shown to increase the sensitivity of unbound androgen receptors increasing the amount of serum testosterone. Studies have shown carnitine supplementation to have positive benefits on the quality of workout while enhancing recovery.

10. **Quality protein shake and BCAA's:** Catabolic vs anabolic state. Which would you prefer? After a hard workout, the body can fall into a catabolic state with a rise in catabolic hormones and a drop in anabolic hormones. With certain supplements such as Branch Chain Amino Acids (BCAA's) or quality whey/casein protein shakes the body can quickly return to an anabolic state after a workout. The ingestion of BCAA's pre/during or after a workout can keep testosterone levels from dipping too low, while keeping cortisol levels from elevating too dramatically. The same goes for a post workout Quality protein shake.

These can also have beneficial effects on protein degradation during workouts as well as increasing protein synthesis in the hours/days after the workout.

11. **Greens Powders/Drinks:** Alkalizing agents. Antioxidants. Digestive nutrients. Healthy bacteria. The benefits to a quality greens drink are many, especially for those not ingesting proper amounts of healthy green vegetables or high antioxidant fruits and berries. These simple drinks may restore and in some cases enhance immune health and PH levels.

Fat Burning/Blocking supplements

After your optimal health supplement regimen is in order, perhaps you may be thinking about investing in some sort of fat burning/fat blocking supplement. Now that you have a clearer picture of how fat metabolism works, let's take a brief look at some supplement ingredients that are known for their potential fat burning/blocking properties.

1. Guarana (Paullinia Cupana)

You're saying, "I know I have seen this any somewhere. Oh, yeah, those energy drinks I have been drinking." Well here is the "skinny" on this fat mobilizing herb. Native to the Amazon, Guarana is loaded with a substance very similar to caffeine called guaranine, which is known as an energy enhancer, and potential fat cell mobilizer. This herb can be used as a caffeine substitute as it seems to lack the jittery side effect.

2. Yerba Mate (Ilex Paraguariensis)

This antioxidant-laden shrub is loaded with vitamins and minerals including magnesium, selenium, and Vitamin E. Yerba Mate has been shown to have positive effects on both brain boosting and fat burning. Be careful with what you read about Yerba Mate as there has been research on the correlation between Yerba Mate and cancer. One of the studies found a positive correlation. Interesting enough the correlation was not between the Mate leaves and cancer, but smoke from the wood used to create the fire to dry the leaves and cancer. Much of the other research has found the antioxidant capacities to be anti-carcinogenic.

3. Green Tea

Hard to believe that something this simple has such strong effects on fat metabolism. When ingesting a green tea drink or supplement, not only are you getting the thermogenic and brain stimulating effects from the caffeine, but you are also getting the calming effects of the amino acid Theanine as well. As an added bonus, the EGCG (Epigallocatechin gallate) catechin content may also provide a one two punch against muscle soreness, inflammation, and cancer. Be sure to drink green teas that have no sugar or artificial color or flavoring.

4. Carnitine

Not exactly an amino acid, but close, this nutrient is associated with fatty acid transport to the mitochondria to be used as energy. In other words, it brings the fat cells to the furnace where they can be used as fuel. Some of the side benefits of carnitine include sensitizing of unbound androgen receptors and cognitive functioning.

5. Bitter Orange (Citrus aurantium)

This Chinese herbal has long been used for its health promoting benefits. The research is a little unclear on the usage as a single ingredient, as the synephrine has been shown to have similar effects to the currently banned ephedrine. A "calmer" version of Ephedrine, Synephrine is known as an appetite suppressor as well as adrenal stimulator. It may be wise to consult with a knowledgeable Chinese Medicine Practitioner or Functional Medicine doctor prior to trying this one out.

6. GuggalSterone (Guggul Lipid)

Guggul Lipid is the sap from the bark of a tree. How come in the US the sap we get from our trees is turned to maple syrup and makes us fat, while the sap from the Mukul myrhh tree found in Africa, Asia and India has the exact opposite effect. Not only has Guggul been linked to cardiovascular benefits, but some of the studies (performed on animals) show that it may enhance thyroid hormone metabolism, which in turn can raise metabolism.

Sample Pre-Workout Stacks

Another option may be a quality pre-workout stack to promote fat loss, optimize energy production, and increase mental acuity. An effective pre-workout supplement strategy may be beneficial in getting you through your fat loss plateaus. Though there are many supplement concoctions on the market proclaiming miraculous results in just weeks, it may be a bit of a stretch to achieve such drastic changes without dietary changes and proper training. Below are a few pre- workout supplement strategies that may help increase workout energy levels and promote fat cell utilization.

a. **The poor man's pre-workout concoction:** Coffee (black with Stevia or Cinnamon) + L-Tyrosine. The caffeine in the coffee gives you the pick me up, as well as may increase muscle contractility and fat cell mobilization. The amino acid L-tyrosine is a pre-cursor to the catecholamine hormones (noradrenaline and adrenaline) as well as the rate limiting enzyme in the synthesis of dopamine, which increases heart rate dilates blood vessels, increases blood flow, and affects cognition. Dopamine may also increase levels of testosterone while decreasing galactin levels.

b. **The Anti-Catabolic Stack:** Branch Chain Amino Acids, Carnitine, and Green Tea. When taken before a workout, branched chain amino acids have been shown to keep post workout testosterone levels elevated and decrease the protein degradation from strength training. The combination of BCAA's, carnitine and Green Tea can have positive effects on strength and energy as well as enhanced recovery from workouts.

   The carnitine plays a beneficial role in testosterone binding sites and energy production. The green tea provides the caffeine and the potential to decrease DOMS (delayed onset muscle soreness). Among their many benefits, BCAA's can decrease protein degradation and aid in maintaining healthy catabolic/anabolic hormone ratios during and after the workout.

c. **Chinese Herbals:**

   1. **Tongkat Ali:** This potent herb may increase dopamine levels, increase testosterone levels and decrease sex hormone binding globulin levels and leaves you with higher levels of free testosterone.
   2. **Mucuna Pruriens Extract:** Another dopamine stimulator, probably due to the fact that is contains l-dopa, which is a precursor to dopamine.

3. **Epimedium (horny goat weed):** Found in many "enhancement" supplements, this Chinese herb may increase testosterone as well as increase nitric oxide production. The name comes from Chinese legend in which a goat herder noticed a dramatic increase in his flocks' sexual activity after eating this weed.

4. **Cnidium:** Another Nitric oxide enhancer, Cnidium is a potent herb in increasing sexual function and circulation.

d. **The Grocery store Stack**: Sugar free energy drink with Guarana, Ginseng, Ginkgo, and Echinacea and organic coconut oil. The coconut provides the pre-workout amino acid fix, along with medium chain triglycerides for energy/mental function.

If you really want to get down and dirty: Green Tea + Vinpocetine + a testosterone boosting Chinese herb + slap in the face from your ex-girlfriend. Vinpocetine can enhance circulation and oxygen utilization in the brain. The green tea will give the caffeine energy kick without the jitters, while the Chinese herb may raise dopamine levels giving you a little extra "oomph" in your workout.

Supplements may not always be essential, as sleep patterns, recovery from workouts, and stress reduction also play key roles in energy production and vigorous health. But, if you find you are lacking in any of these departments, a "pick me up" or energy boost prior to your workout may be a viable option.

CHAPTER IX

OLYMPIC WEIGHTLIFTING, 2 A DAY WORKOUTS AND GLUCOSE TOLERANCE

The ability for your body to not only burn calories during workouts, but also burn them outside of workouts is a critical element in fat loss and increased metabolic rate. Keeping the insulin sensitivity ramped up can be the difference between storing calories in the muscle and liver tissue vs the fat cells.

Creating a furnace fueled by fat should be the goal of any body composition venture. Increasing the efficiency of glucose uptake and fat cell utilization are priority. Optimizing growth hormone secretion and androgen/cortisol ratios while maintaining insulin sensitivity glucose transporter expression can be effective methods in the battle of the bulge. Let's look at a few strategies for achieving optimal fat metabolism.

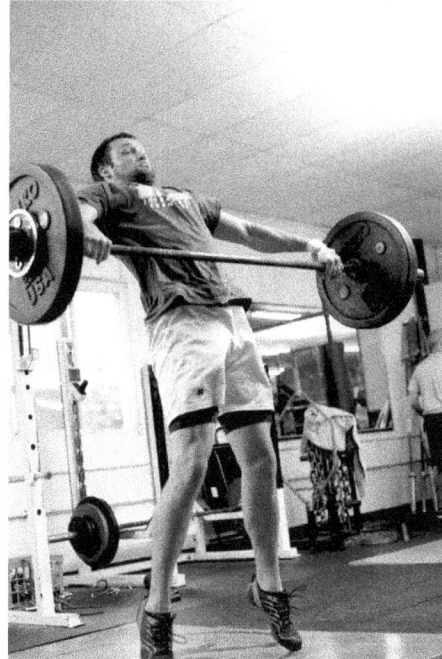

Glucose Tolerance

Shuttling glucose into muscle and liver tissue is a priority in order to get or stay lean. GLUT transporters are transport proteins found in soft tissue cells, particularly fat and muscle tissue. When the body consumes calories, insulin is secreted to signal the cells to begin absorption of glucose in the bloodstream. With regards to glucose transport we are interested in the GLUT 4 transporter. One of 13 sugar transport proteins, GLUT 4 is primarily responsible for glucose, while GLUT 5 and GLUT 11 are hypothesized to be fructose transporters.

At the surface of muscle, liver, and fat cells is an insulin receptor responsible for the activation of the GLUT 4 transport proteins found inside the cells. These transport proteins act as shuttles by transporting the glucose from the outside of the cell to the inside of the cell where it is then stored as Glucose-6-phosphate. GLUT 4 proteins are only activated in the presence of insulin.

When blood insulin levels decrease, the GLUT 4 proteins leave the surface of the cell. If they do not leave the surface, cellular uptake of glucose will continue. Likewise, if one is insulin resistant or diabetic, the insulin secretion may be too great for the GLUT 4 proteins to handle, eventually leading to a decreased expression of these proteins.

Increasing the expression of these proteins can lead to greater sensitivity of insulin. For instance working out has been shown to increase GLUT 4 protein expression as well as insulin sensitivity. A 2002 study found that those subjects with insulin resistance had better glucose transport and increased insulin sensitivity after working out. The research found an increase in the expression of GLUT-4 transport proteins is associated with bouts of acute exercise [13]. This may be one of the reasons the body becomes more carbohydrate tolerant after an intense exercise bout.

Hormones and Training

Besides enhanced glucose tolerance, weight training has also been shown to have positive effects on androgen hormone responses. In 1988, researchers studied nine elite weight lifters over a two-year period, measuring endocrine and neuromuscular characteristics. Over that time, androgen hormones rose significantly, indicating a positive hormonal response to the training. The researchers concluded that the intensive training over prolonged periods of time could lead to increases in androgen hormone production [7].

It is important to distinguish between resistance training and endurance training. Excessive endurance training has been shown to not only be less effective at increasing insulin sensitivity, but also more detrimental in increasing inflammatory biomarkers. A 2003 study found that with excessive eccentric training, ie; marathon running, a state of insulin resistance can be induced for up to 48 hours after the exercise bout. Possible rationale includes the dramatic inflammation resulting from this form of training. On the other side of the coin, a smart approach to exercise, including proper resistance training, can lead to an increase in glucose tolerance while decreasing the expression of the inflammatory biomarkers associated with excessive eccentric endurance training [17].

Regarding the hormonal response to different types of exercise, in 2004 a research team studied and compared the physiological characteristics of weightlifters, cyclists, and controls. 41 subjects were broken down into the three groups, with the researchers testing serum hormone levels, strength, power, muscle mass, and endurance. The researchers found on average 50% higher power values in the weightlifters, while the muscle mass and strength values were not as significant. Of particular interest though were the testosterone levels among the three groups. The weightlifters had significantly higher testosterone levels than the other two groups, while the untrained individuals actually had higher testosterone levels the elite amateur cyclists [15].

In looking at the results, the higher power output and strength values seen in the weightlifters may be due to the positive hormonal response resulting from their training methods. One could argue that athletes with higher testosterone levels gravitate toward the strength sports, but the study did provide insight on the fact that untrained individuals actually had higher T levels than their high volume, endurance training counterparts.

So which is better, relative strength work or hypertrophy specific training? Each has their benefits. Depending on the individual needs of the athlete, both may be necessary, as each elicits a different endocrine response. Research has compared the hormonal responses of 10 sets of 10 hypertrophy training versus 20 sets of 1 relative strength training. The 10 sets of 10 elicited a much greater growth hormone response, while the 20 sets of 1 led to more positive increases in testosterone [8].

Strength training is very important, not only for its effects on body composition, bone mineral density, cardiovascular health, but also for its positive effects on the endocrine system. Let's look at possible strategies for ensuring fat loss success.

Two a day training

Understanding that resistance training increases glucose tolerance and insulin sensitivity after a workout, just imagine what the effects of two workouts in one day might be. The possibility of an optimal hormonal profile and the compounding effect of increasing GLUT 4 expression and insulin sensitivity twice in one day exist.

Many national teams have taken the two a day approach with great success by combining several short duration, high intensity workouts throughout the day. The shorter workouts allow the body to keep cortisol levels at bay while keeping testosterone optimal. Multiple workouts also allow the athletes to train and eat without gaining excessive bodyfat due to the positive glucose tolerance and increased insulin sensitivity.

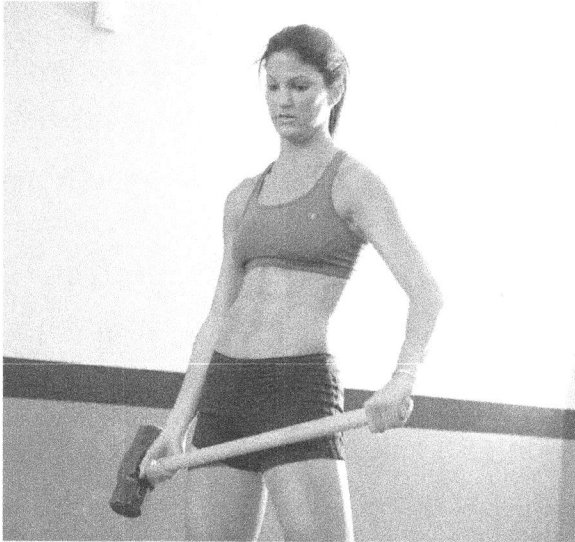

In 2007, researchers compared the effects of one a day and twice a-day training in ten nationally ranked competitive weightlifters. After the three week study period, the two a day training group had twice the gain in EMG muscle activation results, as well as much more favorable increases in testosterone and testosterone/cortisol ratios [12].

On an acute level, the effects of twice a day training can be just as important as the long term effects. Research out of Finland tested those effects. After two high intensity-training sessions in one day, the researchers studied various strength, EMG, and hormonal parameters in the subjects. Though decreases in EMG and isometric strength were seen, increases in testosterone were measured during the second workout of the day, followed by a drop in these hormones post workout. The researchers concluded that acute hormonal and neuromuscular responses could be elicited with two a day high intensity training [5].

The same research team then studied the same eight weightlifters through one week of two a day training sessions, monitoring the same physiological variables. Once again, decreases in EMG and isometric strength were seen, while significant increases in free and total testosterone were seen during the second training session of each day. One of the most interesting findings of this study was the testosterone rebound that occurred. The researchers found the T levels to gradually decrease as the week went on, but after only one day of rest, the T levels had rebounded back to the baseline levels measured before the training started. If the study had been longer, with T level measurements during the rest and recovery periods, the T levels could have potentially rebounded to even greater levels. It is for this reason that phases of hard training followed by proper recovery can lead to dramatic gains in strength, power, and hypertrophy (6).

We know relative strength training and hypertrophy training elicit different hormonal responses. We have seen that two a-day training can be of benefit for lean muscle accumulation and optimal hormonal profile. We know that glucose tolerance and insulin sensitivity are highly important factors in minimizing body fat accumulation. What else can we do?

Training Efficiency and Olympic Weightlifting

Olympic weightlifting has gained popularity the past few years with the growth of many cross training workout regimens and centers. The Olympic lifts consist of the Snatch and the Clean and Jerk. Related exercises include variations from various start and catch positions. Athletes and strength coaches have used these exercises for decades due to their explosive characteristics and ability to develop triple extension: extension of the hips, knees and ankles. Explosive triple extension may be one of the single greatest movement characteristics separating athletes on the field.

Another great quality of Olympic weightlifting is its ability to actively recruit a large number of motor units/muscle fibers with just one lift. It may be the most compound of compound exercises. When done properly, the muscles of the posterior chain (glutes, hammies, low, mid and upper back, calf musculature) are all activated to initiate the pulling movement. Upon completion of the second pull, the catch involves a deep squat, requiring the muscles about the core, back, shoulders, quadriceps, and hips to eccentrically load the weight and then concentrically drive the weight upward in a front squat.

An excellent study from 2007 compared the metabolic effects of exercises with high contraction speeds versus those with low contraction speeds. The researchers had 9 subjects perform squat variations at different contractions speeds with different loads. Blood lactate samples were collected every 15 minutes for one hour after the workout, while expired air was taken before, during, 60, and 90 minutes post workout. The researchers found higher blood lactate levels after the slow contraction training, but the energy expenditure rates were significantly greater during and after the workout with the explosive training group [20].

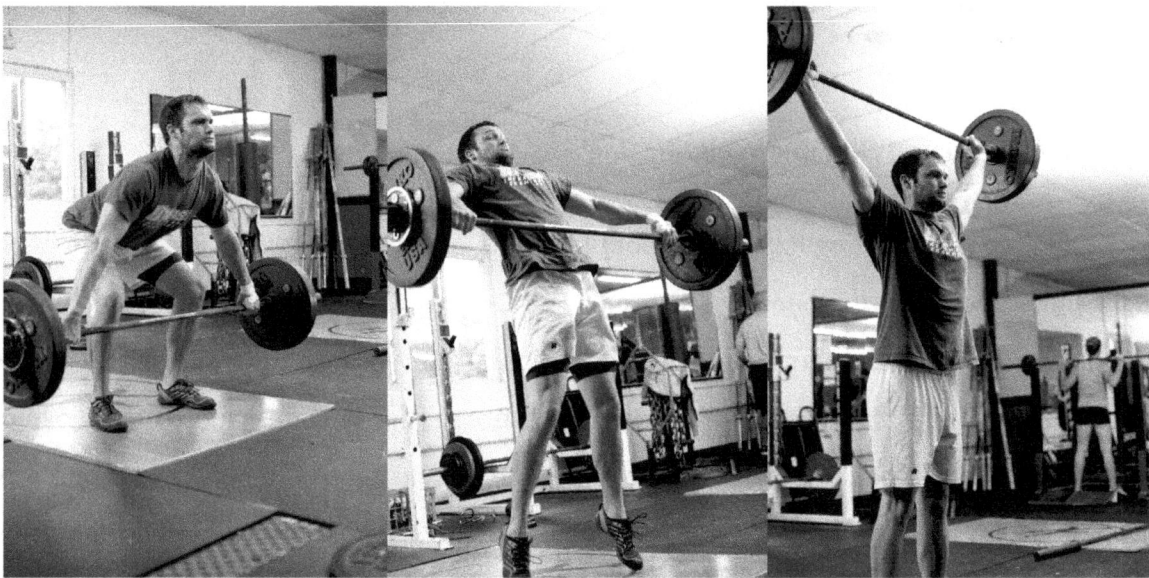

Not only have Olympic lifts been associated with dramatic increases in strength and power, but their effects on metabolism and androgenic hormone production may be under appreciated. Studies have shown Olympic lifts to have positive effects on androgen hormones and strength gains. From their maximization of motor unit recruitment, to their eccentric-less movement, Olympic lifts are one of the most efficient methods of optimizing strength, power and metabolism.

Another overlooked element of the Olympic lifts is their ability to create and improve flexibility. From the initial starting position, which requires hamstring flexibility and low back mobility, to the catch which requires flexibility about the hips, shoulders, and back, these lifts are an excellent method of actively training transferable flexibility.

Olympic Weightlifting Technique:

The best way to learn correct Olympic weightlifting technique is to hire an Olympic Weightlifting or USAW certified coach. It can be difficult to learn technique or correct technical flaws when learning from videos, books, and internet websites.

Putting it Together

- Focus on eating carbohydrates when insulin sensitivity and GLUT 4 expression are high.
- Weight training increases glucose tolerance and insulin sensitivity.
- Two a-day training keeps glucose tolerance elevated.
- Olympic weightlifting is an efficient method for increasing metabolism, strength, and power.
- Combining these can potentially lead to increased gains in fat metabolism, strength, and hypertrophy.

Sample 2-a-Day Programs

4 Day Per Week Sample Program

Split Routine Day 1 Am Workout

Exercise	Rep Range	Sets	Tempo	Rest Interval
A1: Barbell Bench Press	2-3	8	51X0	180s
A2: Chin Ups	2-3	8	51X0	180s
B1: Dips	3-5	4	31X2	120s
B2: Bent Over Barbell Rows	3-5	4	31X2	120s
C1: Dumbbell Trap 3 Lift	6-8	3	3011	45s
C2: Cable External Rotator	6-8	3	3011	45s

Split Routine Day 1 Pm Workout

Exercise	Rep Range	Sets	Tempo	Rest Interval
A1: Neutral Grip Dumbbell Bench Press	10-12	3	4010	20s
A2: Pushups	15-20	3	1010	60s
A3: Neutral Grip Chin Ups	10-12	3	3010	20s
A4: Seated Cable Rows	15-20	3	2010	60s

Split Routine Day 2 AM Workout

Exercise	Rep Range	Sets	Tempo	Rest Interval
A: Olympic Cleans from above knee	2-3	5	X0X0	180s
B1: Front Squats	3-5	6	31X0	120s
B2: Kneeling Hamstring Curls	3-5	6	40X1	120s
C: Reverse Hyperextensions	4-6	3	3011	90s

Split Routine Day 2 PM Workout

Exercise	Rep Range	Sets	Tempo	Rest Interval
A1: Dumbbell Split Squats	10-12	3	4010	60s
A2: Box Step Ups	10-12	3	1010	60s
B: Walking Lunges	10-12/leg	3	3010	60s
C: Leg Press	25-30	3	2010	60s

Split Routine Day 3 Am Workout

Exercise	Rep Range	Sets	Tempo	Rest Interval
A1: Close Grip Bench Press w/chains	3-5	6	3010	120s
A2: Fat Grip Barbell Curls	3-5	6	3010	120s
B1: EZ Bar Skull Crushers	3-5	5	3010	120s
B2: EZ Bar Preacher Curls	3-5	5	3010	120s

Split Routine Day 3 Pm Workout

Exercise	Rep Range	Sets	Tempo	Rest Interval
A1: Overhead EZ Bar Tricep Extensions	10-12	5	4010	20s
A2: Rope Tricep Pressdowns	10-12	5	3010	60s
A3: Incline Dumbbell Curls	10-12	5	3010	20s
A4: Standing Dumbbell Curls	10-12	5	3010	60s

Split Routine Day 4 Am Workout

Exercise	Rep Range	Sets	Tempo	Rest Interval
A1: Olympic Snatch from mid thigh	2-3	5	X0X0	180s
B1: Back Squats	3-5	6	31X0	120s
B2: Swiss ball hamstring curls	3-5	6	40X1	120s
C: Glute Ham Raise	4-6	3	3010	90s

Split Routine Day 4 Pm Workout

Exercise	Rep Range	Sets	Tempo	Rest Interval
A1: Dumbell Step Forward Lunges	10-12/leg	4	3010	20s
A2: 1 ¼ dumbbell squats	20	4	3010	60s
B1: Walking Lunges	10-12/leg	4	2010	20s
B2: Backward Sled Drags	40yds	4		90s

3 Day Per Week Sample Template

Cross-Training Total Body Day 1 Am Workout

Exercise	Rep Range	Sets	Tempo	Rest Interval
A1: Power Clean from hang above knee	2-3	5	X0X0	120s
B1: Deadlifts	2	5	2010	60s
B2: Standing Overhead Press	4-6	5	3010	60s
C1: Tire Flips	3-5	3	X0X0	45s
C2: Gymnastic Ring Dips	8-10	3	2010	60s
D1: Hand Stand Pushups	N	2	2010	20s
D2: Landmine	20	2	1010	20s
D3: Backward Sled Drag	40yds	2		60s

Cross-Training Total Body Day 1 Pm Workout

Exercise	Rep Range	Sets	Tempo	Rest Interval
A1: Front Squat	5-6	12m	3010	0s
A2: Wide Grip Pull ups	8-10	12m	3010	0s
B1: Snatch Grip Deadlifts	5-6	12m	3010	0s
B2: Parallel Bar Dips	10	12m	2010	0s

12m is 12 minutes. Alternate between the two exercises for 12 minutes

Cross-Training Total Body Day 2 AM Workout

Exercise	Rep Range	Sets	Tempo	Rest Interval
A: Power Snatch from hang above knee	2-3	5	X0X0	120s
B1: Atlas Stones	2-4	4		45s
B2: Split Jerk	3-4	4	X0X0	60s
C1: 60s Heavy Bag Round	60s	5		0s
C2: Gymnastic Ring Jacknifes	10	5	2010	0s
C3: Plank Crunches	10	5	2010	0s
C4: Lateral Med Ball Slamdowns	10	5	X0X0	90s

CHAPTER X

ONE SIZE DOES
NOT FIT ALL

In order to get in the best shape, many still believe they need to:

1. **Run on the treadmill at least 1 hour per day**

2. **Eat a diet consisting of zone numbers (40/30/30) regardless of the sources of those calories**

3. **Drink 4 protein shakes a day (because they read that the muscle competitor in the newest muscle magazine does this)**

4. **Perform 3 muscle endurance circuit workouts per week in order to lose weight/bodyfat.**

Let's discuss each of these recommendations and determine if they are viable options for attaining our "best shape".

Hormones and Endurance Training

Knowledge of the fact that hormones play a critical role in both exercise and supplement prescription and dietary recommendations is critical. A practical approach might be to not assume you are not like every other gymgoer. You may have individual differences and needs.

For example, you may have elevated cortisol levels, which can lead to impaired insulin sensitivity. This can disrupt the balance between cortisol, insulin and testosterone [21]. This imbalance can then lead to a decrease in the production of anabolic hormone precursors or a disruption in the conversion of these anabolic precursors. The recommendation of 1 hour of long, slow, distance training on the treadmill might elevate those cortisol levels even higher [5,14] and lead to a greater imbalance between the anabolic and catabolic hormones [7,13].

Studies have shown that exercise stress can also disrupt other hormones, including leptin [6], which plays a role in your body's satiety mechanism. With the endocrine system in a less than optimal state, excessive endurance exercise or prolonged physical activity can impair the body's ability to mobilize fat cells (6), leading to an inability to utilize free fatty acids as a fuel source. *In essence, all that excessive endurance training may actually make you fatter!*

GLYCEMIC LOAD

Next, the zone diet recommendation (40/30/30) may be too heavy on the carbohydrates for a person with compromised insulin sensitivity. Never mind the fact that many of these calories may be coming from processed foods that contain additives and chemicals that add to toxic burden. Different foods can have different effects on insulin secretion (18).

Sparked by the low-fat food craze and obesity epidemic that came along with it, researchers from Harvard University created the Glyemic load. The Glycemic Load is a ranking system taking into account the portion size along with the Glycemic index of food.

By calculating the grams of carbohydrates per serving and multiplying it by the Glycemic index of the food, then dividing by 100, you can get an accurate depiction a single serving of a food actually has on your blood sugar levels. This can be useful in the management of insulin spikes and the regulation of blood sugar (4). The Glycemic load is a useful tool in combatting obesity (10,12), regulating diabetes (9), normalizing HDL and

> **Glycemic Load Calculation:**
>
> # of grams of carbohydrates per serving X glycemic index of food, then divide by 100.

triglyceride (4), and decreasing heart disease risk factors (8). Anything below 10 is considered low, while anything above 20 is considered high Glycemic load.

Liquid Meals and Insulin

The next to consider is the 4 protein shakes per day. For the purposes of staying lean, liquid protein shakes, or post workout recovery shakes, may be best used for recovery (2,3). That is recovery from a physical workout, particularly weight training in which protein breakdown occurs.

Liquid meals are assimilated by the body much faster than a solid meal (1,15). Understanding this concept, and the fact that whey protein is insulinogenic, it is easy to see how a liquid meal elevates your insulin levels much faster than a protein containing solid meal (52).

What happens to the excess calories? They are shuttled to your liver, broken down into fatty acids, and shuttled back to the bloodstream. These can then be absorbed by fat cells.

"I Don't Want To Get Big and Bulky"

Three muscle endurance workouts per week? Let's put one myth to rest. Women produce almost 10-20 times less testosterone than men (11), yet they still believe that heavier weight training is going to build bulky muscles. Most men wish it was that easy.

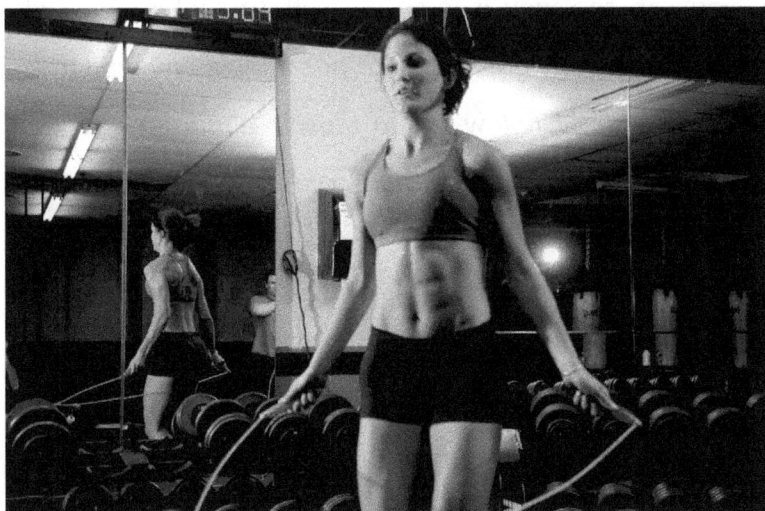

At any local gym, diehard males will perform set after set of heavy bench presses and curls (minus proper nutrition, rest and recovery) only to find they look the same as they did when they started. So, if these men can't put on big and bulky muscle, how can a woman whom produces 10-20X less testosterone expect to do it? Don't be mistaken with proper training, nutrition, and recovery, one is definitely capable of putting on quality lean muscle tissue. This takes us back to the muscle endurance workouts.

You have to love it when you hear "you need high repetitions to tone your muscles". Is this saying that lower repetitions or diet won't tone muscles, and only high repetition training will tone muscles? With that in mind, you have to wonder why sprinters are muscular and ripped while marathon runners are typically skinny with little muscle tone. A quick review of the two types of hypertrophy, myofibrillar and sarcoplasmic, may provide some insight.

Each type of hypertrophy plays a role in the development of lean muscle tissue (along with proper nutrition, time under tension, and rest periods). When you add lean muscle to your frame there is an increase in metabolic rate.

Remember that the sarcoplasmic hypertrophy (*and to some extent myofibrillar*) is gained through progressive hypertrophy specific training protocols (*ie:7-12 repetitions, increased time under tension, shorter rest periods, higher volume*), while myofibrillar hypertrophy is gained through progressive strength (maximal or relative) based protocols (*ie; 1-6 repetitions, longer rest periods, less time under tension*).

With these factors in mind, you can see why it is so difficult to "get toned" while utilizing high repetition muscle endurance protocols only. You are not adding any lean muscle to your frame! *And many people who constantly follow group muscle endurance protocols wonder why their body aches, and has not changed since the Dukes of Hazzard went off the air on Friday nights.*

Knowledgeable Professionals

Finding quality professionals to teach and guide you through your journey toward optimal heath can be of tremendous benefit. Surrounding yourself with a team of go to people should be imperative. For example when/if you get injured, it all starts with a good doctor. From there you will need a good physical therapist, perhaps a good soft tissue/ART practitioner, then a good trainer or strength coach to get you back to performance. If diet is an issue, a quality nutritionist can go a long way.

As can be seen, there are many pieces to the puzzle, each playing an important role in maintaining stability of your overall health. The following information may be a good place to start when looking for certain cogs in the wheel of optimal health:

Functional Medicine Doctors: www.acamnet.org

www.functionalmedicine.org

Nutritionist: www.westonaprice.org

www.nanp.org

Soft Tissue Work: www.activerelease.com

www.thefitinstitute.com

Physical Therapy: www.apta.org

Strength and Conditioning: www.charlespoliquin.com (Look for PICP)

www.nsca.com (Look for CSCS)

www.weightlifting.teamusa.org (Look for USAW Coach)

CHAPTER

XI

GETTING UNSTUCK

Advertising on television would have us believe cereals are good for our health because they are fortified with vitamins, minerals, and calcium. We get sucked into the belief that we need to take a heavily marketed fat burning supplement because the people in the commercial got such good results. Through savvy advertising, we are given the impression that it is the fat in our diets that is making us fat while snacking on chips and drinking diet soda will keep us thin. On and on the list can go..

Stepping outside the box and digging a little deeper into the actual science surrounding our health choices can be enlightening. For instance, there is an abundance of propaganda made readily available on how important grainy carbohydrates are in our everyday diets, but you have to dig a little deeper into the literature that may tell us otherwise. The following are a few of the myths that may need a second look.

Myth 1: You need to eat your grains

6-11 servings of grainy carbohydrates per day! It is interesting to note that as the carbohydrates increased in our diets (209 g/day in 1988-1990 to 241 g/day in 2003-2004)[11], so too did our waist sizes, bodyfat percentages, obesity rates, use of cholesterol lowering drugs, rate of type II diabetes as well as increased rates in metabolic syndrome. It is almost as if the Food Pyramid that was recommended to us back in 1992 was made to make us look like pyramids.

There is much controversy surrounding the role of food lobbyists and their role in the development of recommended portion sizes for their respective clients (ie; the companies with the highest profits have the most lobbyists, therefore the most servings).

A 2004 study out of the *American Journal of Clinical Nutrition* drew direct parallels between the increased consumption of refined carbohydrates and the increasing rates of type II diabetes. In this study the researchers concluded that there was a direct parallel between the prevalence of type 2 diabetes in the US during the 20th century and the intake of refined carbohydrates, particularly those that were corn syrup based [11].

A similar 2009 study out of Emory University in Atlanta [32] looked at the changes in our nutrient intake over a 17-year period. What the researchers found is nothing short of astonishing, especially in this day in age in which cholesterol has become the evil villain. They found that the diets highest in fructose based carbohydrate intake also had the highest C-peptide concentrations, while those with lower carb diets had almost 14% lower concentrations of the same biomarker. In other words C-peptide concentrations (which are reflective of insulin resistance and the development of type II diabetes) were much higher in those consuming larger quantities of refined carbohydrates. Perhaps Bell and Sears were on track when they proposed an approach to dieting that reflected science, not the other way around [6,33].

· *Did you know that in the past 25 years prevalence of obesity in children aged 2–5 years has more than doubled (5.0% to 12.4%), nearly triple for those aged 6–11 years (6.5% to 17.0%), and more than triple for those aged 12–19 years (5.0% to 17.6%)[21,22,31]?*

· *Did you know that as of 2005-2006, 34% of Americans are now obese, 32.7% are overweight, and just under 6% are considered morbidly obese [11,22, 36,38], compared to 33% overweight, 22.9% obese and 2.9% morbidly obese between the years 1988-1994?*

· *Did you know that new diagnoses of type 2 diabetes nearly doubled as it rose from 4.8 per 1,000 people (1995 to 1997) to 9.1 per 1,000 people (2005 to 2007) [32,36,38]?*

In this day and age we have grainy carbohydrate cereals and snack bars claiming to be "heart healthy". Even soy milk has information on the internet regarding its beneficial effects on heart health. Perhaps one or two of the ingredients in the cereals and snack bars have been found to be beneficial to one's heart health, but what happens to the healthy benefits during the refining process?

So which macronutrient has been shown to have a more positive impact on our ability to stay lean and maintain overall health: fats or carbs? I am sure there are plenty of studies that have shown both, but here are a few eye openers that may not have made their way into the Saturday morning TV commercial time slots. (*I can see it now, commercials for avocados and grass fed organic beef*!)

Research has shown that those incorporating lower carbohydrate diets into their lifestyles realize better weight loss and bloodwork results. An interesting study from 2004 compared the blood lipid profiles of subjects partaking in the National Cholesterol Education Program Diet to those on lower carb, high protein/quality fat diets. The subjects on the low carb diet had more favorable lipid profile levels than their National Cholesterol Education Program counterparts (4).

I can hear it now, "but you still need to eat your grainy carbohydrates. You just can't get rid of an entire food source." (A quality rebuttal: We have essential amino acids. We have essential fatty acids. There is no such thing as an essential carbohydrate.)

This is a blanket statement that seems to be thrown out there quite often by many of those giving us nutritional advice. Does the same go for adding an entire food source, as many, if not most populations seem to have done with the addition of grainy carbohydrates to their diets? Paleolithic diets consisted of food sources that could be picked, fished, or hunted.

Looking at more modern times, Eskimos lived off of high protein/fat diets, with little or no consumption of grainy carbohydrates, as their environment is a difficult one to cultivate any sort of grains. Another population is the aborigines of Western Australia, who were the subjects of scantily publicized but very important studies on the Westernized diet and the development of diabetes.

The addition of a food source came in the form of the Westernized diet, known for its rather large consumption of processed foods and refined carbohydrates. In 1982 a research team set out to Western Australia to research the effect diet had on metabolic risk factors in a group of overweight, diabetic, and middle aged aborigines. These ten individuals moved out of their natural habitat and into a more westernized environment years before. With that move came the westernized lifestyle and diet to go with it.

All of these individuals then developed metabolic syndrome symptoms, heart disease risk factors, and diabetes soon after. The team was determined to see if these negative health consequences could be reversed just by bringing these individuals back to their natural environments and diets.

Amazingly enough, after only 7 weeks back in their natural environment, the Aborigines had significant improvements in nearly all measures of human health. From drops in blood pressure to serum triglyceride levels that now fell into the normal range, these individuals saw dramatic increases in all metabolic and cardiovascular risk factors associated with diabetes and heart disease. After only 7 weeks of eating according how they were genetically programmed to eat. Oh, before I forget, they also lost an average of 17.9lbs over that 7-week period (24,25,26,27,28,29,30)!

Myth 2: Deep Squats are bad for the knees

We are taught in our educational institutions and by many medical professionals to never let the knees go over the toe during weight bearing exercise. But, what happens when we walk up or down a staircase. Doesn't the knee cross over the toe plane with each step? Or what about squatting? Many personal trainers and therapists insist the deep/full squat is bad for the knees as it causes excessive shearing stress on the knee capsule. Have you ever watched a baby when they first learn to stand? They are constantly deep squatting to maintain balance so they do not fall.

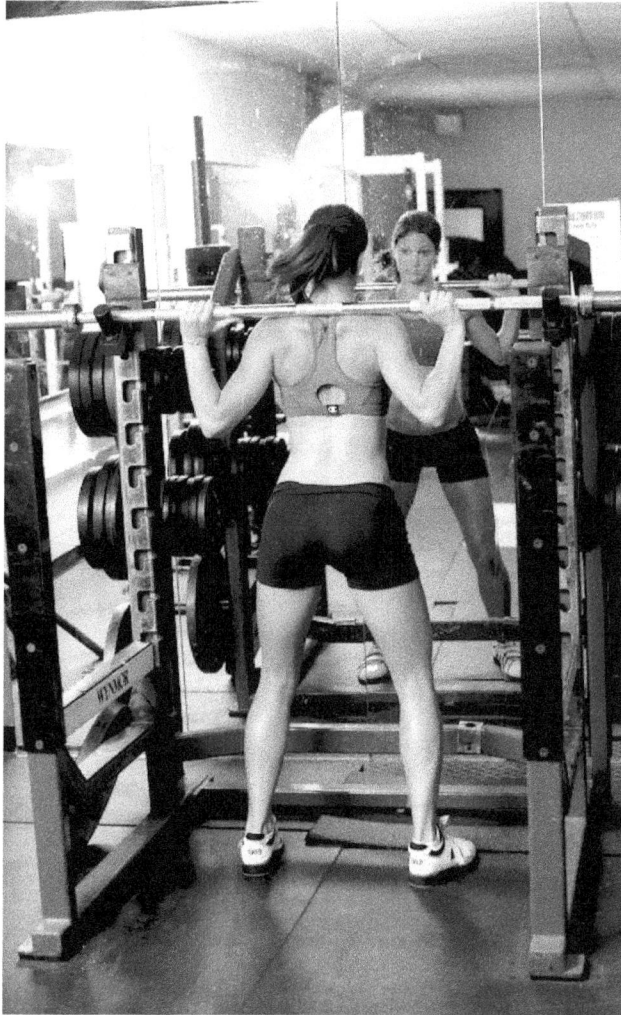

A study out of 2002 provides valuable insight into squat depth and muscle activation. In this groundbreaking study, the researchers found glute activation during full squat to be greater than twice that of partial squats (35.4% compared to 16.9%), hamstring activation to be similar, while quadriceps activation dominated during the partial squats only [8]. Understanding the importance of this can be a critical element in protecting oneself from injury, while achieving desired training outcomes.

Let's examine the fundamental biomechanics of the squat for a moment. Basically we have hip flexion/extensions, knee flexion/extension, plantar/dorsiflexion and spinal pressurization/stability.

What muscle groups are we trying to work in the squat? The quads yes. But also the glutes, hamstrings, adductors, deep and superficial musculature about the hip and "core" and spinal stabilizers and extensors. Half/parallel squats, as seen in the above study provide mostly quad dominance, while deep squats provide complete activation of the rest of the musculature about the legs, hips, core, and low back.

Thinking about the fact that muscles exert their force by pulling on bones we can gain a better understanding of how proper technique deep squatting can actually protect the knee. With greater activation/recruitment from a larger number of muscle groups, the knees are better protected during both the eccentric and concentric phases of the motion. For example, in the correct deep squat position (knees pulled out to the sides, slight lean in the torso, lordotic/neutral posture), the adductors on the inside of the thigh and hamstrings on both sides of the knee stabilize the knee to negate the anterior forces of the quadriceps. This combined with greater VMO activation at the bottom 15 degrees of motion and the knee can be kept strong and stable throughout the movement.

So where did this half squat phenomenon come from anyway? It appears to have originated back in 1961 with a study done by Kenneth Klein. In his study Klein pre-qualified 128 competitive weightlifters and compared their knee ligament stability to that of 360 college students with little or no training experience. Bias could have become an issue in this study as the subjects were pre-qualified into two groups, weightlifters and students.

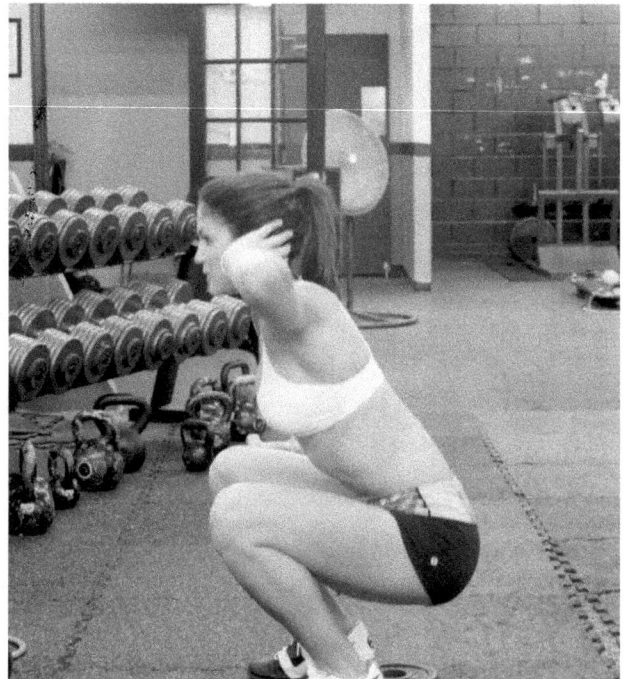

The ligament stability test was performed with manual force application, rather than a measurable/quantifiable force. Apparently the subjects would be pre-qualified (lifter or not) then the testers would determine how much force to apply to their knee structure. The combination of pre-qualification and non-quantifiable manual pressure application, could potentially lead to biased and/or flawed results (15).

The story goes that once the study was made public, the news spread like wildfire, and soon deep squats became public enemy number one in the physical therapy and medical side of physical fitness. Bodybuilders, Olympic Weightlifters, and Powerlifters seemed to trust their gut instincts and stick with what worked for them, and has since been proven to work now.

Other studies have followed the Klein effort, but with dramatically different results. For instance, 10 years after Klein's study, Meyers et al reproduced the study using the same mediolateral collateral ligament testing instrument to measure collateral ligament stability with completely different findings. In this 8 week study, sixty-nine subjects were randomly assigned different groups involving variations of the deep and parallel squat. The researchers found no significant differences in collateral ligament instability and knee joint flexibility within any of the treatment groups (19). Contradictory to Klein's oft-referred study, the study by Meyers et al found that neither deep squat nor parallel squat were detrimental to knee stability.

Other studies have had similar findings (9,34). In fact, a study from the *American Journal of Sports Medicine* performed in 1986 compared the knee health of powerlifters to that of college basketball players and 10K recreational runners. The researchers found an increase in posterior/anterior knee laxity in the runner/basketball player group, not the weight training group (39).

Contradictory to popular belief, research has shown that properly executed deep squats (for those with good lower extremity health) do not increase knee laxity/instability, but can actually increase muscle recruitment, which can lead to increases in performance on the field. So, if deep squats don't cause knee instability then what could some of the possible culprits be? In 1989 a group of researchers tested the knee laxity of 20 recreational long distance runners before and after running. The researchers found an increase in ligamentous laxity post exercise (14).

Myth 3: If you want to have a 6 pack you need to do lots of horizontal based abdominal exercises

Do you really need to do all those crunches or sit-ups to develop a washboard stomach? Is it possible to develop your abs without even directly training abs?

Did you know that in a study performed in 2007 a research team compared the abdominal activation of horizontal core exercises versus squats and deadlifts? The researchers found the squats and deadlifts to have significant abdominal activation when compared to the targeted core training exercises. This study showed there is significant activation of the abdominals while performing standing exercises that do not directly target the abdominal musculature (12).

Is there a way to further enhance abdominal activation? Loaded exercises while walking have been shown to have considerably greater activation than standing exercises. Walking with an asymmetric load held at waist height in front of you has been shown to elicit 132% greater abdominal activation than standing loaded exercises (2). Standing compressive loaded exercises (ie; squats and deadlifts) have been shown to be more effective/efficient than horizontal targeted ab exercises (12), whereas loaded walking exercises have been shown to elicit even greater abdominal muscle activation than their standing counterparts (2).

In a more recent study, performed by world-renowned low back/core specialist, Dr. Stuart McGill and his team, researchers studied the EMG activation of different trunk musculature in strongman events. They found the greatest number of peak muscle contractions of the rectus abdominis, and internal/external obliques during the walking phases of the Farmer Walk, Super Yoke Walk, and Suitcase carry (18).

Trainees wants to make sure they are getting the most bang for their buck by utilizing the most effective methods which will lead to positive outcomes in the shortest periods of time. Performing exercises that not only strengthen other parts of your body from a functional upright position, but also have greater muscle activation needs to be a priority.

Here is a quick peek at some examples of both effective and efficient abdominal training methods:

1. **Super Yoke Walk:** If you do not have access to a Super Yoke, you can set up a chain Yoke that involves setting up some lifting chains on both sides of a barbell. Weights or Kettlebells can be looped into the chains, hanging roughly 6" from the ground. Begin by unracking the bar from a squat rack, with the bar in proper back squat position across the shoulders. Keeping the torso stable, with significant intra-abdominal pressure to maintain stability, begin walking a pre-determined distance. Try to walk a straight line with little lateral or anterior/posterior movement of the chains. Be sure you do not let yourself lean or bend at the torso, as this may lead to increased injury potential.

2. **Farmer Carry:** If you do not have access to farmer carry handles, barbells can do the trick as they require not only great levels of forearm strength/control, but with their 7' length, the core activation to control the bar can be significant. Similar to the super Yoke, predetermine a distance, maintain torso rigidity/stability, and go.

3. **Overhead Slosh Stick Walks:** A Slosh stick is basically a large PVC pipe, roughly 8 feet long, partially filled with water (the degree of difficulty depends on how much water you want to add). Due to the fact that the water will "slosh" from side to side inside the pipe, it is very difficult to lift this tool, never mind holding it stable above your head while walking. That said, the core activation and spinal stabilization requirements are tremendous.

4. **Keg Carry:** Holding an asymmetric load at wrist or waist height in front of you while walking has been shown to have significant rectus abdominis muscle activation.

5. **Squat and Deadlift Variations:** Besides the highly effective conventional squat and deadlift techniques, an unconventional method for more advanced athletes is the asymmetric loading method. This method basically involves loading only one side of the bar (or loading more onto one side) while maintaining upright posture and spinal stability. Not only is this tremendously challenging, but elicits significant activation of the internal/external obliques, as well as the rectus abdominis.

6. **Chin Up/Pull Up variations:** When stabilizing the lower extremities and torso properly, the abdominal and core musculature are heavily active. After a high volume of chin ups/pull ups, you may notice a little soreness across the midsection the next couple of days.

7. **Hanging Knee/Leg Raises:** Done from either hanging from a chin-up bar, captains chair, or decline bench, we have seen from the San Diego State University study that abdominal exercises which involve movement of the legs have a high degree of muscular activation.

8. Ab Rollouts: There are many variations to this including ab wheels, barbell rollouts, single arm rollouts, resisted rollouts, standing rollouts, and many more.

9. 45 degree incline cable crunches: Try setting up a 45 degree incline bench facing away from a high cable pulley. Attach a triceps rope to the cable. Place a Bosu trainer on the low back portion of the bench. Sit down on the bench with feet curled under you and heels apart. Have a partner hand you the rope. With fully extended arms and spine, look back at the cable and begin pulling the rope toward your shoulders, with arms at each side of the head. Once your hands are resting at the anterior portion of your delts, begin crunching your torso while exhaling as much as possible. Only crunch to the position in which you can maintain abdominal contraction. Once concentric contraction is completed, perform the eccentric contraction by slowly uncurling the body back to the full extension start position.

Myth 4: A calorie is just a calorie is just a calorie etc……….

Ever wonder why you hear this statement from those who deal with excessive bodyfat issues while defending their appetite for point system based brownies and microwavable dinners? If a calorie were just a calorie, then why don't most people get fat when eating a high calorie diet consisting of quality fats, proteins, and vegetables, while their counterparts snacking on potato chips, frozen fudge bars, and bagel sandwiches seem to balloon up quicker than a Thanksgiving Day parade Homer Simpson float.

Have you ever wondered what the negative health impacts/consequences may be in eating microwavable plastic meals for every lunch and dinner? Or what effects some of the chemical ingredients used for processing and enhanced shelf life may have on your physical health? Never mind the fact that calories from different macronutrients can have different effects on your body's hormonal balance.

Did you know that a caloric consumption of roughly 20-30% below your daily requirement can raise cortisol, decrease testosterone, and interrupt thyroid hormone effectiveness? Now that is over just a short period of time, such as a couple of days. With chronic excessively low caloric consumption your body may actually begin to eat away at muscle tissue as it needs energy from somewhere in order to survive.

With chronically low calories cortisol levels may also begin to rise. Cortisol is the stress hormone that signals the body into storage mode in order to protect itself from a famine. Your body may begin to store fat as a protective mechanism the longer you semi-starve yourself. It is for this reason that many of these diet programs no longer work after 1-2 months, as the dieter has to keep dropping caloric consumption in order to continue weight loss.

When we think of our food, we typically think of those ingredients put in our food by Mother Nature. Thanks to savvy marketing, we seem to overlook the fact that much of the food in our grocery store aisles is processed with the majority of ingredients being made up of chemicals. Sadly the original food is stripped of the good stuff, milled, processed to increase shelf life, then injected with synthetic vitamins, minerals, and other ingredients.

Let's look at the ingredients of a lean microwavable meal and compare them to the ingredients of something simple like sardines.

Microwavable Chicken Club Ingredients

Flatbread Part

Enriched wheat flour ***See Below****

Water

Soybean Oil****See Below*****

Isolated Oat Product***???***

Yeast

Glycerine

Dough Conditioner (Guar Gum, Calcium carbonate, Datem, Wheat flour, Ascorbic Acid, Enzymes) **Calcium Carbonate may lead to plaque buildup**

Salt

Sardines Ingredients

Sardines

Water

Calcium Propionate **can be toxic to humans with side effects ranging from migraines and stomach aches to depression and irritability**

Sugar,

Dough Conditioner (Monoglycerides, Calcium Sulfate, Guar Gum, Sodium Metabisulfate, Ascorbic Acid)

Dough Conditoner (Wheat Starch, calcium carbonate, L-Cysteine HCL)****See below for some info on L-Cysteine****

Whole Wheat Flour

Cooked White Meat Chicken

White Meat Chicken

Water

Isolated Soy Protein **Good hiding spot for MSG****!!!! See below for some details on thyroid dysfunction, endocrine disruption, growth of tumors, etc......*****

Soy Lecithin

Rice Starch

Sodium Phosphates

Salt

Glazed with: Water, Seasoning (modified food starch, salt, dried garlic, spices, dried onion, citric acid, parsley, hydrogenated soybean and cottonseed oil)**Hydrogenated Oils (AKA: Trans Fats) Funny because they weren't listed on the label. ****

Canola Oil

Maltodextrin

Caramel Color****Sounds good. But how bad can "Caramel" color really be. See below for details******

Reduced Fat Mozzarella Cheese

Cultured Milk and nonfat milk

Modified Cornstarch*****See below********

Salt

Vitamin A Palmitate***One would think it is vitamin A, but is it really. See Below*******

Enzymes (An ingredient not in regular mozzarella cheese)****Can you be more vague*****

Tomatoes, Water, Seasoning:

Nonfat Milk Creamer (Sunflower Oil, Corn Syrup Solids, Sodium Caseinate , Potassium Phosphate) ***Sodium Caseinate may contain MSG!!!

Buttermilk (Buttermilk, Whey, Sodium Caseinate, Lactic Acid)***Sodium Caseinate may be a good hiding place for MSG!!!

Modified Cornstarch Cream (Cream, Soy Lecithin)**Modified cornstarch, again. See Below******

Whey

Buttermilk Flavor (Maltodextrin, Lactic Acid, Modified food starch, vinegar, buttermilk solids)

Sugar

Flavor (Salt, Maltodextrin, Modified Food Starch, Natural Flavor (contains sunflower oil, smoke) Canola Oil

Dried Garlic

Corn Syrup Solids***Don't worry it is not high fructose corn syrup, but….. See Below****

Yeast Extract****Yet another additive which is known to contain MSG*****

Potassium Chloride

Salt

Xanthum Gum

Spice***Can you be more vague!! Once again another possible culprit for MSG!!!****

Lactic Acid

Flavor***Another possible disguise for MSG!!!****

Soybean Oil***More Soybean oil…You may feel your estrogen rising just reading this****

Parsley

Light Pasteurized Process Cheddar Cheese

Cultured Milk

Water

Potassium Citrate

Salt

Sodium Citrate

Whey

Sorbic Acid

Cream

Apo Carotenal and Beta Carotene Color*** Additional food colorings****

Enzymes***It is amazing that there is no requirement to provide more detail****

Sodium Phosphate

Lactic Acid (ingredient not in regular pasteurized process cheddar cheese)

Green Onion, Bacon

Water

Salt

Sugar

Sodium Phosphate

Sodium Erythorbate

Sodium Nitrate***Potential Carcinogen****(See Below)

Vinegar

Isn't it reasonable to expect that the foods we eat contain, well, food? For instance doesn't it make sense that the ingredients of peanut butter just say peanuts (and in some cases salt) rather than hydrogenated vegetable oil and dextrose. Take for instance the ingredients list of Bison Steak Medallions. It is one ingredient long: 100% American Bison. Compare this to the ingredients encyclopedia that is the microwavable steak dinner, with complex carbs. A degree in chemistry may be recommended to understand the ingredients list. You shouldn't need a degree in chemistry to figure out what you are eating!!!! Let's look for a moment at just some of the ingredients of the microwave meal.

Enriched Wheat Flour

Enriched flour is basically flour in which most of the natural vitamins, minerals and natural elements have been extracted. Manufacturers do this to give the bread longer shelf life, improved texture and deter insects. When you strip the good stuff (germ, bran, vitamins, minerals) the absorption capacity of the wheat is altered. It becomes a highly insulinogenic food, causing a flood of sugar to ones bloodstream. Much of this may be absorbed as in the fat cells, creating the potential for obesity and obesity related diseases.

Calcium Propionate

Calcium Propionate is a mold growth inhibitor used on breads. Manufacturers use this chemical to increase product shelf life. The problem is this chemical can have some side effects in humans including cancerous tumors, depression, irritability, migraines, stomach issues, skin rashes and sinus problems.

Calcium Carbonate

Calcium Carbonate is a non-soluble form of calcium that has very low if any bio-availability. This type of calcium may lead to buildup of plaque in the arteries restricting blood flow. Arthritis, kidney and gallstones, as well as other major health issues have been linked to the plaque buildup caused by non-soluble forms of calcium.

Isolated Soy Protein

Isn't Soy supposed to be good for us? Improperly fermented or processed soy has been linked to biological defects, thyroid dysfunction, endocrine disruption, growth of tumors, impaired immune function, breast cancer, and maturation issues. Makes you want to go out and buy a soy bar!

L-Cysteine

Not a chemical, but can come from surprising sources such as animal fat or human hair.

Hydrogenated Oils (Trans Fats)

Basically a reconfiguring of the hydrogen/carbon bonds which creates a more viscous oil and a fat that can be held solid at room temperature. This makes for a much easier cooking experience. But at what cost? These fats are believed to increase LDL while lowering HDL, increase the potential for clogging of the arteries that may increase the risk of heart disease, and increase potential for insulin resistance. Stick with butter.

Caramel Color

Did you know that caramel coloring has been used to suppress immune function in mice by disrupting white blood cell production?

Modified Corn Starch

What do you do if you want to make a food harder to break down in the stomach and intestines? Simple, you modify it. Modifying basically refers to chemically treating it to alter the physical properties so it can be used as a food thickener or moistener, basically to improve texture. Besides ingestion of treatment chemicals, modified starches may lead to gastrointestinal or bloating issues.

Vitamin A Palmitate

Not to be confused with the healthy vitamin A found in cod, liver, and cold water fish, Vitamin A Palmitate requires a very healthy gut mucosal villi surface to break down and absorb.

MSG

Monosodium Glutamate. Did you know that when scientists need to make a mouse or rat fat for an experiment they inject them with a chemical form of MSG? It can cause a threefold increase in the production insulin. If it has this effect on rats, what is the human cost?

As the public has become more aware of the dangerous effects of MSG, it still seems to find it's way into foodstuff under different identities or by disguising itself. Rather than using the name Monosodium Glutamate, it may fall under the disguises of Hydrolyzed Plant Protein or Plant Protein Extract, Yeast Extract or Sodium (or calcium) Caseinate.

Corn Syrup Solids

Manufactured from corn syrup liquid, this is a precursor to high fructose corn syrup, minus the enzymatic process that converts the dextrose to fructose.

Sodium Nitrate

Sodium nitrate is used for dried cured meats. It breaks down into nitrite, which can then lead to the formation of nitrosomes, which are potential carcinogens.

One of the best things we can do for our health is to learn where your food comes from and what is actually in it. Learning how to decipher the label can go a long way in reaching our weight loss goals and achieving optimal health.

MYTH 5: YOU NEED TO DO LONG SLOW DISTANCE CARDIO TO LOSE FAT

Besides the fact that it burns muscle rather than builds it, decreases testosterone rather than elevates it, increases catabolic hormones rather than depresses them, and has been the culprit of tens of thousands of chronic lower extremity injuries, excessive long slow distance cardio training is not that bad.

Can't weight training be considered cardio? Does increasing heart rate, blood flow, oxygen demand, and breathing rate qualify an exercise as being cardio? In a 2008 study comparing the fat loss effects of strength and endurance training, the researchers found that both training modalities increased insulin sensitivity, but of greater significance were their findings regarding fat loss. Of the two modalities, only strength training led to significantly greater reductions in both trunk and limb body fat (nearly double the fat loss), while increasing total lean mass (16).

When utilizing weight training for fat loss/body composition purposes, the body has a tendency to build muscle, increase fat cell mobilization, and keep stress hormones at manageable levels.

Believe, Work, and……………….Become!

CHAPTER

XII

EXERCISE

DESCRIPTIONS

90/90 Crunches with Med Ball

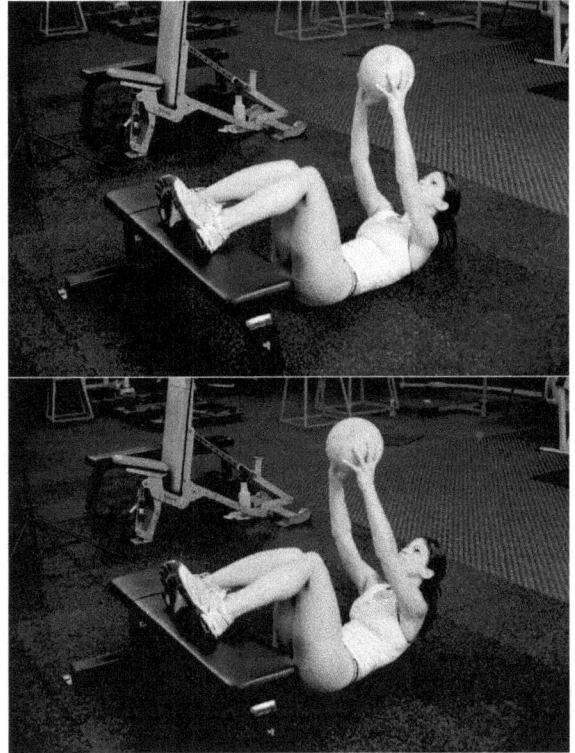

Exercise Prerequisites: Avoid if you have low back, neck, or abdominal pain.

Movement: Lay on floor with your back flat and feet propped on bench 18-24" high. Your calves should rest on top of the bench with your knees and hips bent to 90 degrees each. Hold the med ball with your arms straight directly over your chest. You're your heels down into the bench, activating your hamstrings. Looking upward, begin to exhale and slowly raise your shoulder blades off the floor reaching upward with the med ball. Make sure your heels do not come off bench throughout the movement. Once you reach the top of your range of motion, slowly lower back to start and repeat.

Keys to Movement:

1. Lay flat with feet elevated on bench and 90 degree angles at hips and knees.
2. Crunch upward while holding med ball with extended arms.
3. Do not allow your heels to come off the bench throughout the movement.
4. Lower slowly back to start.

Back Squat

Exercise Prerequisites: Use caution if you have knee, low back, or neck pain.

Antagonistic Muscles: Hamstrings as flexors of the knee.

Movement: Place hands on the bar slightly wider than shoulder width with thumbs and fingers around the bar. Rest the bar across the rear deltoids and upper trapezius, squeezing your shoulder blades down and together with chest out. Ensure the bar does not rest across the lower neck or spine. Once you have un-racked the bar, assume a stable neutral/lordotic posture, keeping the weight evenly distributed between feet. Place the feet hip width apart or slightly wider, with toes pointing straight ahead or slightly out. Keep your elbows pulled down. As you begin the descent, make sure to maintain lordotic/neutral posture beginning the decent by bending your knees first (a variation is to bend at the hips first). As you sit downward, begin pushing your knees outward, pointing in the same direction as your toes, to ensure maximum hip muscle recruitment. Once your hamstrings touch your calves, or you have gone as low as your flexibility allows, begin to transition to the ascent. Keeping the back arched/neutral with torso rigid, focus on driving the chest up first, keeping the torso upright. Be sure to keep the heels driving into the ground and avoid caving knees and rounding of the back. Make sure to exhale maximally after you have passed the sticking point and ascend all the way to the top. Then perform next repetition.

Keys to Movement:

1. Pinching shoulder blades back and down, rest bar across rear delts and upper trapezius.
2. Place feet hip width or slightly wider with toes pointing slightly outward.
3. Keep the elbows pulled downward.
4. Maintain neutral/lordotic posture while keeping the torso as upright as possible.
5. Bend at the knees first when you begin your ascent (variation is to bend at the hips first).
6. Push the knees outward, ensuring they point in the same direction as the toes throughout the movement.
7. Do not allow the heels to come off the ground or knees collapse inward throughout the movement.
8. Lower down until your hamstrings touch your calves or as low as your flexibility allows.
9. Initiate ascent by driving chest upward at first

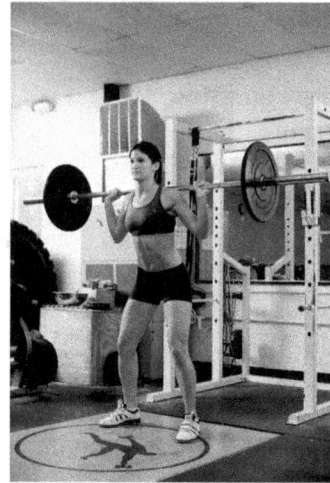

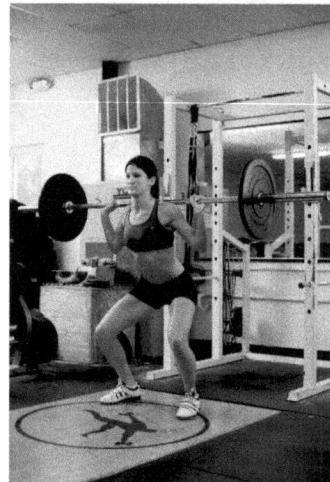

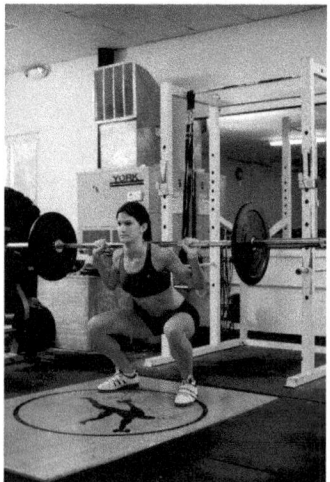

Backward Sled Dragging

Exercise Prerequisites: Use caution if you have neck, knee, or low back pain.

Antagonistic Muscles to movement: Hamstrings as flexors of the knee.

Movement: Facing a sled while holding the handles, lean back with shoulders behind hips and feet hip width apart. Keeping hips extended and shoulders behind hips, begin walking backward focusing on fully extending the drive leg with each stride by pushing through the ball of the foot. Be sure not to reach back more than one foot length with the non-working leg as this can put unnecessary stress on the knee. The hips locked at 90 degrees sled drag is another option.

Keys to Movement:

1. Position feet hip width apart.
2. Lean back with hips extended and shoulders behind hips.
3. Focus on driving through the ball of the foot.
4. Extend the leg with each step.
5. Be careful not to step too far back and this can put excessive pressure on the knee.

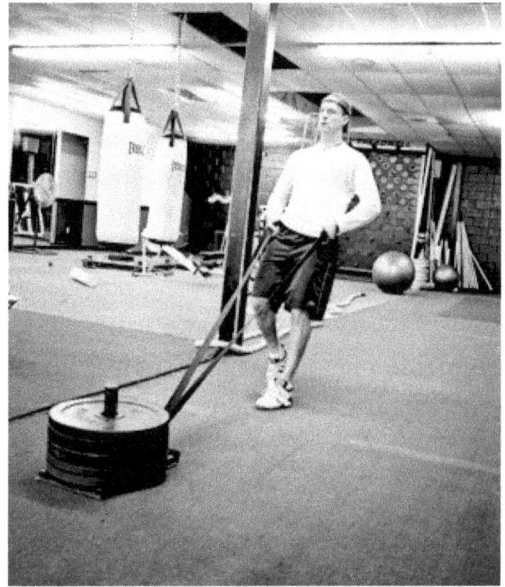

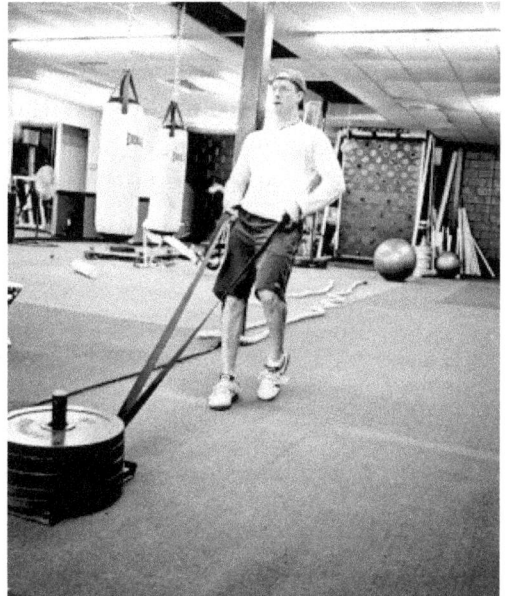

Barbell Bench Press

Exercise Prerequisites: Use caution exercise if you have low back, shoulder, neck, or elbow pain. If upper crossed syndrome is an issue, perform corrective movements.

Antagonistic Muscles: Rhomboids, Mid Trapezius Musculature, External Rotators

Movement: Lie on a flat bench with feet flat on the floor (variations for foot positioning include up on toes with feet pulled under or feet up on a low box if you have persistent back problems). Grasp the bar with a pronated grip roughly shoulder width apart (variations include wide grip, close grip, supinated grip, neutral grip, etc), keeping the angle between the upper body and upper arm roughly 45 degrees or less. Pinch your shoulder blades back, squeezing the bench, while expanding your chest upward.

Begin by lowering the bar straight down. Lower the bar down until it touches your chest. Without bouncing the bar off the chest, keep the shoulder blades pulled back, begin the concentric action, retracing the same pattern the barbell was lowered. Breathe out on the way up.

Keys to Movement:
1. Grasp barbell with shoulder width grip, hands in pronated position.
2. Upper arm at roughly 45 degree angle or less relative to the upper body.
3. Pinch shoulder blades back with chest out.
4. Breathe out during concentric movement.

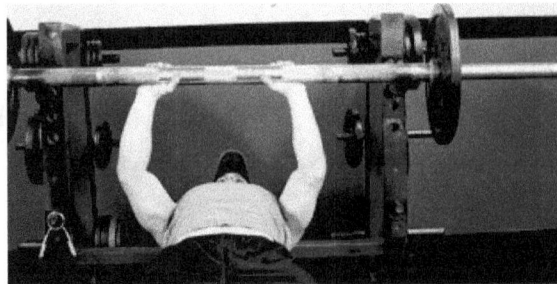

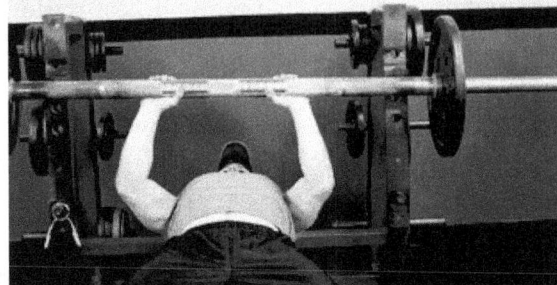

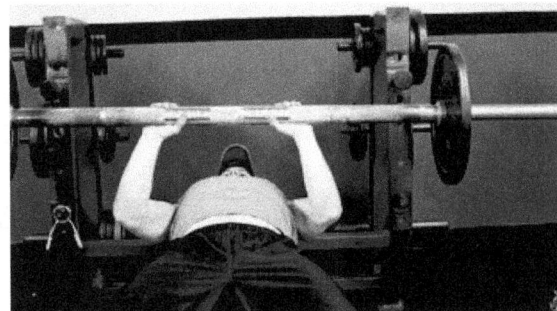

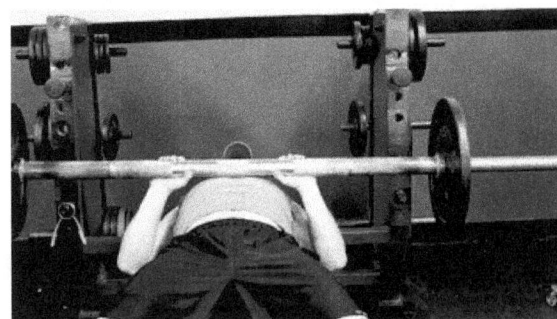

Barbell (Front Rack Position) Split Squats

Exercise Prerequisites: Use caution if you have neck, knee, or low back pain.

Antagonistic Muscles to movement: Hamstrings as flexors of the knee.

Movement: This technique was first taught to me by Charles Poliquin and his Poliquin Institute staff. Position body with feet hip width apart, torso in neutral/slightly lordotic posture, with a barbell across your anterior deltoids and upper pectoral musculature. The "clean grip" is preferred. If you do not have the flexibility for the clean grip, use straps. Maintain upright posture throughout movement. With toes pointing straight ahead, step one foot forward into a lunge position. The distance between your feet is determined by your hip flexor range of motion. If the rear foot is too close, the heel of the front foot will come off during the movement. If the rear foot is too far back, the knee will not cross the heel plane. After you have found the optimal distance between front and rear foot, lower the hips forward and toward the ground maintaining upright posture with no lean forward in the torso. Keeping the back leg as straight as possible, descend until the hamstring comes in contact with the calf on the front leg. It is imperative not to lean forward or allow the front foot heel to come off the ground throughout the movement. As the hamstring comes in the contact with the calf, the knee may cross the toe plane. If the knees are healthy, this can help to strengthen the knee as there is a greater VMO, adductor, hamstring, and gluteal activation with deeper squats and lunges. Initiate the concentric movement through the ball of the front foot by driving the shoulders back with no change in posture and extending the working leg until you have reached the start position. Make sure the front heel never comes off the ground or elevated platform. Perform all reps on one leg, then perform all reps on the opposite leg.

Keys to Movement:
1. Maintain lordotic/neutral posture with torso perpendicular to floor throughout the movement.
2. Determine optimal distance between front and rear foot.
3. Focus on keeping the back leg as straight as possible to ensure maximal tension on front leg and stretching of back leg hip flexor musculature.
4. Lower down until hamstring comes in contact with calf. In healthy knees, the knee may cross of the toe plane as there is a greater recruitment of VMO, adductor, hamstring, and gluteal musculature.
5. Begin ascent by focusing on driving the shoulders/torso back and upward first.
6. Do not allow the front heel to come off during the movement.
7. Do not allow torso to lean over during the movement.

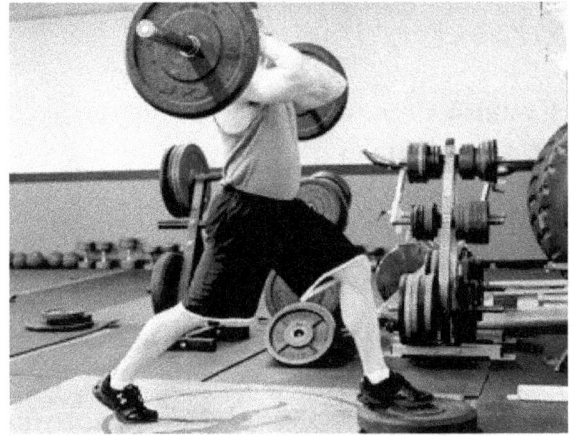

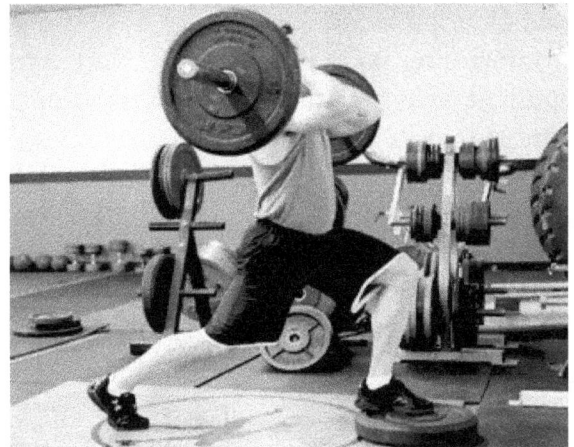

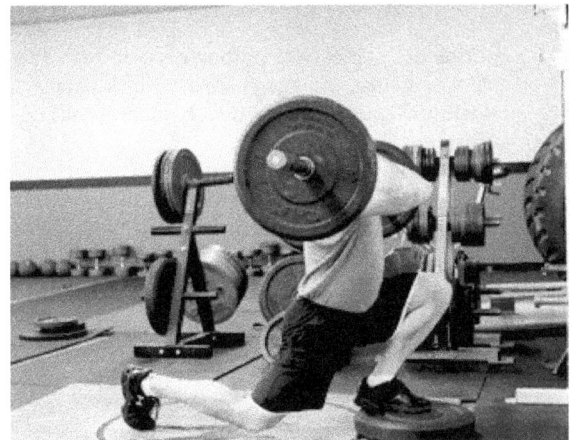

Bent Over Barbell Row

Exercise Prerequisites: Use caution if you have low back, neck, or shoulder pain

Antagonistic Muscles to movement: Shoulder internal rotators, elbow extensors.

Movement: Hold barbell in front of you with pronated grip and hands slightly wider than shoulder width. Bend your knees 20 degrees and lean over until your torso is parallel or near parallel to the floor. Arch your back, with chest out, shoulder pulled back and down, eyes straight down.

Maintaining torso parallel to the floor with lordotic posture, pull the weight toward your sternum/belly button, pulling with the rear delt, rhomboid and lat muscles. To do this, retract your shoulder blades back and down, then focus on pulling back with the elbows until full contraction of the upper back musculature.

Make sure there is no bounce or rounding of the back throughout the movement. Slowly lower the weight back to start and perform next repetition.

Keys to Movement:

1. Position body in correct starting position with knees bent 20 degrees, chest out, back arched, and torso parallel or near parallel to the floor.
2. Initiate movement by retracting shoulders back and down, maintaining torso posture.
3. Focus on pulling elbows back.
4. Do not allow shoulders to shrug upward.
5. Row back until complete contraction of shoulder blades.

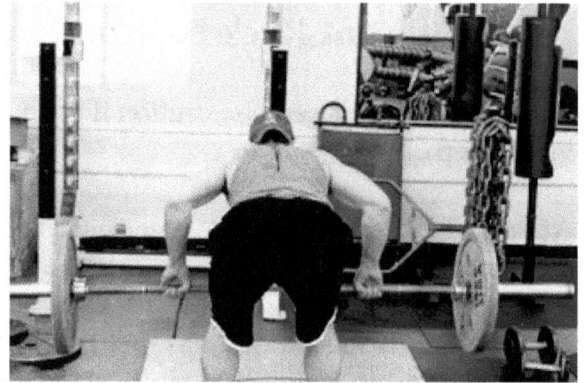

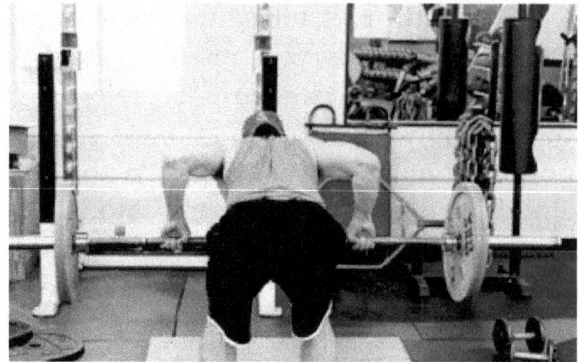

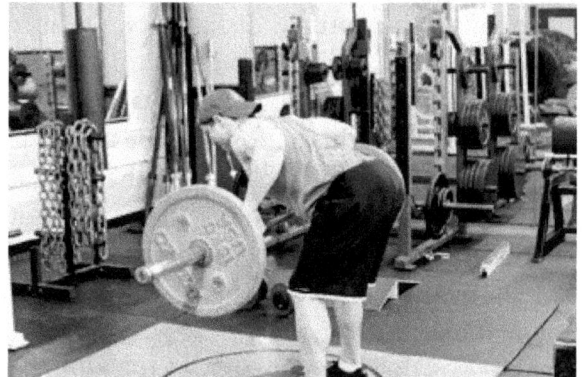

Bicep Curl with Dumbbells

Exercise Prerequisites: Use caution if you have shoulder, elbow, or neck problems.

Antagonistic Muscles to movement: Elbow Extensors

Movement: Standing or sitting at the edge of a bench, retract the shoulder blades down and back while keeping the chin up and looking straight ahead. Start with the arms directly by your sides, with the thumb side of the hand offset closer to the end of the dumbbell. With palms up, arms fully extended, wrists straight or slightly extended, begin curling the weight upward. Be sure not to allow the upper part of the arm to move forward while raising the weight. During the entire range of motion, the shoulder blades are retracted and the head is looking straight ahead with the chin up. Once concentric contraction is completed, lower slowly back down to the full elbow extension start position.

Keys to Movement:

1. Stand or sit with shoulder blades retracted and chest out.
2. Keep elbows at your sides.
3. Do not tuck your chin downward during the movement.
4. Focus on pulling with the pinky side of the hand.
5. Ensure complete range of motion by flexing the triceps at the bottom and flexing the biceps at the top of the range of motion.

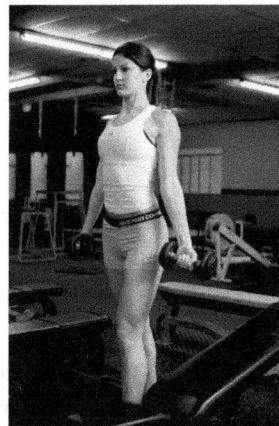

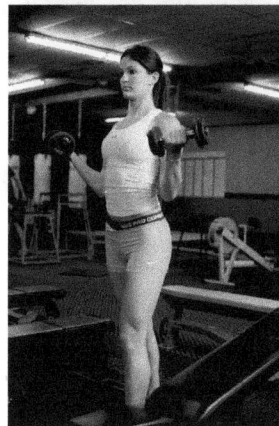

Box Jumps

Exercise Prerequisites: Use caution if you have knee, ankle, or low back problems.

Movement: Stand in front of a box with your feet hip width apart and toes pointing forward. Rapidly bend at the knees, hips, and ankles. Immediately reverse direction, extending knees, hips, and ankles and jump onto the box. Land quietly with feet hip width apart and knees pointing in the same direction as the toes. Ensure that you try to minimize knee and hip flexion during the landing. Step off the box and perform next rep.

Keys to Movement:

1. Feet and knees pointing in the same direction during jump and landing.
2. Keep torso in neutral or slightly lordotic posture throughout.
3. Land quietly.

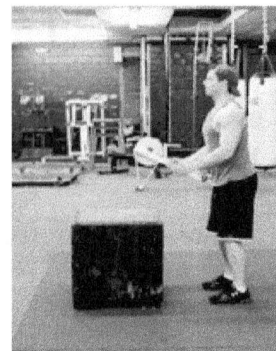

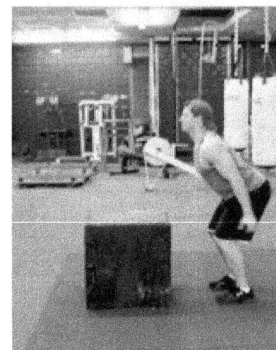

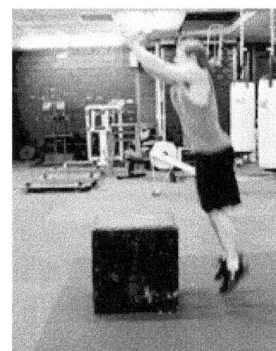

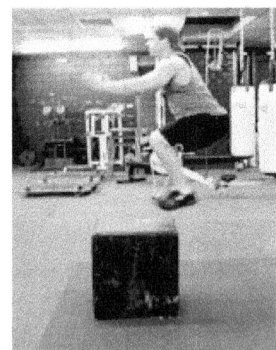

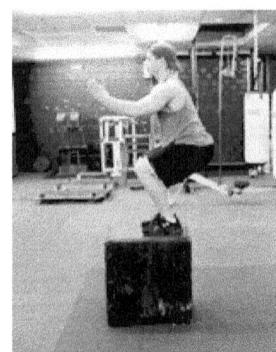

Box Step Ups

Exercise Prerequisites: Use caution if you have knee, hip, or low back problems.

Movement: Choose a box height and stand with neutral posture beside or behind the box. Step one foot up onto the box with the foot flat on the box and the other leg (foot on ground) in extended position. Plantar flexing or dorsiflexing the foot on the ground is a method of ensuring maximal recruitment of the working leg. Holding dumbbells down by your sides or a barbell across your shoulders, begin the movement by driving chest and shoulders up first while minimizing assistance from foot on the ground.

Keeping your torso straight and trying to maintain perpendicular to the ground, focus on driving through the heel of the foot on the box, allowing for hip and knee extensor muscle activation.

Extend the hip and knee of the drive leg until you have reached full extension of each joint. Do not allow the knee to collapse inward (valgus stress) during the movement.

Complete all reps on one leg and then perform reps on the other leg.

Keys to movement:

1. Start with one foot on the box and the other on the floor in fully dorsiflexed or plantar flexed position with knee and hip extended.
2. Begin movement by driving chest and shoulders first, keeping torso perpendicular to the floor.
3. Without assistance from leg on the floor, extend hip and knee of leg on the box.
4. Do not allow the torso to lean or knee to collapse inward.

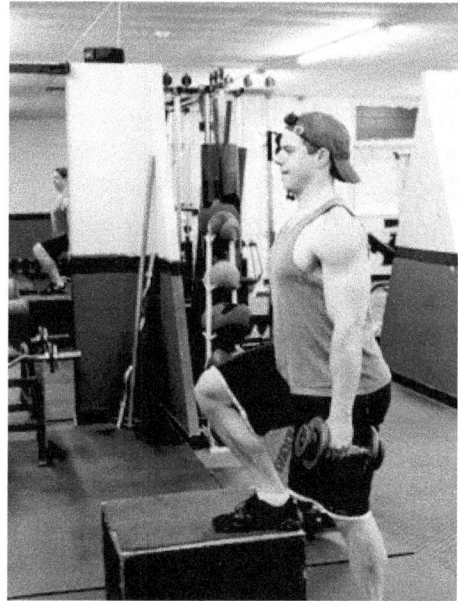

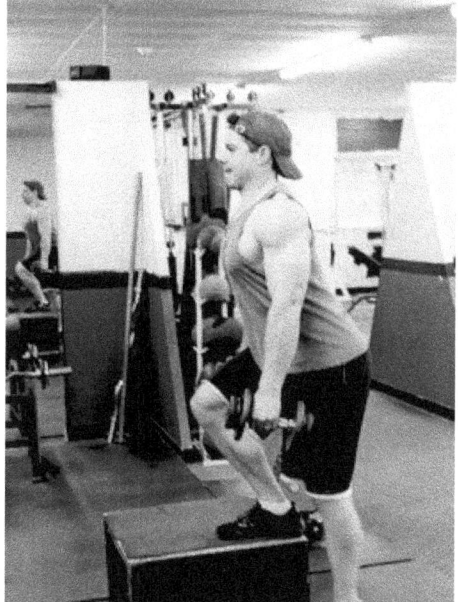

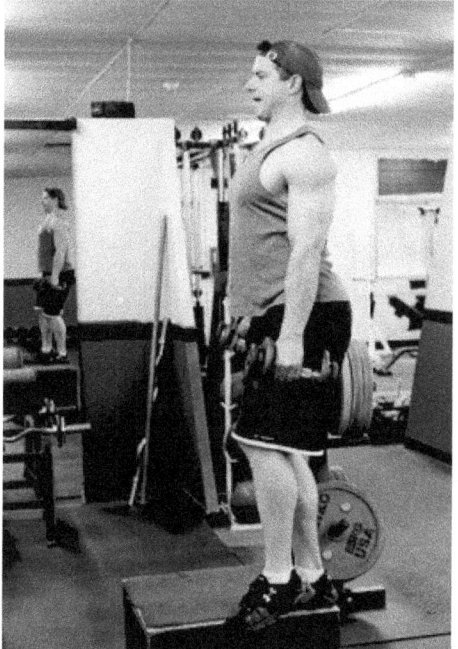

Chin-ups

Exercise Prerequisites: Use caution if you have elbow, shoulder, neck or low back pain

Movement: Grasp a pull-up bar with hands supinated, shoulder width or slightly wider. Hang from the bar, with arms, hips and shoulders in full extension. Initiate movement by retracting shoulder blades back and down. Begin pulling your body straight upward, continuing to pull the shoulder blades back and downward. Do not allow the shoulder to internally rotate as you are pulling upward.
Pull upward, pinching your shoulder blades back until the upper portion of the chest comes in contact with the bar.
Lower the body slowly, retracing the same pattern until you reach full the extension starting position.

If you cannot perform a non-assisted chin-up, you can use the assistance of a partner or a band around the knee or foot.

Keys to Movement:

1. Supinated grip with hands shoulder width or slightly wider.
2. Begin in dead hang position.
3. Retract shoulders back and down prior to and during the movement.
4. Focus on pulling the elbows back and down.
5. Do not allow the shoulders to internally rotate,
6. Pull up until upper part of chest comes in contact with the bar.
7. Lower down until full extension in the elbows and shoulders.

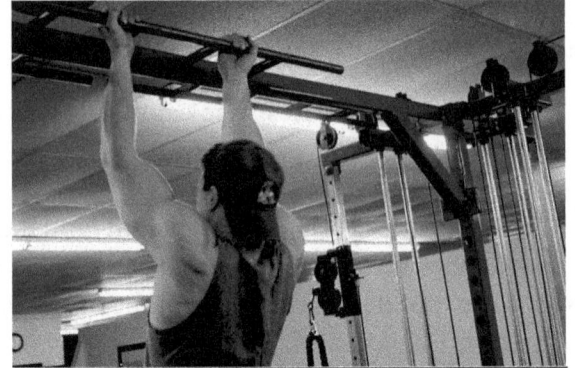

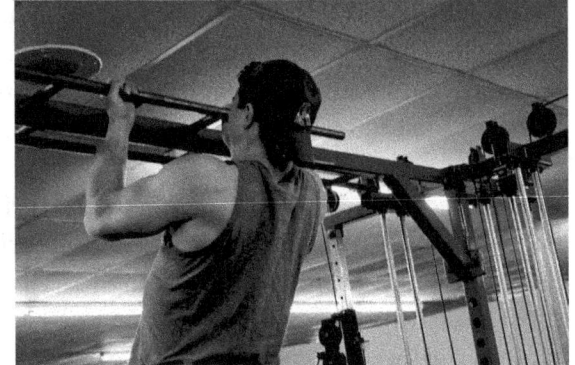

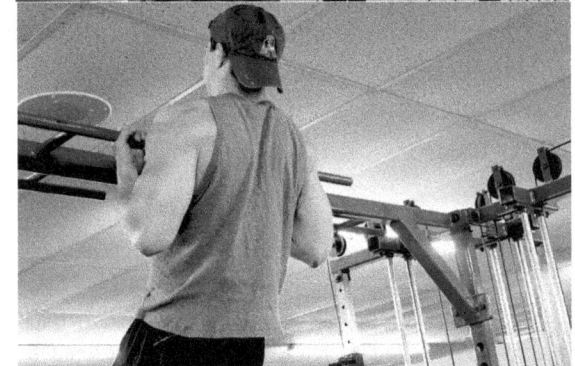

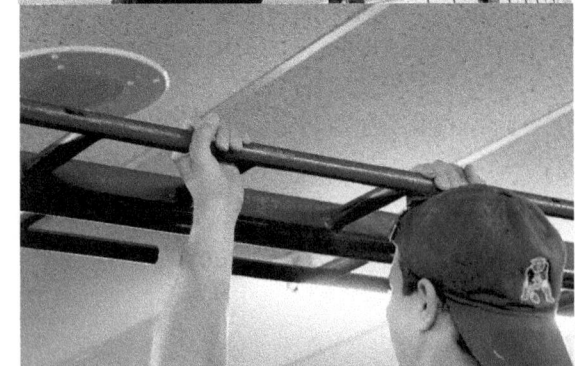

Cuban Press

Exercise Prerequisites: Use caution if you have elbow, shoulder, neck, or low back pain.

Movement: Stand with feet hip width apart, holding a barbell or dumbbell with pronated grip. The width of the grip is determined by the length of your upper arms. The objective is to hold the elbows at 90 degree during the rotational component of the exercise.

Begin by holding a barbell using pronated grip with the upper arms are out to your sides and parallel to the floor. Externally rotate the forearms/barbell upward until it is over your head. Once over your head, overhead press the bar and lower back to start.

Keys to Movement:

1. Grasp the barbell with pronated grip, hands roughly the width of upper arms extended out to sides.
2. Upright row the barbell, focusing on driving the elbows upward.
3. Once the upper arms are parallel to the floor, externally rotate the forearms/barbell until it is above your head.
4. Press overhead. Bring the head through as the barbell passes your forehead and focus on active shoulders at the top of the press.

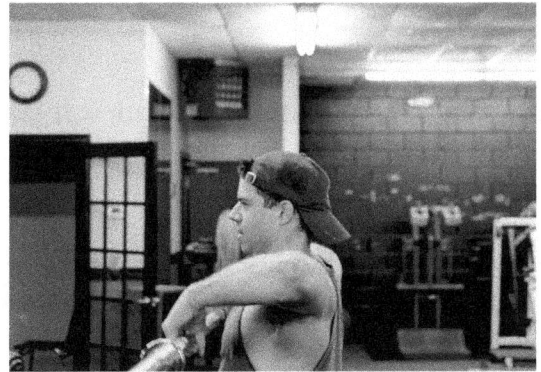

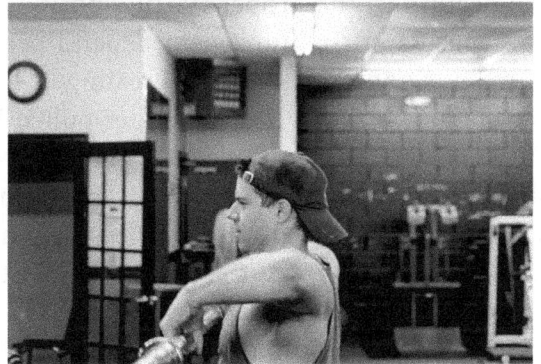

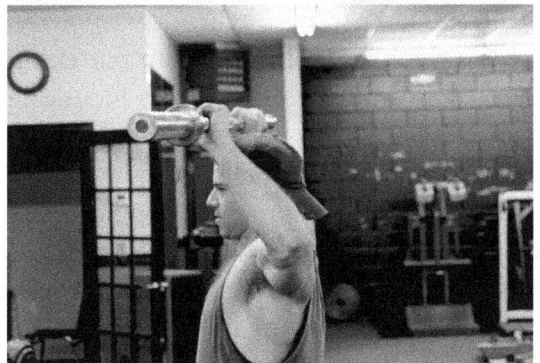

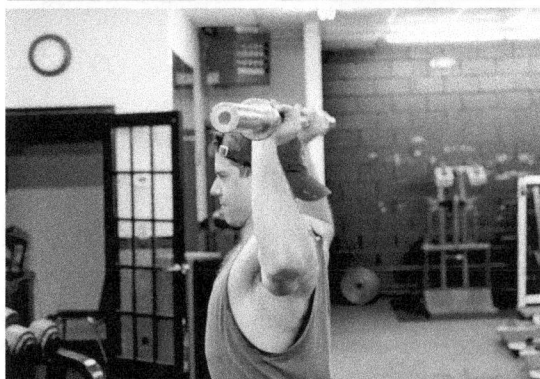

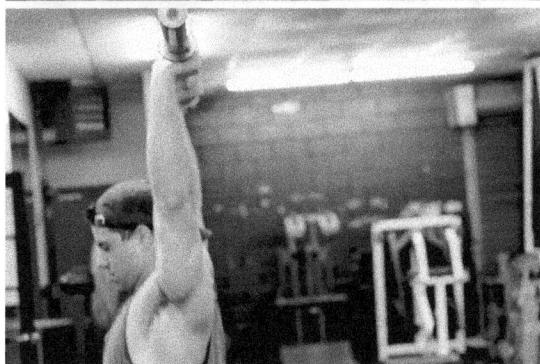

Deadlift

Exercise Prerequisites: Use caution if you have neck, knee, or low back pain or lack flexibility to assume proper starting position.

Movement: You can use an Olympic bar or a Hex deadlift bar. Pronated grip is preferred for higher repetitions while mixed grip may be effective for lower reps. It is important to begin the deadlift in the proper starting position as the mechanics and success of the movement depend heavily on this initial body positioning. Begin by creating a lordotic posture in the spine, with chest out, shoulder pulled back, eyes straight ahead. Lean the torso over to roughly 45 degrees and with shins touching the bar o roughly 1 inch away. Maintaining the same torso angle relative to the floor, begin bend at the knees to grasp the bar. Keep the weight shifted to the heels (think about wiggling your toes in the start position). Once in the correct start position, begin the lift by pulling the shoulders up first, trying to maintain torso angle and rigidity. Try not to raise the hips first as this can put excessive strain on your low back ligaments. As you raise, focus on pulling the bar into you, clearing your knees so the bar can travel in a straight a line upward. Extend the hips and knees, increasing the torso angle, until the bar comes in contact with the bottom part of the upper thigh. Once you have reached complete extension of the hips and knees, retrace the movement pattern during the eccentric part of the movement.

Keys to movement:

1. A weightlifting belt may be preferred for this lift.
2. Proper start position with roughly 45 degree angle of torso relative to ground.
3. Bar in contact with shins or one inch away in starting position.
4. Back arched with weight through the heels.
5. Mixed grip for low reps and pronated grip for higher reps.
6. Focus on raising the shoulders first, keeping the same angle at the torso throughout the movement.
7. Try not to raise the hips first..
8. Retrace the same movement pattern during the eccentric part of the movement.

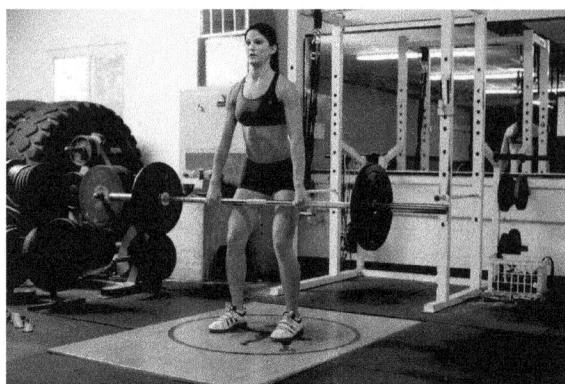

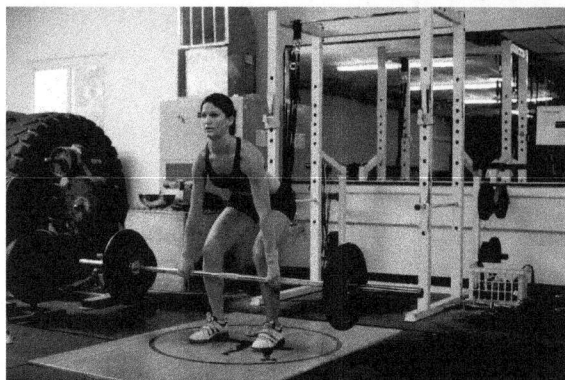

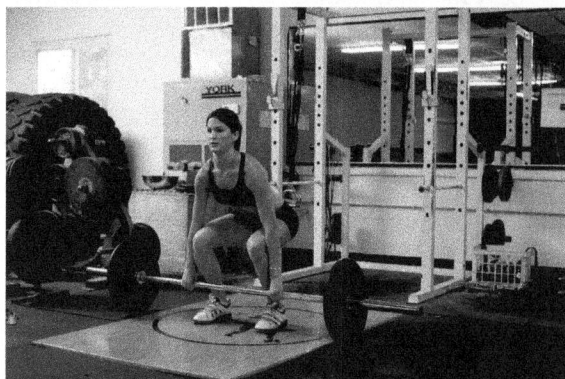

Dips

Exercise Prerequisites: Use caution if you have shoulder, neck, or elbow pain.

Movement: Start with hands on dip bars, arms in extended position with chest high, hips extended, and elbows pointing back. Begin lowering your body with elbows pointing 45 degrees or less. Allow the body to lean slightly forward for greater pectoral recruitment. Lower until the brachioradialis makes contact with the bicep.

Once you complete the range of motion, begin the concentric contraction by focusing on driving the chest up first while keeping the elbows pointing back or out to 45 degrees or less. Press until arms are straightened.

In his book Target Bodybuilding, Author Per Tesch states "All three head of the triceps brachii are markedly used as you raise and lower the body. (1)"

In strength circles one of the best methods of improving the bench press in the structurally balanced trainee is to improve performance in dips. Other benefits of dips include minimal equipment requirements and maximal variation options. Dip variations include Gironda dips, elbow in, elbows out, isometric pauses at top of concentric or bottom of eccentric, torso perpendicular to the floor, torso slightly leaned forward, fat grip dips, and V bar dips.

Keys to the Movement:

1. Start with the eccentric contraction first
2. Begin with elbows pointing back or upper arms at roughly 45 degrees or less from the body.
3. Keep chest high.
4. Lower until biceps touch brachioradialis.
5. Initiate concentric motion by focusing on driving the chest up first.
6. End concentric contraction once elbows are extended.

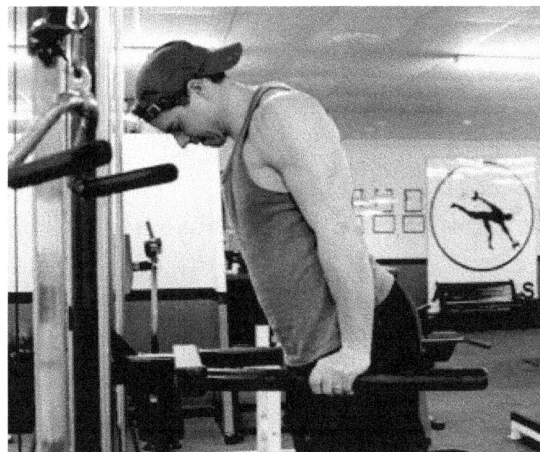

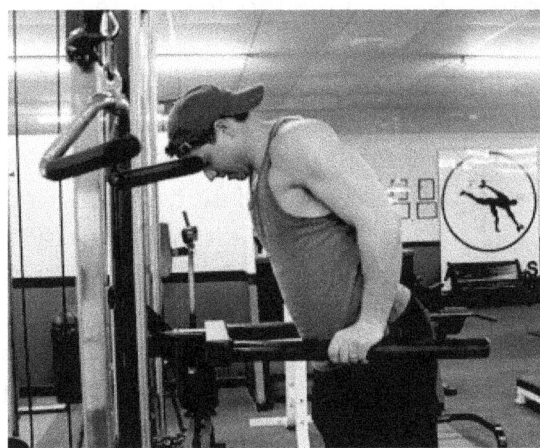

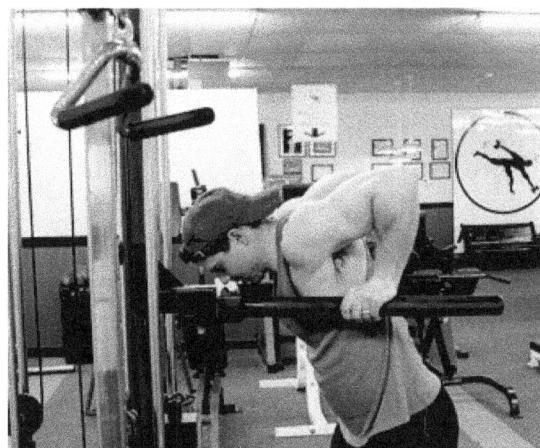

Drop Lunges

Exercise Prerequisites: Use caution if you have neck, knee, or low back pain.

Antagonistic Muscles to movement: Hamstrings as flexors of the knee.

Movement: Another great exercise learned from Coach Poliquin and his staff. Stand on a 3-6" elevated platform. Position body with feet hip width apart, torso in neutral/ slightly lordotic posture, with dumbbells held at your sides or barbell across the shoulders or in font squat rack position. Maintain upright posture throughout movement. With toes pointing straight ahead, take a large step forward. Lower the hips forward and toward the ground maintaining upright posture with no lean forward. Keeping the back leg as straight as possible, descend until the hamstring comes in contact with the calf of the front leg. It is imperative not to lean forward or allow the front foot heel to come off the ground throughout the movement.

As the hamstring comes in the contact with the calf, the knee may cross the toe plane. If the knees are healthy, this can aid in strengthening the knee due to VMO, adductor, hamstring, and gluteal activation associated with deeper squats and lunges.

Initiate the backward/upward movement through the ball of the front foot by driving the shoulders back with no change in posture back to the start position. Perform all reps on one leg, then perform on the other leg.

Keys to Movement:

1. Stand on a 3-6" platform.
2. Maintain lordotic/neutral posture with torso perpendicular to floor throughout the movement.
3. Take a large step forward keeping the front heel in contact with the ground throughout the movement.
4. Focus on keeping the back leg as straight as possible to ensure maximal tension on front leg and stretching of back leg hip flexor musculature.
5. Lower down until hamstring comes in contact with calf..
6. Begin ascent by focusing on driving the shoulders/torso back and upward first.
7. Do not allow the front heel to come off during the movement.
8. Ensure the torso does not lean over during the movement.

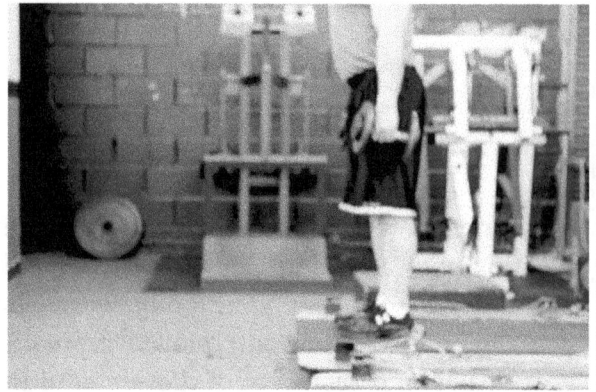

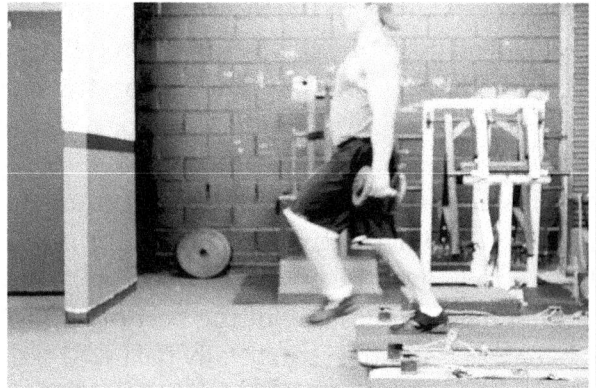

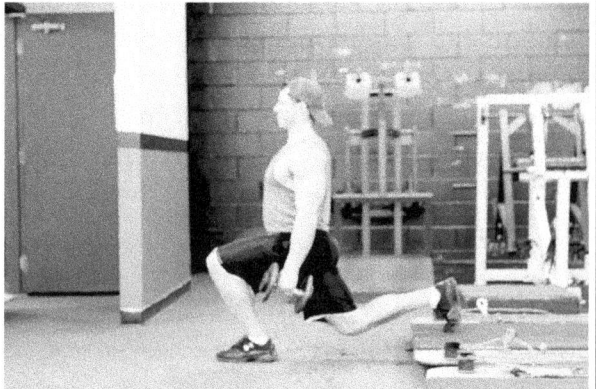

Dumbbell Split Squats

Exercise Prerequisites: Use caution if you have neck, knee, or low back pain.

Antagonistic Muscles to movement: Hamstrings as flexors of the knee.

Movement: Position body with feet hip width apart, torso in neutral/slightly lordotic posture, with dumbbells held at your sides. Maintain upright posture throughout movement. With toes pointing straight ahead, step one foot forward into a lunge position. The distance between your feet is determined by your hip flexor range of motion. If the rear foot is too close, the heel of the front foot will come off during the movement. If the rear foot is too far back, the knee will not cross the heel plane. After you have found the optimal distance between front and rear foot, lower the hips forward and toward the ground maintaining upright posture with no lean forward in the torso. Keeping the back leg as straight as possible, descend until the hamstring comes in contact with the calf on the front leg. It is imperative not to lean forward or allow the front foot heel to come off the ground throughout the movement. As the hamstring comes in the contact with the calf, the knee may cross the toe plane. If the knees are healthy, this can help to strengthen the knee as there is a greater VMO, adductor, hamstring, and gluteal activation with deeper squats and lunges. Once the back knee is 1-2" above the ground initiate the backward movement through the ball of the front foot by driving the shoulders back to the start position with no change in posture. Make sure the front heel never comes off the ground or elevated platform. Perform all reps on one leg, then perform all reps on the opposite leg.

Keys to Movement:
1. Maintain lordotic/neutral posture with torso perpendicular to floor throughout the movement.
2. Determine optimal distance between front and rear foot.
3. Focus on keeping the back leg as straight as possible to ensure maximal tension on front leg and stretching of back leg hip flexor musculature.
4. Lower down until hamstring comes in contact with calf. In healthy knees, the knee may cross of the toe plane as there is a greater recruitment of VMO, adductor, hamstring, and gluteal musculature.
5. Begin ascent by focusing on driving the shoulders/torso back and upward first.
6. Do not allow the front heel to come off during the movement.
7. Do not allow torso to lean over during the movement.

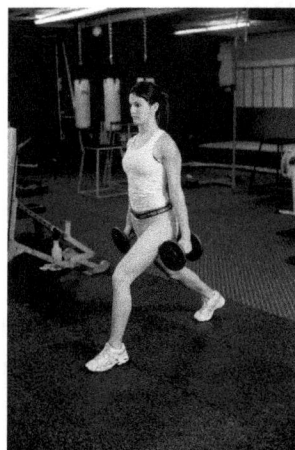

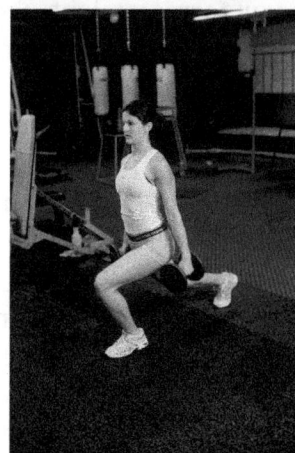

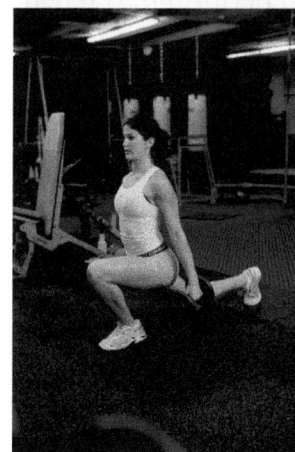

Dumbbell Squat

Exercise Prerequisites: Use caution if you have chronic neck, knee or low back pain.

Antagonistic Muscles to movement: Hamstrings as flexors of the knee.

Movement: Hold dumbbells by your sides with arms extended. Assume a stable neutral/lordotic posture, keeping the weight balanced between feet. Position the feet hip width apart or slightly wider, with toes pointing straight ahead or slightly out. Keeping your arms straight, begin the descent by bending your knees first (a variation is to bend at the hips first), making sure to maintain lordotic/neutral posture.

As you sit downward, push your knees outward to ensure maximum hip muscle recruitment. Once your hamstrings touch your calves, or you have gone as low as your flexibility allows, begin to the ascent.

Keeping your back arched/neutral with torso rigid, focus on driving the shoulders up first, maintaining the torso upright. Be sure to keep the heels driving into the ground and avoid caving knees and rounding of the back. Be sure to exhale through the sticking point and complete the rep all the way to the top. Then perform next repetition.

Keys to Movement:

1. Hold dumbbells by your sides with arms straight.
2. Place feet hip width or slightly wider with toes pointing slightly outward.
3. Maintain neutral/lordotic posture while keeping the torso as upright as possible.
4. Bend at the knees first when you begin your ascent (variation is to bend at the hips first).
5. Push the knees outward, ensuring they point in the same direction as the toes throughout the movement.
6. Do not allow the heels to come off the ground or knees to collapse during the movement.
7. Lower down until your hamstrings touch your calves or as low as your flexibility allows.

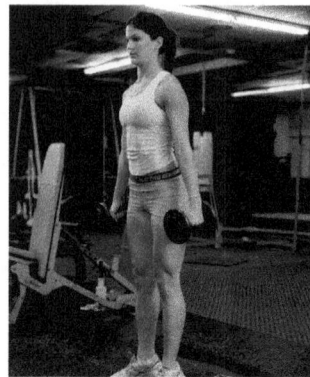

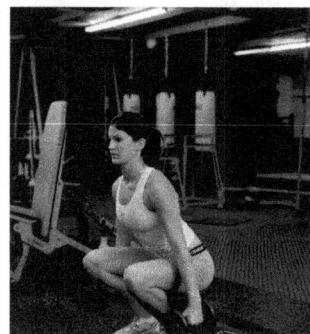

Forward Sled Dragging

Exercise Prerequisites: Use caution if you have neck, knee, shoulder, or low back pain.

Movement: Facing away from a sled, holding the straps by your sides with arms extended. Lean forward to about 45 degree angle relative to the floor. Feet should be feet hip width apart. Keeping the same torso position with arms straight by your sides, begin walking by driving the knee upward and landing in a modified lunge. From here focus on pulling with the hip extensors of the lead leg until the leg is straight. Drive the opposite knee high and repeat.

Keys to Movement:

1. Position feet hip width apart.
2. Lean over with torso roughly 45 degrees relative to the floor.
3. Keep arms extended by your sides.
4. Lunge step outward, driving the lead leg knee high.
5. Focus on driving forward using the lead leg hip extensor musculature.

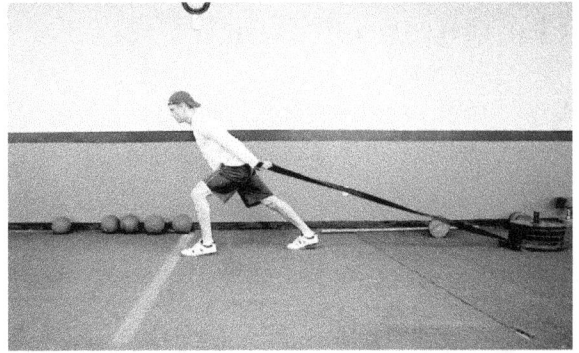

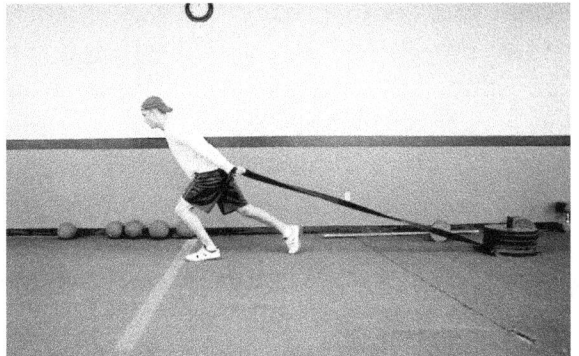

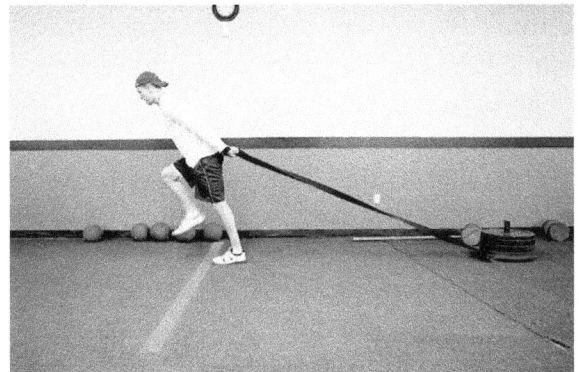

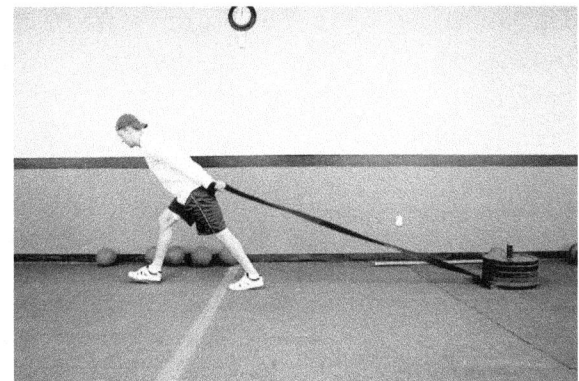

Flat Dumbbell Bench Press

Exercise Prerequisites: Use caution if you have neck, shoulder, elbow, or low back pain.

Antagonistic Muscles: Rhomboids, Lower Trapezius Musculature, External Rotators

Movement: The purpose of the neutral grip flat dumbbell bench press is to enhance pectoral stretch and recruitment while protecting the shoulders and enhancing triceps activation. Lie on a flat bench with feet flat on the floor (if low back problems, elevate your feet on a low box). Utilizing a neutral grip with dumbbells parallel to each other and parallel to the floor, keep the angle of the upper arms relative to the torso to 45 degrees or less. Pinch your shoulder blades back, hugging the bench, while expanding your chest upward.

Beginning with the dumbbells in the arms extended position, begin by lowering the dumbbells straight down. Keep the dumbbells parallel to the floor and parallel to each other, while keeping the upper arm angle relative to the body at 45 degrees or less.

Lower down to your sides until the handgrips of the dumbbells are parallel to the chest, with the pectoral musculature in a stretched position.

Keeping the shoulder blades pulled back, begin the concentric phase of the repetition by retracing the direction the dumbbells were lowered. Breathe out on the way up, while focusing on pectoral muscle recruitment.

Do not allow the dumbbells to rotate or the elbows to flare outward during the pressing movement. Also, ensure the low back is pressed firmly against the bench to avoid neck or low back strain.

Keys to the Movement:
1. Ensure dumbbells are kept parallel to each other and parallel to the floor throughout the movement.
2. Upper arm at 45 degree angle or less relative to the upper body.
3. Keep low back firmly pressed against bench.
4. Pinch shoulder blades back with chest out to minimize shoulder injury potential.
5. Breathe out during concentric part of the repetition.

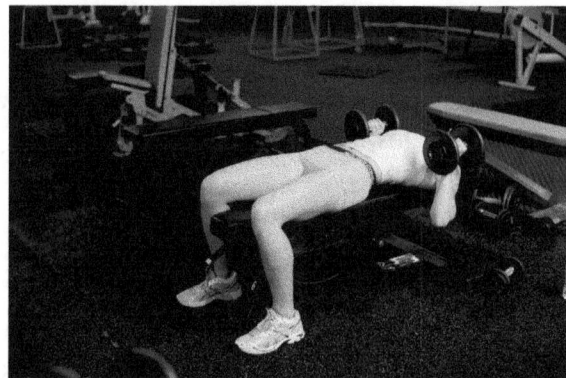

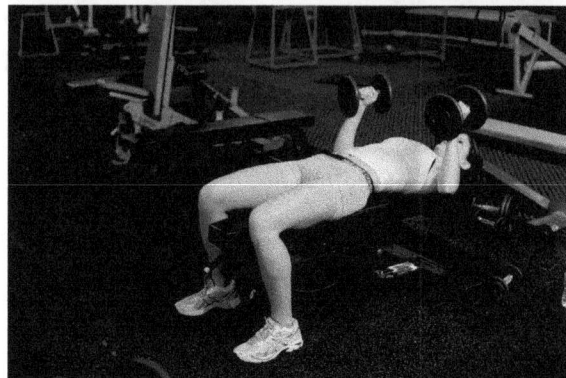

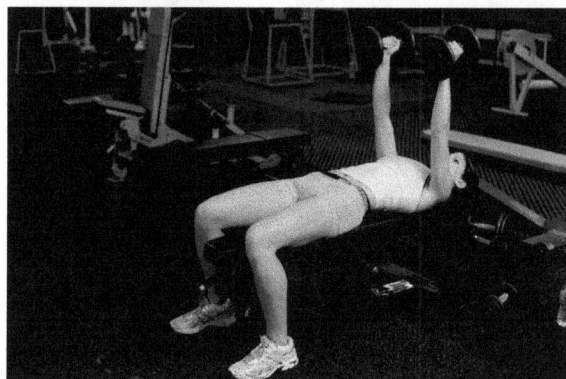

Front Squat

Exercise Prerequisites: Use caution if chronic knee, low back, or shoulder pain.

Antagonistic Muscles to movement: Hamstrings as flexors of the knee.

Movement: Position hands in power clean/Olympic clean rack position, with barbell resting across upper chest, clavicles, and anterior deltoids. Keep upper arms parallel to the floor with elbows pointing straight forward. Once you have un-racked the bar, assume a stable neutral/lordotic posture, keeping the weight balanced between feet. Position the feet hip width apart or slightly wider, with toes pointing straight ahead or slightly out. Keep your elbows up. As you begin the descent, make sure to maintain lordotic posture. As you sit downward, push your knees outward. Once your hamstrings touch your calves, or you have gone as low as your flexibility allows, begin driving the bar upward.

Keeping the back arched/neutral with torso rigid, focus on driving the elbows up first. Be sure to keep the heels driving into the ground, and avoid caving knees and rounding of the back. Exhale through the sticking point and ascend all the way to the top. Then perform next repetition.

Keys to Movement:

1. Place bar in "clean" rack position across the upper chest and anterior deltoids.
2. Place feet hip width or slightly wider with toes pointing slightly outward.
3. Keep the elbows pulled upward and pointing straight ahead.
4. Maintain neutral/lordotic posture keeping the torso as upright as possible.
5. Push the knees outward, ensuring they point in the same direction as the toes throughout the movement.
6. Do not allow the heels to come off the ground or the knees to collapse throughout the movement.
7. Lower down until your hamstrings touch your calves or as low as your flexibility allows.

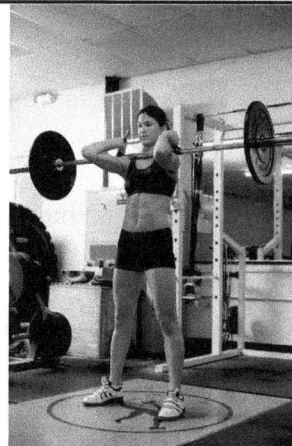

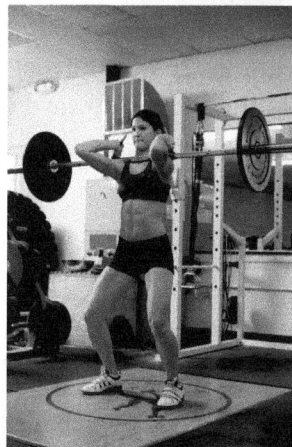

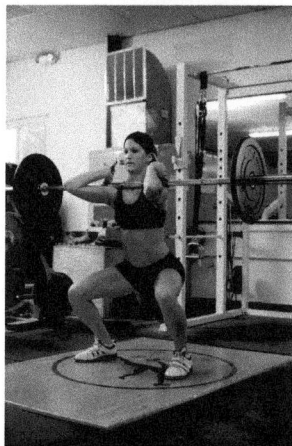

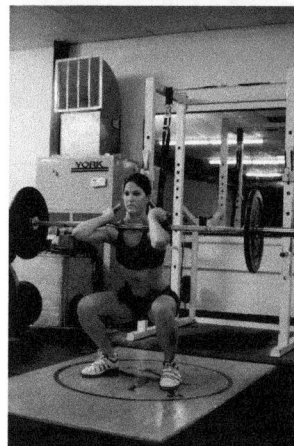

Glute Ham Raise

Exercise Prerequisites: Use caution if you have knee, neck, or low back pain.

Movement: Lie on a glute ham raise machine with heels locked into pads, feet against foot plate, and quads across support pad. Lock your torso rigid, maintaining neutral/slightly lordotic posture throughout. Extend your legs and lower your torso downward by flexing at the hips only. From here, contract the glutes, keeping your torso rigid as you begin hip extension (do not shoot your butt back first by bending at the hips). After your hips have reached full or near complete extension, begin flexing the knees, similar to a hamstring curl. Curl your extended torso upward until you are perpendicular to the floor. Lower back to start.

Keys to Movement:

1. Keep neutral/slightly lordotic posture throughout movement.
2. Extend legs at the bottom end range of the movement.
3. Do not bend at the hips when pulling yourself upward.
4. Contract the glutes for greater stability and hamstring activation.
5. Pull with your hamstrings until you are perpendicular to the floor.

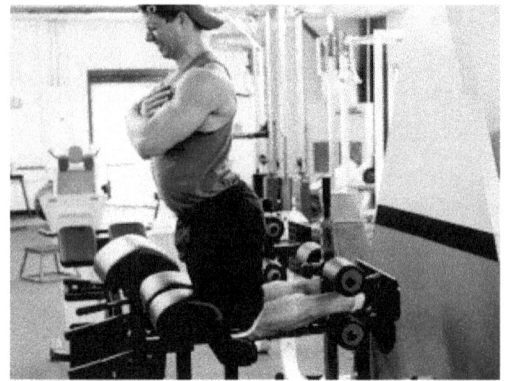

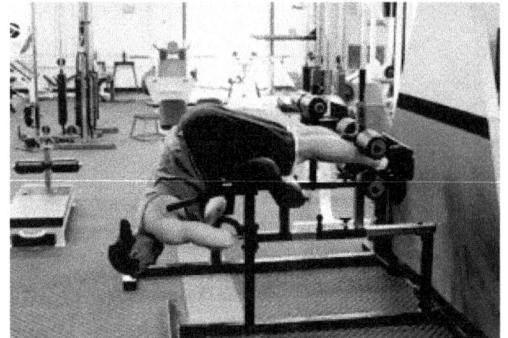

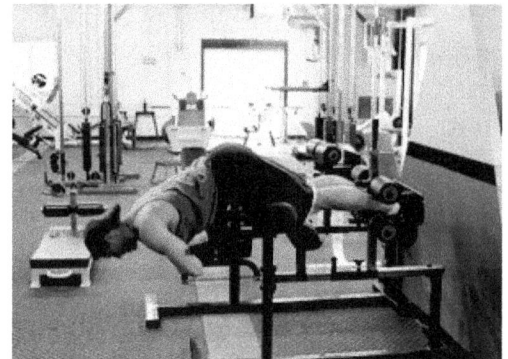

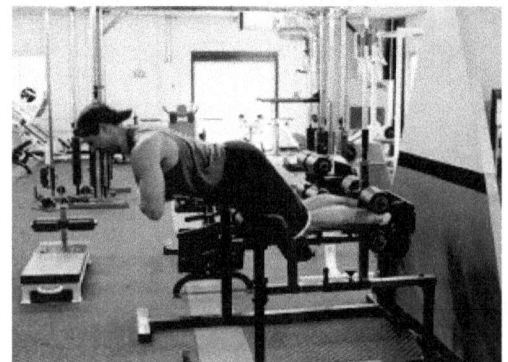

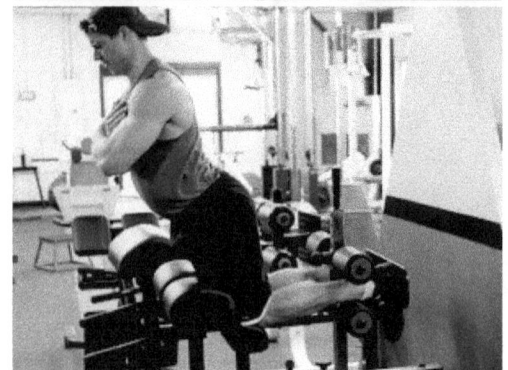

Hamstring Curls (Kneeling)

Exercise Prerequisites: Use caution if you have neck, knee, or low back pain.

Antagonistic Muscles to movement: Knee Extensors

Movement: Hamstring curl options include:
- Prone hamstring curl machine
- Seated hamstring curl machine
- Kneeling hamstring curl machine
- Standing hamstring curl machine
- Swiss Ball Hamstring Curl

Each of these machines isolates the hamstrings in a slightly different manner. For those with structural imbalances of the hamstrings, unilateral training may be the best option for correcting these imbalances. For each hamstring curl option, control of the torso, position of the upper leg, and direction the foot is pointing are all critical. During any of these, do not allow for a swinging motion in the torso, rather. maintain a rigid posture throughout. Maintain the same femur position relative to the torso throughout the movement.

Adjusting the direction the toes point during hamstring curls can aid in correcting structural imbalances. Feet inverted, everted, or neutral are all options. Also, plantar flexing the ankle can aid in minimizing gastroc recruitment.

Keys to Movement:

1. Rigid torso position throughout the movement. Do not allow the torso to swing or generate momentum.
2. Femur position is locked. Do not allow to swing backward to generate momentum.
3. Structural imbalances can be corrected by changing the direction the toes are pointing.
4. Plantar flexion can aid in minimizing gastroc recruitment.

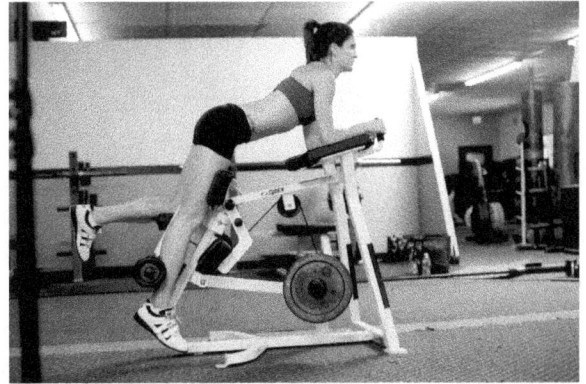

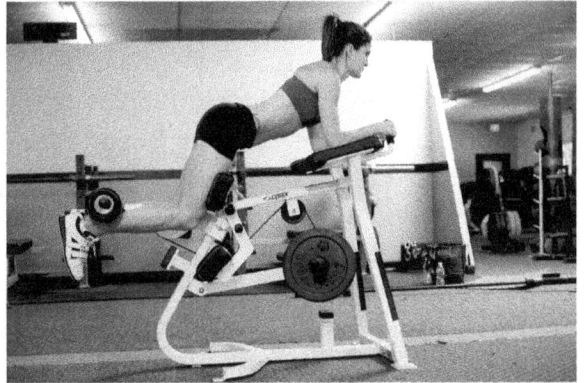

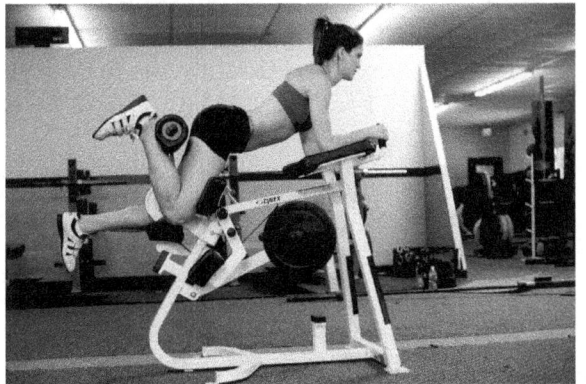

Heels Elevated Dumbbell Squat

Exercise Prerequisites: Use caution if you have chronic knee or low back pain.

Antagonistic Muscles to movement: Hamstrings as flexors of the knee.

Movement: This another exercise variation learned from Charles Poliquin and his Poliquin Institute staff. Hold dumbbells by your sides with straight arms. Stand with heels elevated on a ramp or weight plate. Keep the weight distributed between the feet with a stable neutral/lordotic posture. Position feet hip width apart or slightly wider, with toes pointing straight ahead or slightly out. Keep your arms straight. As you begin the descent, maintain lordotic posture. As you sit downward, push your knees outward, ensuring they point in the same direction as the toes throughout the exercise. Lower down until your hamstrings touch your calves or you have gone as low as your flexibility allows.
Keeping your back arched/neutral with torso rigid, begin the ascent. Keeping the torso upright, drive the heels into the ground while avoiding caving knees or rounding of the back. Make sure to exhale through the sticking point and ascend back to the start position. Then perform next repetition.

Keys to Movement: Hold dumbbells by your sides with arms straight.
1. Place feet hip width or slightly wider with toes pointing slightly outward or straight ahead.
2. Maintain neutral/lordotic posture while keeping the torso as upright as possible. Push the knees outward, ensuring they point in the same direction as the toes throughout the movement.
3. Do not allow the heels to come off the ground or knees collapse throughout the movement.
4. Lower down until the hamstrings touch your calves or as low as your flexibility allows.

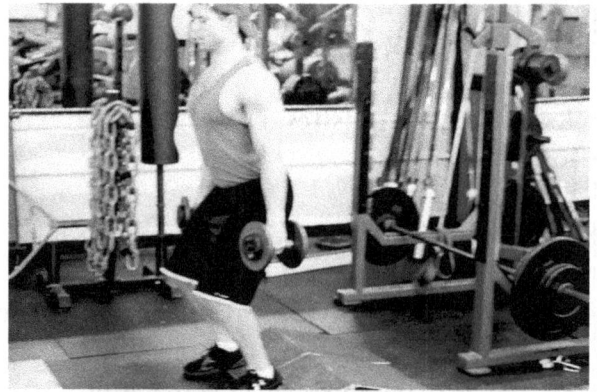

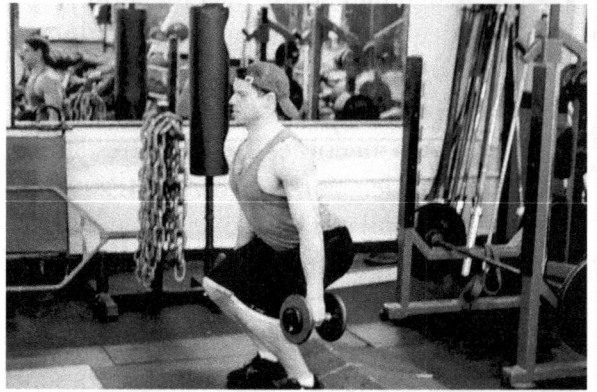

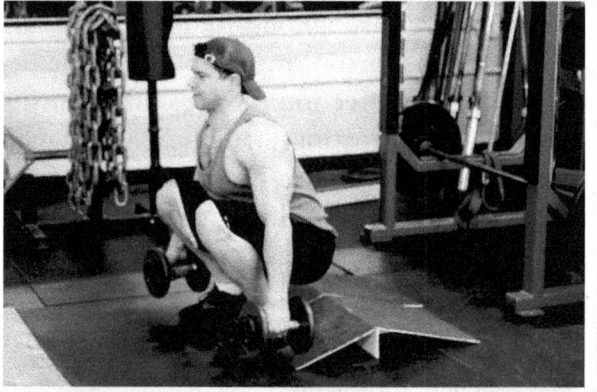

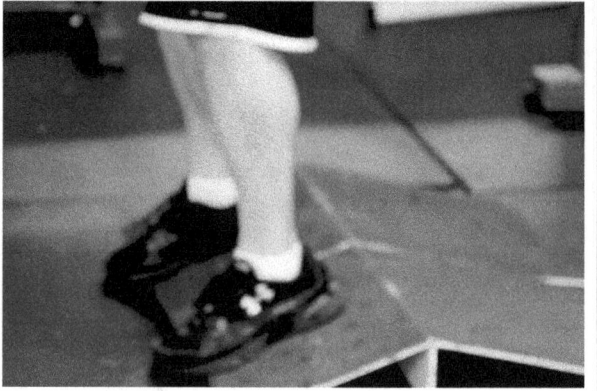

Incline Dumbbell Bench Press

Exercise Prerequisites: Use caution if you have shoulder, neck, elbow, or low back pain. If upper crossed syndrome is an issue, perform corrective movements.

Antagonistic Muscles: Rhomboids, Mid Trapezius Musculature, External Rotators

Movement: Lie on an incline bench with feet flat on the floor (or up on a low box/platform if you have low back issues). Utilizing a neutral grip with dumbbells parallel to each other and parallel to the floor, pinch your shoulder blades back, hugging the bench, while expanding your chest upward. Beginning with the dumbbells in the arms extended position, lower the dumbbells straight down. Try to ensure the dumbbells remain parallel to the floor and parallel to each other, while keeping the upper arm angle relative to the body at roughly 45 degrees or less.

Lower down to your sides until the handgrips of the dumbbells are parallel to the chest. Keeping the shoulder blades pinched back, begin the concentric action, retracing the same pattern the dumbbells were lowered. Breathe out on the way up, while focusing on pectoral muscle recruitment. Try to ensure the dumbbells to rotate or the elbows to flare outward during the pressing movement.

Keys to the Movement:

1. Try to keep the dumbbells parallel to each other and parallel to the floor throughout the movement.
2. Upper arm at roughly 45 degree angle or less relative to the upper body.
3. Keep low back firmly pressed against bench.
4. Pinch shoulder blades back with chest out to minimize shoulder injury potential.
5. Breathe out through the sticking point.

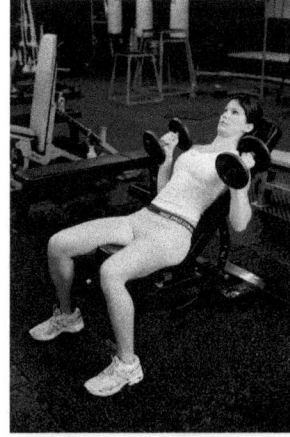

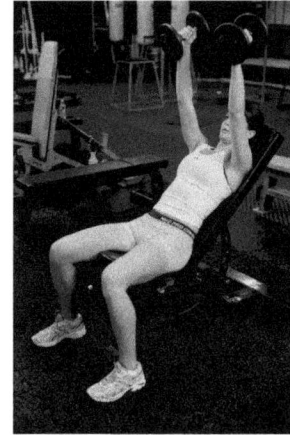

Inverted Row

Exercise Prerequisites: Use caution if you have low back, elbow, shoulder, neck pain

Movement: Position fixed Olympic bar 2-3 feet off the ground. Lay on your back with your heels resting on the floor or on a Swiss ball. Grab the bar with pronated grip slightly wider than shoulder width. Extend hips and push chest locking the body into neutral/slightly lordotic posture. Pull chest to bar by retracting the shoulder blades and driving the elbows back. Once your chest makes contact with the bar slowly lower back to start without breaking posture.

Movement Mechanics:

1. Grasp the bar with a pronated grip and hands slightly wider than shoulder width.
2. Extend hips and maintain lordotic/neutral posture.
3. Do not allow the hips to bend throughout the movement.
4. Retract shoulder blades and pull chest to the bar.
5. Lower back to start position.

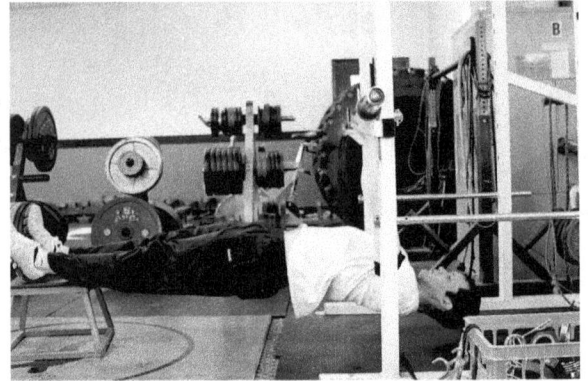

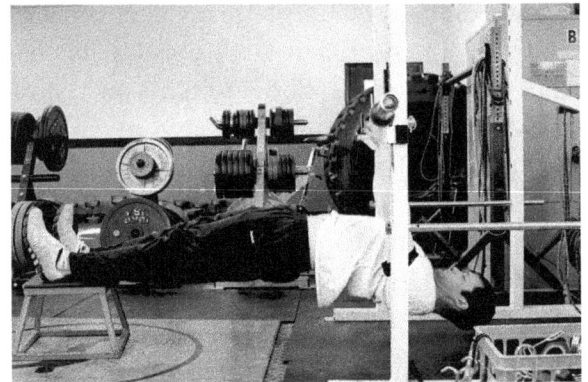

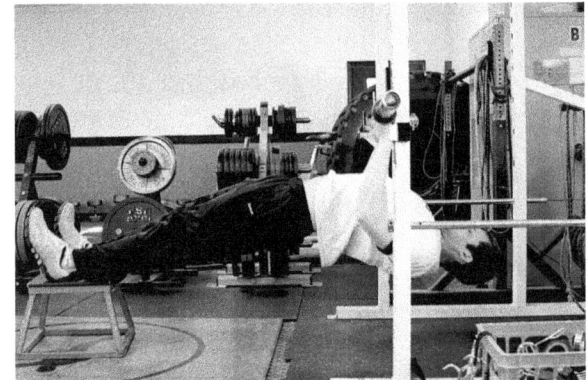

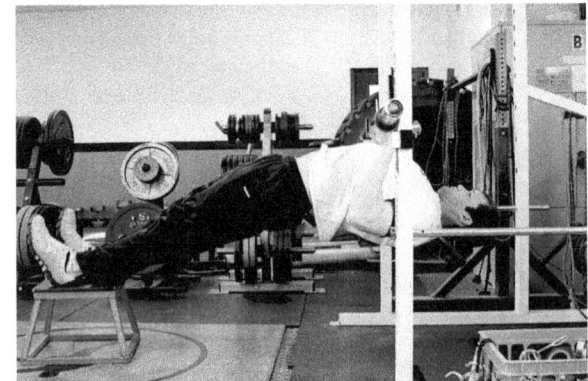

Kettlebell Swing

Exercise Prerequisites: Avoid exercise if you have low back, knee, neck, or shoulder problems.

Movement: Begin with a lordotic posture in the spine, chest out, shoulder pulled back, eyes straight ahead, and knees bent roughly 20 degrees to activate the hip extensor mechanism. Try to keep the weight over the rear of the foot. Bending at the waist rather than low back, can ensure muscle tension in the glutes and hamstrings. Hold the kettlebell with two hands, palms down. Swing the bell between the legs, just above mid shin height. At the point of full tension on the glutes and hamstrings, and the bell back behind the knees/shins, begin the upward acceleration.

The upward pull is initiated through the glutes and hamstrings, while keeping the torso in lordotic/neutral posture. Begin by swinging the weight outward and upward, raising and extending the hips, extending the knees, increasing the torso angle, and bringing the bell in an arcing movement to chin height or up above your head, while keeping the arms extended. A good tip is to contract glutes to ensure proper hip extension. At the top of the movement, stabilize the bell and allow it to swing downward in the same arcing manner. At the point of full tension in the glutes and hamstrings (bell behind the knees/shins) try to immediately change the direction again, accelerating into an upward explosive swing.

Keys to Movement:

1. Hold a lordotic posture in the spine with roughly 20 degree bend or more at the knees.
2. Initiate the swing by extending the hips and knees, creating momentum for the kettlebell to swing upward.
3. Once he kettlebell has reached chin height or above, allow it to swing downward.

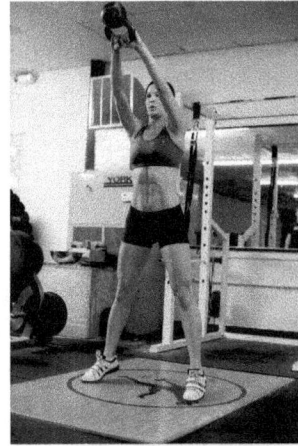

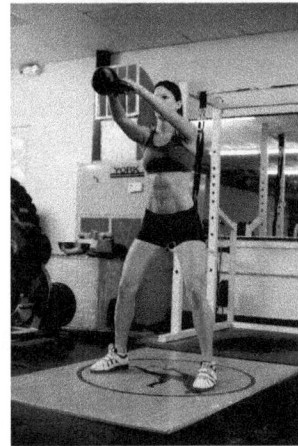

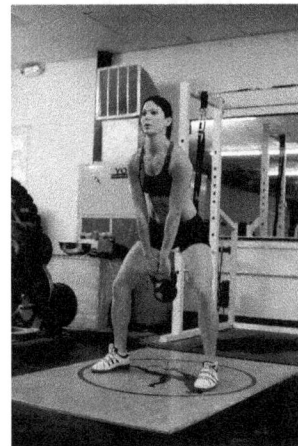

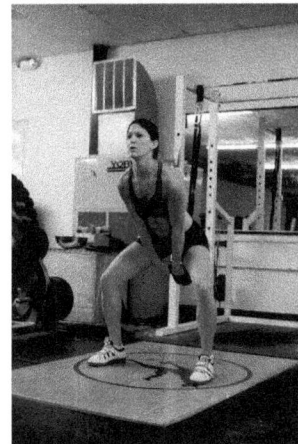

Kneeling Cable Crunch

Exercise Prerequisites: Avoid if you have persistent neck, shoulder, or elbow problems.

Movement: Holding a rope cable attachment, kneel down in front of a high cable column with your knees roughly hip width apart. With hips extended and arms extended overhead, begin by pulling the rope handles downward, initiating the movement by flexing at the hips and spine. As you pull downward allow your hands to come on both sides of your head with your elbows coming toward your sides. Ensure that you do not allow your hips to shoot backward. Focus on keeping your thighs perpendicular to the floor at all times. Continue crunching downward until your elbow touch the floor or your head nears the floor. Slowly allow back to start.

Keys to Movement:

1. Hold on to a rope cable attachment while kneeling down in front of a cable column.
2. Keeping your thighs perpendicular to the floor, begin crunching downward pulling the rope toward your head. .
3. Crunch downward until your elbows or head come close to the ground.

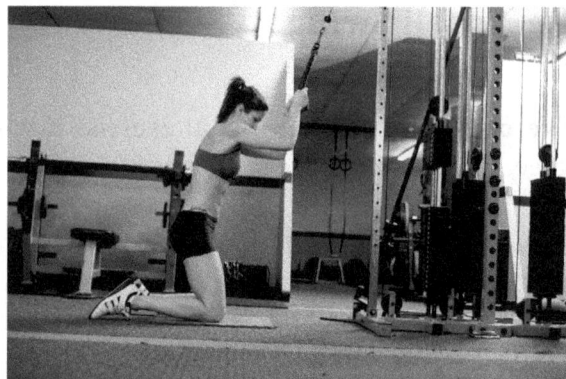
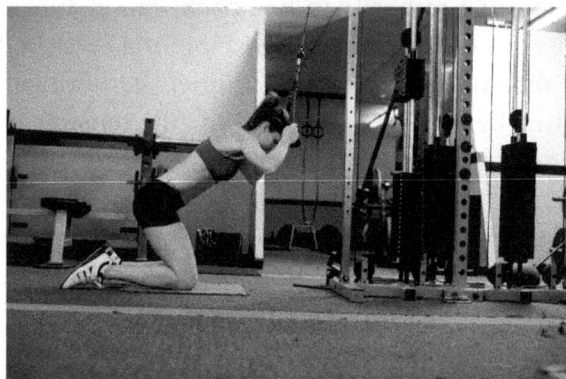
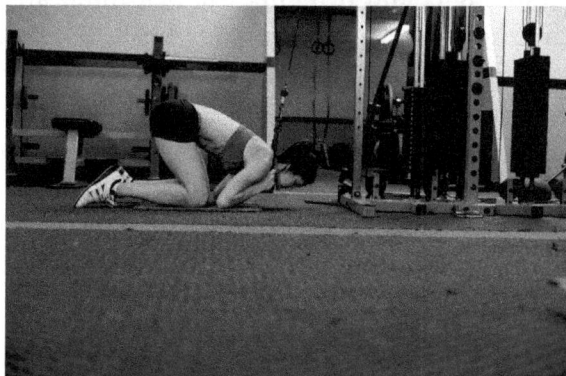

Lateral Med Ball Slamdowns

Classification: GPP and low back

Exercise Prerequisites: Avoid if you have persistent, low back, neck, or shoulder pain.

Movement: Start by standing next to a non-bounce med ball with feet slightly wider than hip width. Reach down pick up the med ball, pivoting the back foot. Lift the ball swinging it upward and outward in a rainbow arcing motion. Keeping the momentum, slam the ball down on your opposite side. Pick it back up and retrace the movement back slamming it down to the other side.

Keys to Movement:

1. Start with feet roughly hip width apart and ball next to one foot.
2. Lift the ball in an arcing motion upward and slam it down to the opposite side.
3. Perform for speed or conditioning.

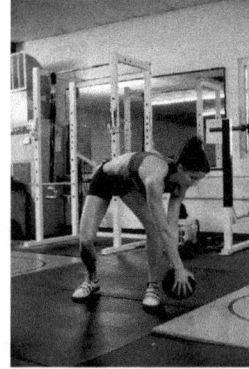

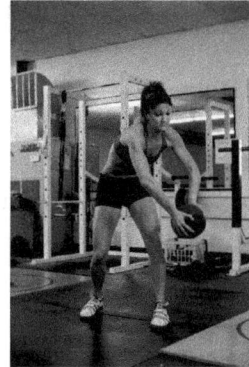

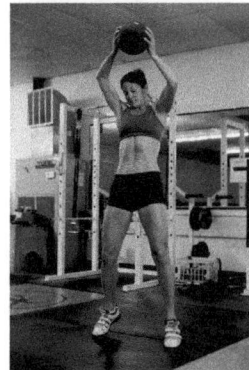

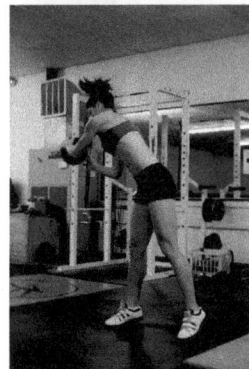

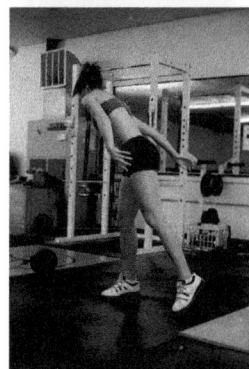

Leg Press

Exercise Prerequisites: Use caution if you have neck, knee or low back pain

Antagonistic Muscles to movement: Hamstrings as flexors of the knee.

Movement: Lay on a 45 degree leg press machine. Position feet hip width apart with weight evenly distributed throughout the feet. Do not allow the butt to come off the pad. Ensure the glutes, hamstrings, and adductors are active throughout the movement by driving through the heels. Keeping your head back, low back pushed firmly against the back of the machine, extend the legs. Be cautious of pushing the back of your head too hard into the pad as this can lead to neck injury or strain. Lower down to the point where the upper thigh is parallel or just below parallel to the foot plate. You can go lower if you have optimal hip mobility, knee health and the low back does not round or come off the bench. Repeat for the required repetitions.

Keys to Movement:

1. Press low back firmly against pad.
2. Ensure that knees are pointing in the same direction as the toes throughout the movement.
3. Keep the heels in contact with the foot plate.
4. Lower to the point where the upper thigh is parallel to the foot plate or as low as your hips allow you to travel without the low back rounding or coming off the pad.

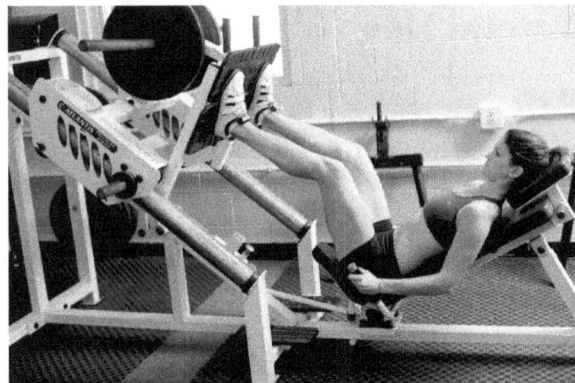

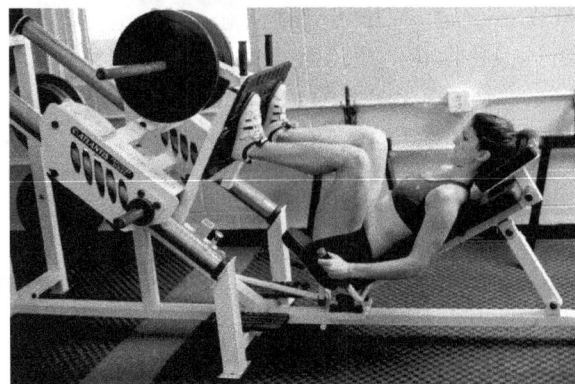

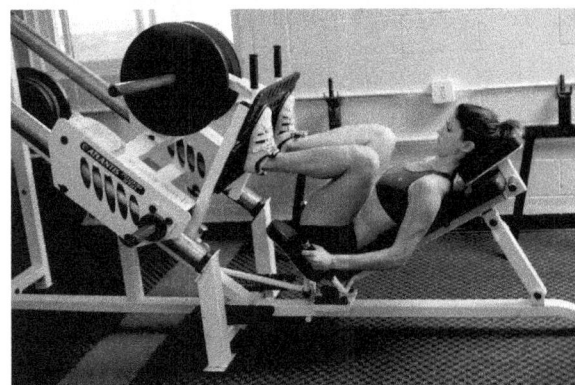

45 Degree Low Back Extension

Exercise Prerequisites: Use caution if you have persistent neck, knee, or low back pain.

Antagonistic Muscles to movement: Hip Flexors

Movement: Position yourself on a conventional hyperextension machine or a 45 degree back extension machine. Make sure the thighs are prone on the pad with the calves or Achilles tendons under the brace pads. Holding a lordotic/neutral spine, lower your body down until reaching roughly 90 degree hip flexion or until you cannot hold lordotic posture. Initiate the upward movement by contracting the glutes and hamstrings while maintaining lordotic/neutral posture. Raise until your torso reaches neutral position. Do not hyperextend.

Keys to Movement:

1. Hold lordotic/neutral posture throughout movement.
2. Lower down until you can no longer hold lordotic/neutral posture.
3. Initiate upward movement by engaging the glutes and hamstrings.
4. Raise until you reach neutral starting position. Do not hyperextend.

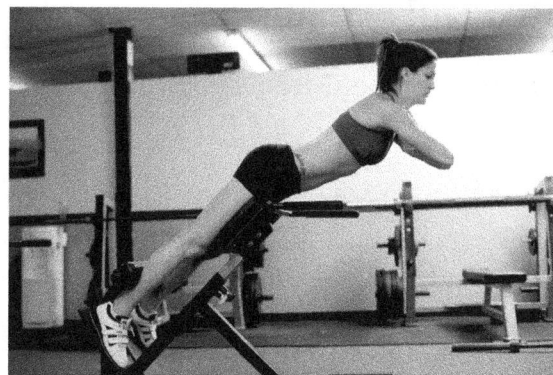

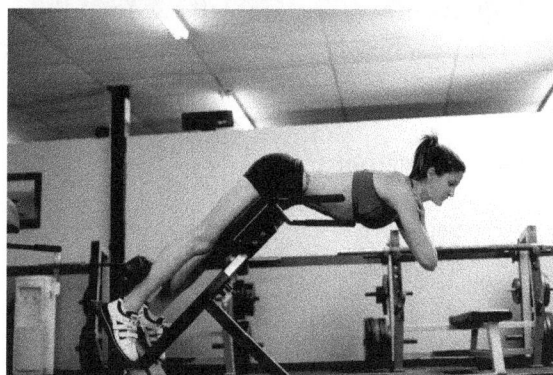

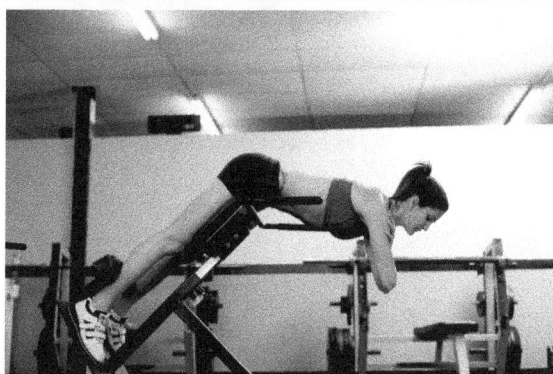

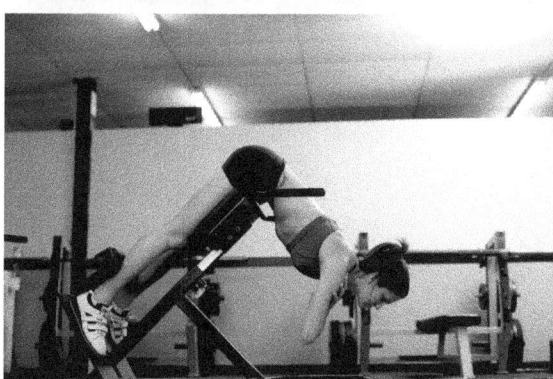

Med Ball Slamdowns

Exercise Prerequisites: Avoid if you have persistent neck, knee, or low back pain.

Movement: Stand with your feet hip width or slightly wider and a non-bounce medicine ball between your feet. Reach downward to pick up the med ball and try to lift with a lordotic posture to ensure activation of the glutes and hamstrings. Powerfully extend the hips and knees driving the medicine ball up overhead, without letting go of the ball. Once the med ball has reached max height overhead, change direction and slam the ball downward into the ground in front of you.

Keys to Movement:

1. Feet roughly hip to shoulder width apart.
2. Try to lift with lordotic posture.
3. Once ball reaches maximum height, change direction and slam it down powerfully into the ground.

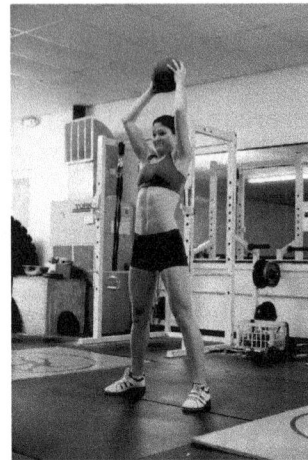

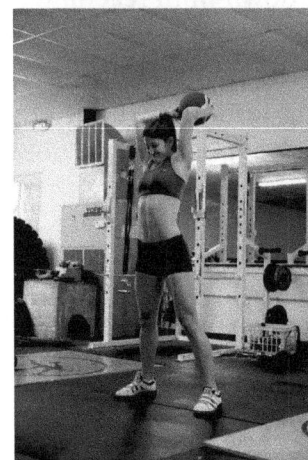

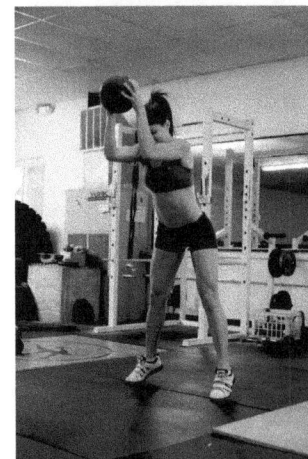

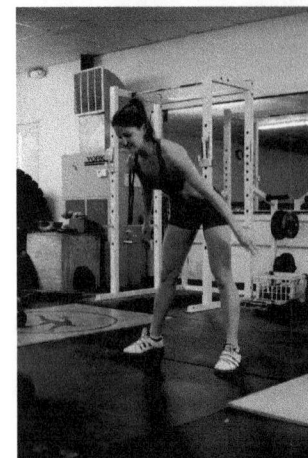

Neutral Grip Chin-Ups

Exercise Prerequisites: Use caution if you have elbow, shoulder or serious low back pain

Movement: Grasp a neutral grip chin-up bar with hands neutral, shoulder width or slightly wider. Hang from the bar, with arms, hips and shoulders in extension. Initiate movement by retracting shoulder blades back and down. Begin pulling your body upward, continuing to pull the shoulder blades back and downward. Try not to allow the shoulders to internally rotate as you are pulling upward.

Pull upward, pinching your shoulder blades back until the upper portion of your chest comes in contact with the bar.

Lower the body slowly, retracing the same pattern until you reach the starting position at the bottom.

If you cannot perform a regular chin-up, you can use the assistance of a partner or a band around the knee or foot.

Keys to Movement:

1. Neutral grip with hands shoulder width or slightly closer.
2. Begin in the dead hang start position.
3. Retract shoulders back and down to initiate the movement.
4. Focus on pulling the elbows back and down.
5. Do not allow the shoulders to internally rotate.
6. Pull up until upper part of chest comes in contact with the bar.
7. Lower down until you reach full extension in the elbows and shoulders.

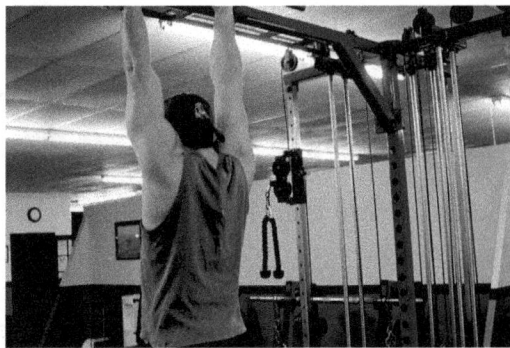

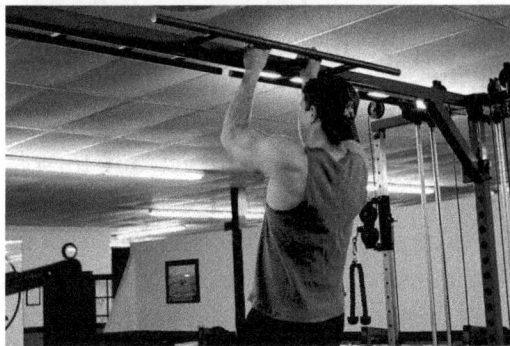

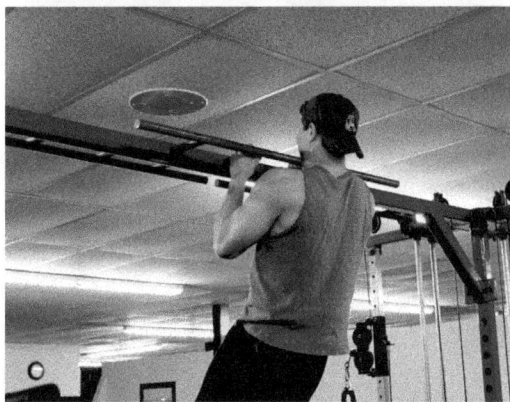

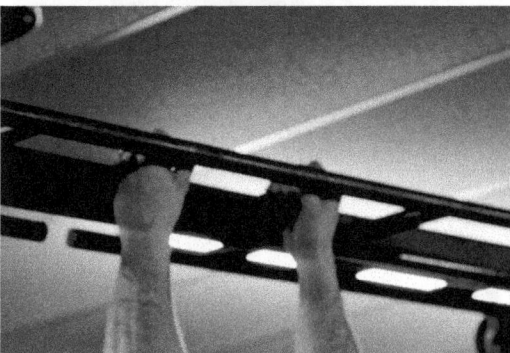

Off Bench Oblique

Exercise Prerequisites: Use caution if you have knee, shoulder, neck, or low back pain.

Movement: More than just an oblique exercise, this exercise strengthens the Quadratus Lumborum muscles of the low back. When strong, these muscles aid in maintaining upright stability in contact sports. Lay down on your side on a bench, with the upper body hanging off the bench and heels/legs anchored under an immovable bar. Fold your arms across your chest (or hands at your ears) and lower your torso/shoulder toward the ground. Once you have lowered yourself as far as your flexibility allows, contract our torso up as high as you can past the start position. Variations to this exercise include feet stacked on top of each other, one foot in front of the other, isometric hold at the top of concentric contraction, or holding a weight in your arms across the chest.

Keys to Movement:

1. Lie on your side with feet anchored (stacked, bottom leg in front, or bottom leg in back).
2. Keep hips squared. Do not allow your hips to rotate forward or backward.
3. Fold arms across your chest (or hands at your ears).
4. Keeping torso parallel to a wall, lower your shoulder closest to the floor.
5. Once you have reached full stretch, pull your torso upward, contracting past neutral posture.

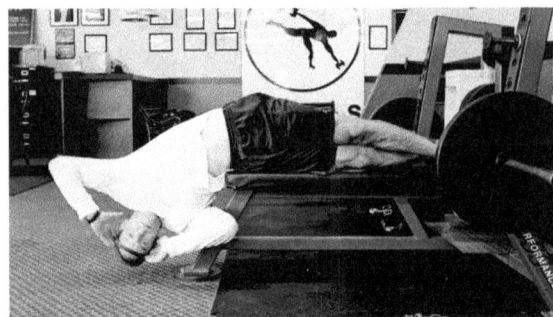

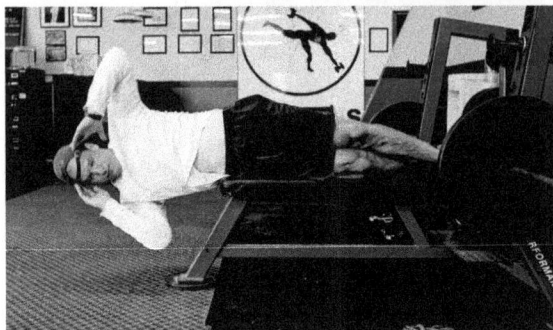

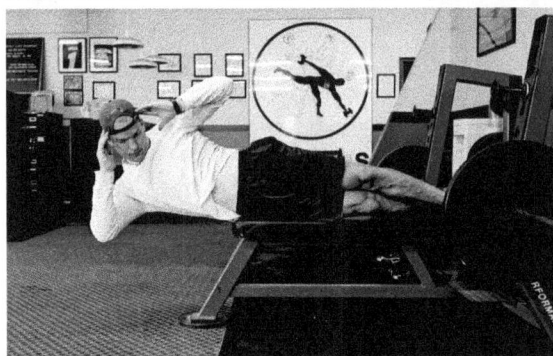

One Arm Dumbbell Row

Exercise Prerequisites: Use caution if you have low back, neck, or shoulder pain.

Movement: Lean torso over until parallel or less than roughly 45 degree angle relative to the floor. Stagger your feet with foot on side of the hand holding the dumbbell in back. Brace the opposite arm against a stable object to aid in holding the torso in position. Hold a dumbbell with neutral grip, knees bent roughly 20 degrees. Arch your back into a lordotic/neutral posture, with chest out, shoulders pulled back and down, eyes straight down.

Maintaining torso position relative to the floor, row the weight toward mid-torso, activating the rear delt, rhomboid and lat muscles. To do this, retract your shoulder blades back and down, focusing on pulling the elbow upward until full contraction of the upper back musculature.

Try not to allow the shoulders to shrug upward as this can take away from the contraction of the mid back/shoulder retractors. Make sure there is no bounce or rounding of the back throughout the movement. Slowly lower the weight back to start and perform next repetition.

Keys to Movement:

1. Position body in correct starting position with knees bent roughly 20 degrees, chest out, back arched, torso parallel or near parallel to the floor, and feet staggered.
2. During the movement retract your shoulders back and down while maintaining torso posture.
3. Focus on pulling elbow upward as high as you can.
4. Try not to allow the shoulders to shrug upward.

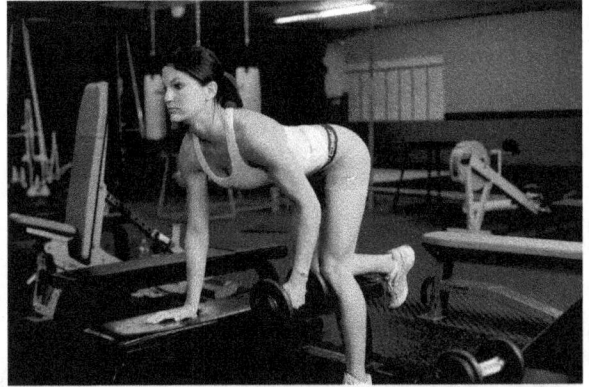

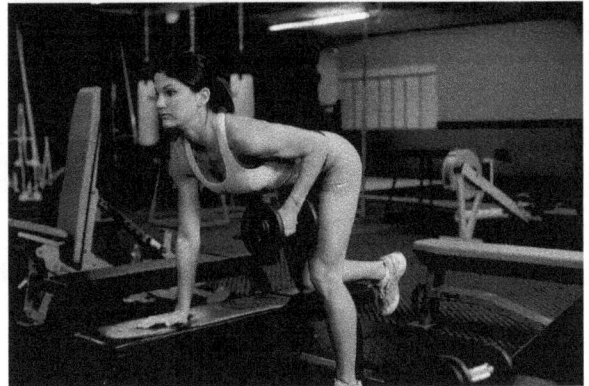

Palloff Press

Exercise Prerequisites: Use caution if you have shoulder, neck, or low back pain.

Movement: Adjust a cable column to sternum height. Stand sideways next to the cable column, roughly three feet from the column. Grasp a D handle with hand furthest from the column on first. The hand on the adjacent side is placed on top. Position your feet hip width or slightly wider with knees slightly bent. Keeping torso upright and rigid, begin the movement with D handle at your sternum. Begin pressing straight outward. Do not allow the resistance from the cable to rotate your torso or pull your arms toward the column. Fully extend your arms and return to start.

Keys to Movement:

1. Stand sideways next to a cable column roughly 3 feet from the machine.
2. Opposite hand grasps the D handle first. Adjacent hand is on top.
3. Position feet hip width or slightly wider.
4. Lock torso, square hips, and bend knees slightly.
5. Press straight outward from sternum height.
6. Do not allow the torso to rotate or arms to be pulled toward the cable column.

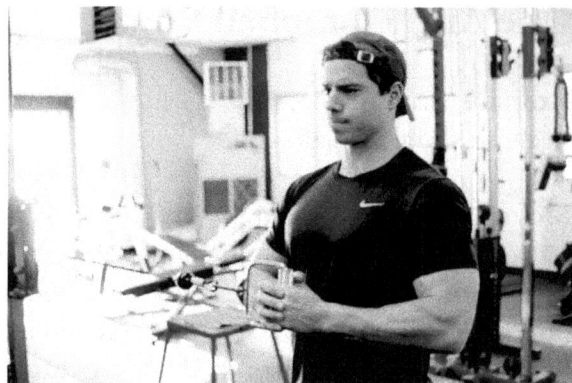

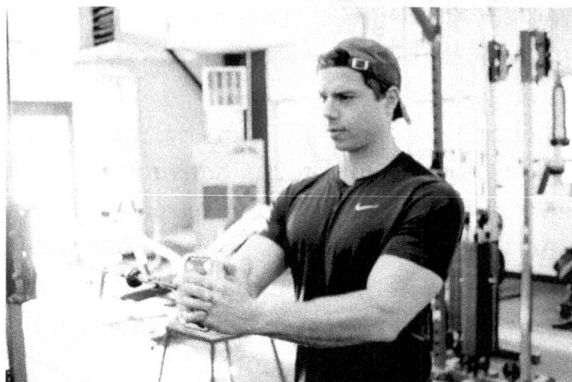

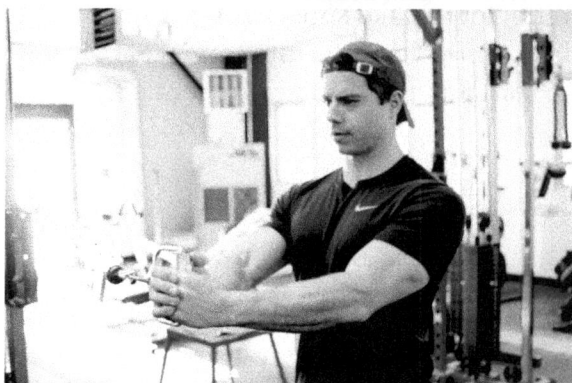

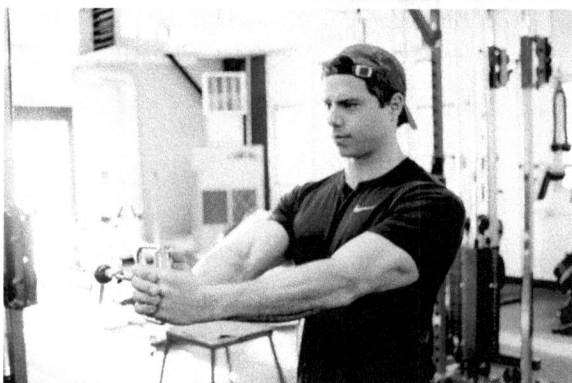

PNF Chop

Exercise Prerequisites: Use caution if you have knee, shoulder, neck, or low back pain.

Movement: Made popular by Functional Movement Screen creator Gray Cook, this exersise is effective strengthening of the core and oblique musculature. Adjust a cable column to a high position. Attach a triceps rope. Offset the rope with the cable attachment ring at the top of the rope and the rest of the rope hanging down. Position your body into a hip flexor stretch position, with your leg opposite the column behind and adjacent leg forward. Keeping your torso upright, grasp the rope with the adjacent hand at the top of the rope directly next to the cable attachment ring. The opposite hand is at the bottom of the rope. Keeping your hip flexor stretched and torso upright, pull the cable toward your sternum with both arms. Your hand adjacent to the column should end up at your sternum while your hand opposite is out and down to your side.

From here press downward to your side until the adjacent hand is parallel to the opposite hip. The other hand should be slightly behind you, roughly glute height. Return to start.

Keys to Movement:

1. Position your body sideways to a cable column in a hip flexor stretch position with opposite leg back and adjacent leg forward.
2. Keeping your torso upright, pull the cable across your body until the adjacent hand is at your sternum and the opposite hand at your side.
3. Press downward until your adjacent hand is parallel to opposite hip. The other hand should be behind your glutes.
4. Make sure to stretch your hip flexor and keep your torso upright throughout the movement.

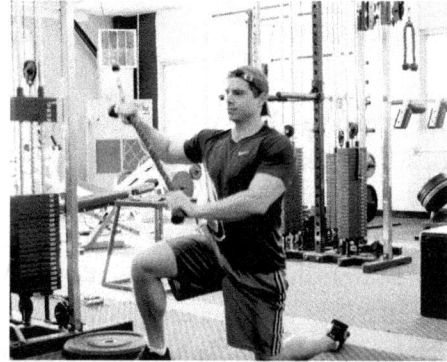

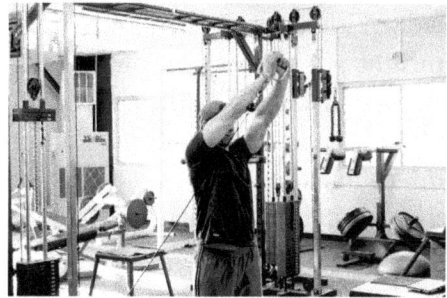

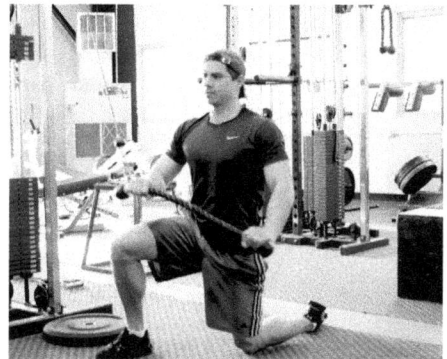

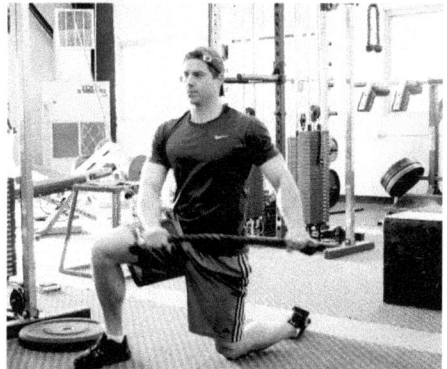

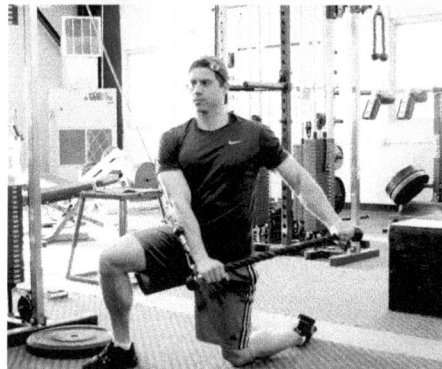

PNF Rotational Lift

Exercise Prerequisites: Use caution if you have knee, shoulder, neck, or low back pain.

Movement: Adjust a cable column to the bottom position. Attach a D handle. Stand sideways next to the column with feet roughly hip width apart. Grasp the D handle with the opposite hand on first and adjacent hand on top with arms extended. With a slight bend in the knees and torso in a rigid upright position, begin pulling the cable in a rotational direction upward. Initiate the pull through the ball of the foot on the foot adjacent to the cable column. Pivot the adjacent foot and rotate the hips until your hips and shoulders are parallel to the column with arms extended outward overhead.

Keys to Movement:

1. Stand sideways next to a cable column with feet hip width apart.
2. Grasp the D handle with the opposite hand first and adjacent hand on top.
3. Initiate the movement by driving through the ball of the back foot.
4. Bring the cable in a circular arcing fashion similar to that of a golf swing.
5. Rotate the hips and shoulders until they are parallel to the column.
6. Finish with the arms extended outward and upward over your head with hips and shoulders squared to the cable column.

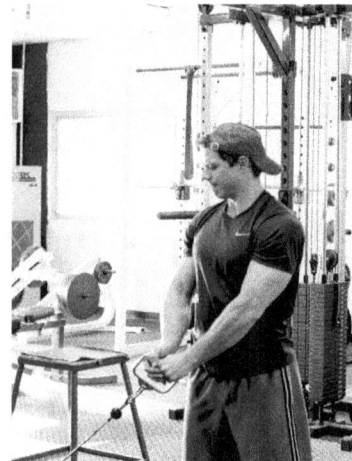

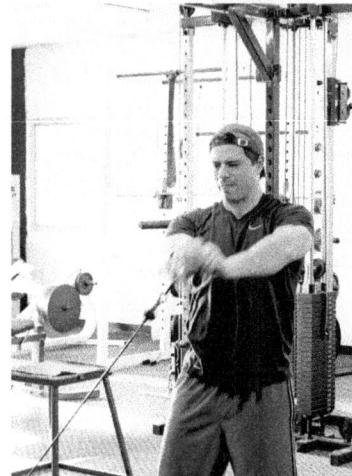

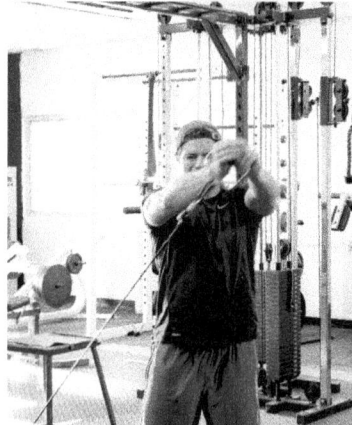

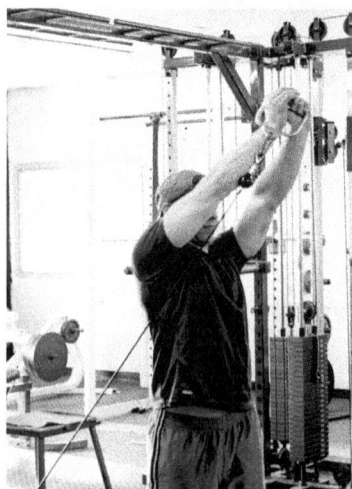

Peterson Step Ups

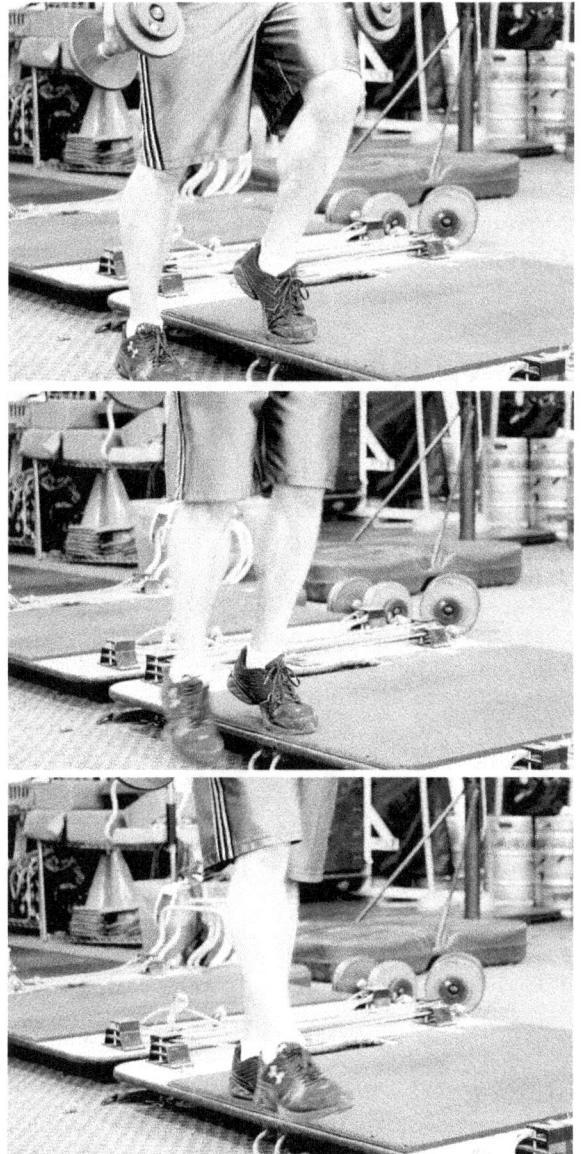

Exercise Prerequisites: Use caution if you have knee or low back pain

Antagonistic Muscles to Movement: Hamstrings as flexors of the knee.

Movement: Stand on a 2-5 inch platform with your working leg heel raised as high as you can and the rest of your foot on the platform, with the weight pushing through the ball of your foot. Extend your hips completely, maintaining a straight line from knee to hip to shoulder on the working leg. Lift the non-working foot off the platform so you are standing on the working leg only. Keeping the non-working leg straight, begin by lowering the foot down toward the ground, maintaining your weight on the ball of the foot of the working leg. Lower the non-working leg by bending the working leg knee until the non-working leg heel comes in contact with the ground. Once the right heel comes in contact with the ground, raise your body up by extending the working leg. Focus on keeping the hips extended to avoid excessive torque and keep the heel elevated as long as you possibly can. Once the leg is near full extension, leg the heel of the working leg drop to the platform and reset for the next repetition.

Keys to Movement:

1. Keep weight on the ball of the foot to ensure recruitment of the VMO
2. Knee points in same direction as the toes throughout the movement.
3. Keep the heel elevated as long as you can.
4. Keep hips extended throughout the movement.
5. Do not use the other foot for assistance.

Power Clean from the Hang

Exercise Prerequisites: Use caution if you have elbow, shoulder, wrist, neck, knee, or low back pain.

Movement:

Start Position:

Feet shoulder width apart with toes pointed slightly out. Feet should be flat on the ground.

Back arched or flat with bar directly over the instep of your foot.

Hips higher than the knees

Shoulders and knees out over or past the bar.

Hands roughly shoulder width with elbows turned out and wrists slightly flexed.

Head should be neutral, focusing on a point straight ahead.

1st Pull
- Maintaining neutral or arched back, the bar is raised by extending the knees, allowing the knees to come behind the bar.
- The shoulders remain over the bar, with elbows turned out and wrists remaining slightly flexed.

2nd Knee Bend
- This occurs between knee and mid thigh, with a re-bending of the knees (this is the second knee bend of the double knee bend) creating a mild "unloading" effect.
- The body is basically re-aligned to position itself for greater vertical force production.
- The bar is pulled to roughly mid thigh.

2nd Pull
- The hips are powerfully extended
- The feet are plantar flexed pushing the toes and balls of the feet into the ground.
- The shoulders are shrugged toward the ears
- Elbows are still rotated outward with wrists trying to hold flexed position.

The Catch
- The body drops under the bar into front squat or partial knee bend front squat position while maintaining a neutral/lordotic posture
- Elbows are high with bar wresting across clavicles
- Feet flat on the ground.
- Eyes looking straight ahead with head neutral.

Variations:
1. "Hang" refers to variations in start ranging from below the knee, above the knee, mid thigh, etc..
2. Power Clean refers to a catch that does not result in deep front squat, with the tops of the thighs above parallel. This exercise is more common in training and testing for sport as it reflects powerful pulling/triple extension rather than flexibility and front squat strength.
3. "From the blocks" refers to a start position directly off a measured box height.

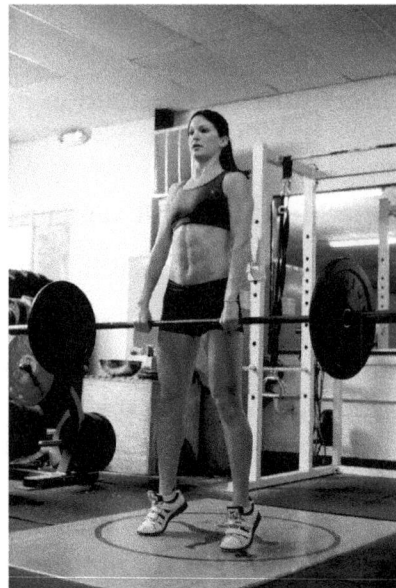

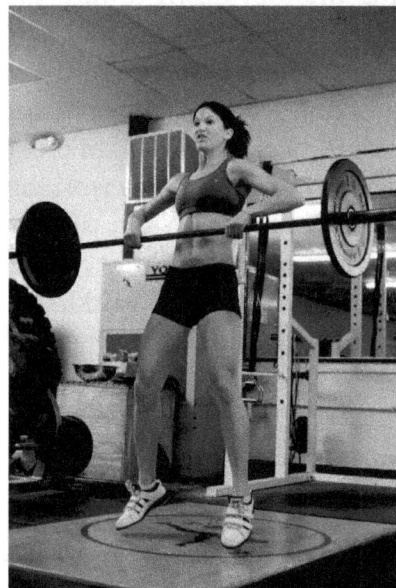

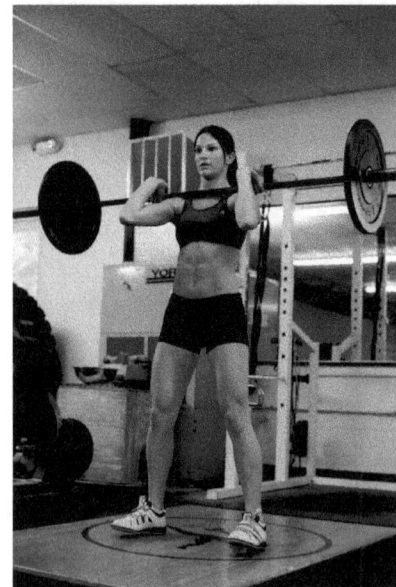

Pull-ups

Exercise Prerequisites: Use caution if you have elbow, shoulder, neck or low back pain.

Movement: Grasp a pull-up bar with hands pronated, shoulder width or slightly wider. Hang from the bar, with arms, hips and shoulders in extension. Begin the movement by retracting shoulder blades back and down. Begin pulling your body upward while continuing to pull the shoulder blades back and downward. Try not to allow the shoulders to internally rotate as you are pulling upward.

Pull upward, pinching your shoulder blades back until the upper portion of the chest comes in contact with the bar.

Lower the body slowly, retracing the same pattern until you reach the starting position at the bottom.

If you cannot perform a regular pull-up, you can use the assistance of a partner or a band around the knee or foot.

Keys to Movement:

1. Pronated grip with hands shoulder width or slightly wider.
2. Begin in a dead hang position.
3. Retract shoulders back and down during the movement.
4. Focus on pulling the elbows back and down.
5. Do not allow the shoulders to internally rotate,
6. Pull up until the upper part of the chest comes in contact with the bar.

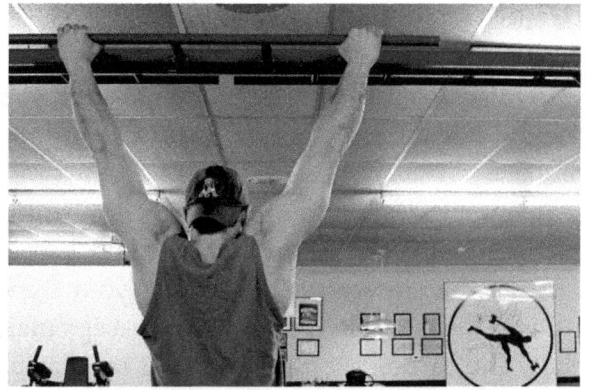

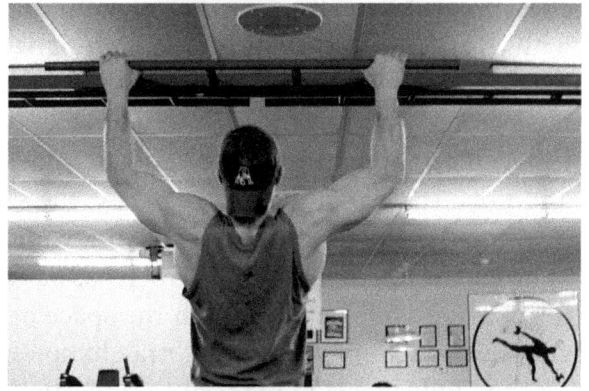

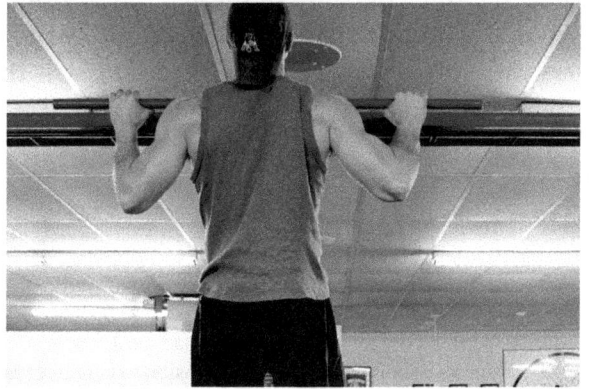

Push Jerk (or split jerk)

Exercise Prerequisites: Use caution if you have shoulder, elbow, wrist, neck, knee, or low back pain.

Movement: Stand with feet in hip width parallel stance or hip width staggered stance. Hold barbell with pronated grip (palms forward). Begin with your upper arms pointing downward/slightly forward with triceps making contact with lats. The barbell should rest across the clavicle area and upper chest musculature. Keeping the pelvis neutral, heels in contact with the floor, torso rigid, and eyes straight, explosively bend knees slightly. Immediately reverse direction, driving through the legs and hips to generate momentum.

Carry the momentum generated through the legs and hips and press the bar straight upward. At the same time you are pressing the bar upward, push the body under the bar by re-bending the knees. Once the barbell has passed the top of your head, bring your head through the space between your arms and the bar. Continue pressing straight upward, until you have reached full extension of the arms and shoulders. Try to bring your shoulders to ear height at the top of the movement. Once you reach top position, you should catch the bar in a knees bent position. Slowly lower back to start.

Keys to Movement:

1. Keep torso upright throughout the entire movement.
2. Hold barbell in pronated grip.
3. Triceps in contact with lats in the start position.
4. Quick knee bend, followed by extension to generate momentum from the legs and hips.
5. Bring your head through once the barbell has passed the top of your head.
6. Do not allow your back to arch as you press overhead.
7. "Active" shoulders at the top.
8. Push yourself under the bar, catching the bar in a knees bent position.

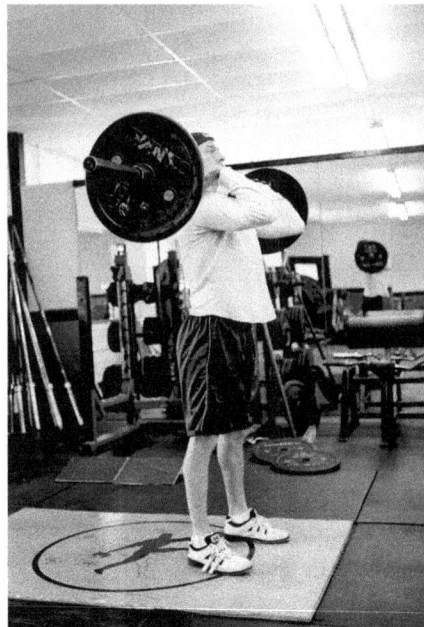

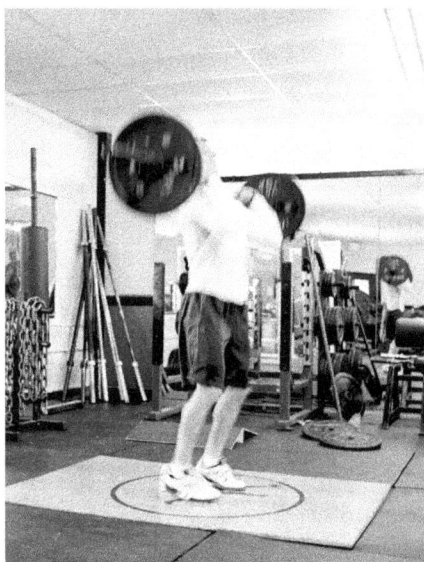

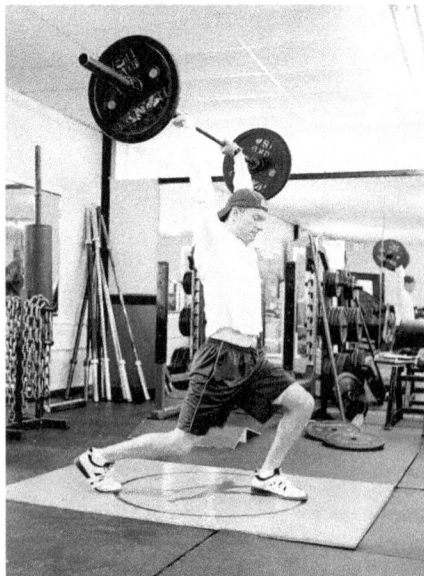

Push Press

Exercise Prerequisites: Use caution if you have elbow, shoulder, wrist, neck, knee, or low back pain.

Movement: Stand with feet in hip width parallel or staggered stance. Hold a barbell across your upper chest clavicle area with pronated grip (palms forward). Begin with your upper arms pointing downward/slightly forward with your triceps making contact with lats. Keeping the pelvis neutral, heels in contact with the floor, torso rigid, and eyes straight, explosively dip down by bending the knees, then immediately reverse direction, driving through the legs and hips to generate momentum.

With the momentum generated the legs and hips, press the bar straight upward. Once the barbell has passed the top of your head, bring your head through the space between your arms (make sure not to hit your head with the bar). Continue pressing straight upward, until you have reached full extension of the arms and shoulders. Try to bring your shoulders to ear height at the top of the movement by reaching upward.

Keys to Movement:

1. Keep torso upright throughout entire movement.
2. Hold barbell in pronated grip.
3. Triceps in contact with lats at the start of the movement.
4. Quick knee bend, followed by extension to generate momentum from the legs and hips.
5. Bring your head through the space between your arms once the barbell has passed the top of your head.
6. Try not to allow your back to arch too far backward as you press overhead.
7. Active shoulders at the top.

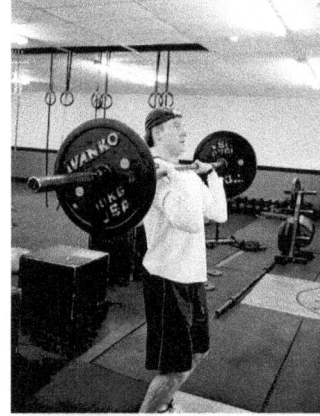

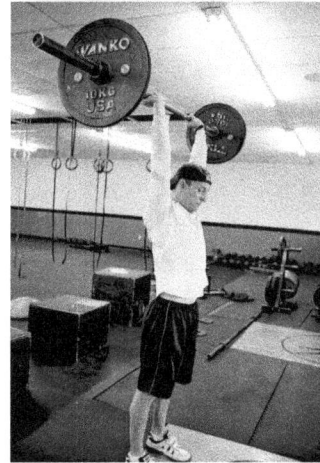

Rack Pull

Exercise Prerequisites: Use caution if you have neck, knee, or low back pain.

Movement: Pronated grip may be preferred for higher repetitions while mixed grip may be preferred for lower reps. Position a barbell across safety pins at roughly knee, upper shin, or other pre-determined height. Walk your legs/shins to the bar and arch your back with chest out, shoulder pulled back and eyes looking forward. Keeping the angle of the torso relative to the floor roughly the same, lean over and bend at the knees to grasp the bar. Keeping the heels on the ground begin by extending the legs and torso at the same time, ensuring not to raise the hips first.

As you extend, focus on pulling the bar toward you so that then bar makes contact with the thigh. Once you have reached complete extension of the hips and knees, retrace the movement pattern during the eccentric part of the movement.

Keys to movement:

1. Proper start position is important.
2. Bar in contact with shins or one inch away in starting position.
3. Back arched with heels maintain contact with the ground.
4. Mixed grip for low reps and pronated grip for higher reps.
5. Try not to raise the hips first.
6. At the top of the movement, be careful of hyperextending if you have low back or neck issues.
7. Some athletes may prefer to look upward during the pull as this may aid in the final lock out.

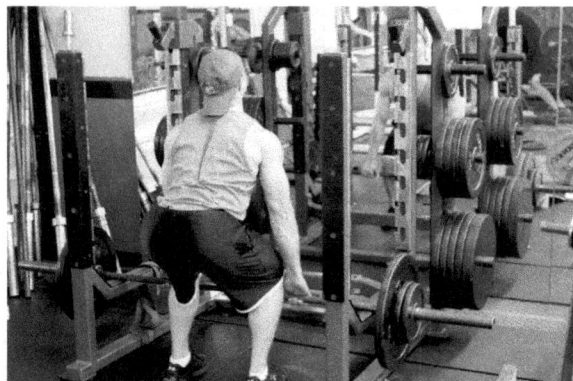

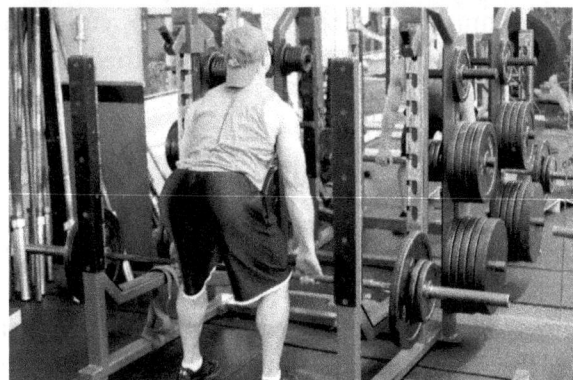

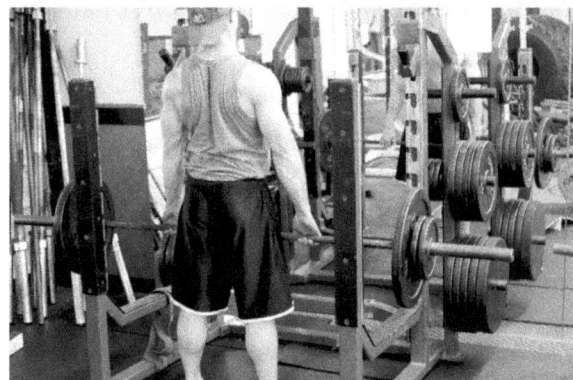

Reverse Hyperextension

Exercise Prerequisites: Use caution if you have low back or neck pain.

Movement: Lay face down on a reverse hyperextension machine. Begin with feet down toward the floor and legs straight. Initiating the movement from the glutes and hamstrings, pull your feet upward toward the ceiling. Extend upward until your legs are parallel to the floor or your low back begins to fatigue or loses posture. Contract your glutes at the top of the movement and lower slowly and perform again.

Keys to Movement:

1. Keep hips flat on the pad. Try not to allow rotation at the pelvis.
2. Keep legs straight and initiate movement from the glutes and hamstrings.
3. Extend hip to the point where legs are parallel to the floor or low back begins to fatigue or feels pain.
4. Contract glutes at the top.

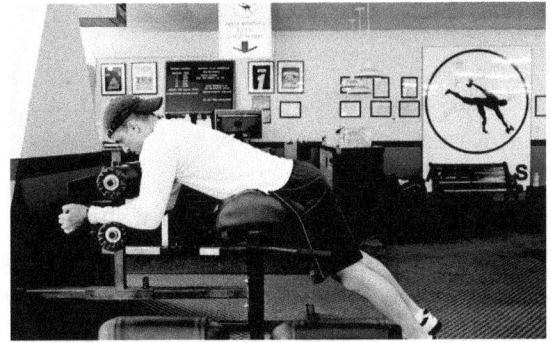

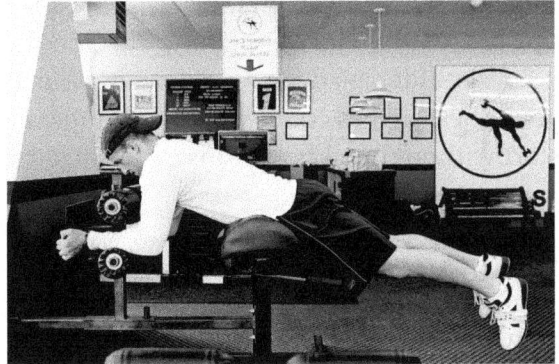

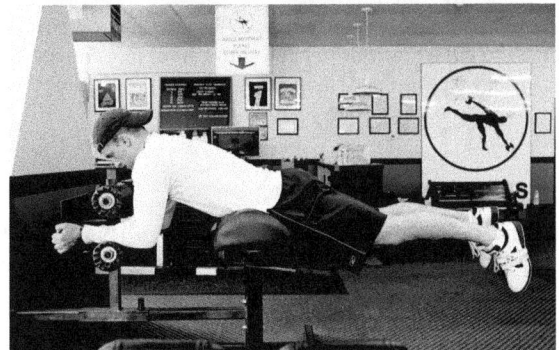

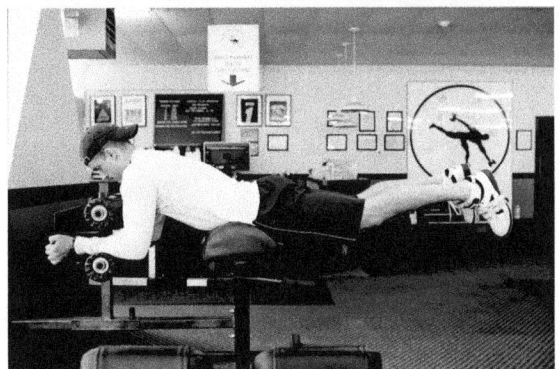

Ring Inverted Row

Exercise Prerequisites: Use caution if you have low back, elbow, neck, or shoulder pain.

Movement: With hands roughly shoulder width apart, grasp a set of low rings with pronated or neutral grip. Lay backward with your heels resting on the floor or on a box. Extend your hips and push your chest out so body is in neutral/slightly lordotic posture. Maintaining this posture, pull your chest upward to the rings, initiating the movement by retracting your shoulder blades while driving your elbows back. Once your chest makes contact with the rings, slowly lower back to start without breaking posture.

Keys to Movement:

1. Grasp the rings with pronated or neutral grip, hands shoulder width or slightly wider.
2. Extend hips and keep back in lordotic/neutral posture.
3. Do not allow hips to bend throughout movement.
4. Retract shoulder blades and pull chest to the rings.
5. Lower back to start position.

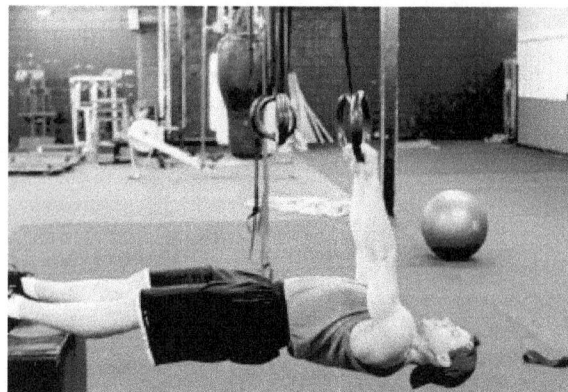

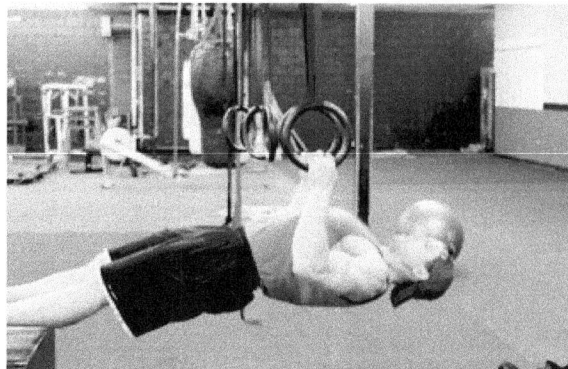

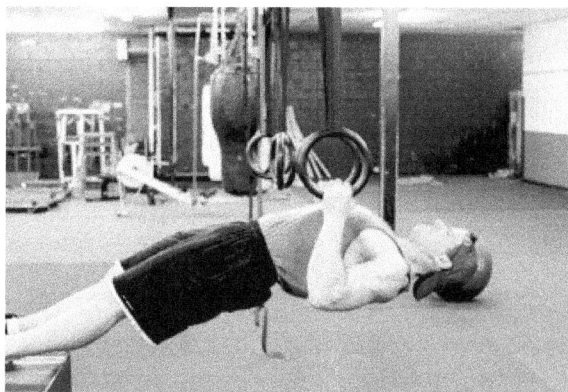

Ring Pushups

Exercise Prerequisites: Use caution if you have shoulder, low back, neck, elbow, wrist, or knee problems.

Movement: Assume correct pushup position with hand on rings and feet hip width or closer. Start with your hands directly below your shoulders with palms facing each other in neutral grip. Squeeze the glutes and try to create intra-abdominal pressure to stabilize the pelvis and spine. Maintaining neutral posture, slowly lower until your chest is parallel to your hands (or lower if you have good shoulder health and mobility). To minimize shoulder problems, try to keep your elbows at 45 degrees or less relative to your torso. Make sure to keep your head looking down and your hips locked. Push up back to start position, keeping neutral posture.

Keys to Movement:

1. Body is rigid with glutes squeezed and head looking down.
2. Keep your elbows at 45 degrees or less relative to the torso.
3. Lower until your hands are roughly parallel to your chest, or as low as your flexibility allows.
4. Try not to allow your hips to dip downward during the movement.

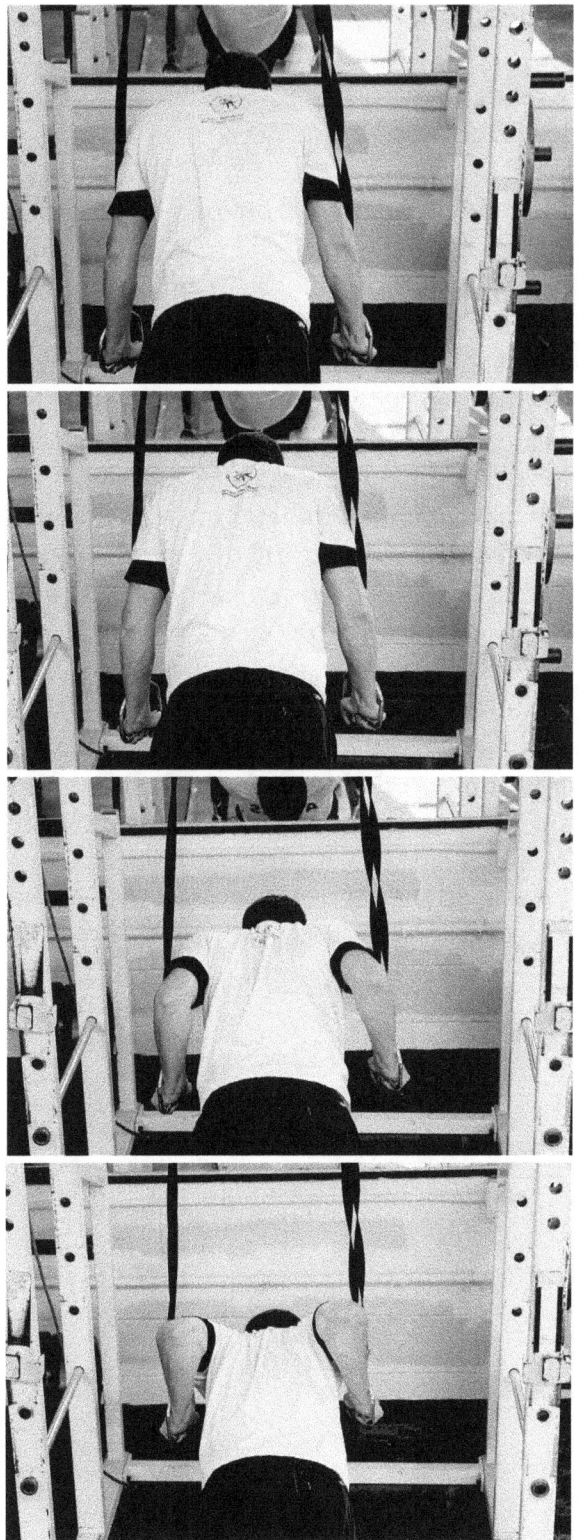

Romanian Deadlift

Exercise Prerequisites: Use caution if you have knee, neck, or low back pain.

Movement: Stand in front of a barbell with your feet parallel and roughly shoulder width apart. Position your torso into a lordotic posture, with chest out, shoulder pulled back, eyes looking ahead, and knees bent to roughly 20 degrees. Your hips should be higher than your knees in the start position. Try to keep the weight distributed over the rear of your feet. Lean over by bending at the hips only, trying to keep the knees locked at the starting angle.

The upward pull is initiated through the glutes and hamstrings. As Olympic weightlifting coach and mentor, Denis Reno states "think big butt" to ensure the powerful glutes are firing during extension of the hip. Extend the hips and bring the bar back up to the start position until the torso is erect with a high chest posture. In the top position, the knees do not extend, rather maintaining the initial start angle throughout. Once at the top position, slowly lower the barbell focusing on maintaining the exact same knee flexion angle and back arch. Lower to the point where your hamstrings are feeling a good stretch. The knee bend should remain the same throughout the movement. Stop if you are feeling low back tightness.

Keys to Movement:

1. Knees bent roughly 20 degrees with feet hip width apart.
2. Back arched with weight shifted toward the heels.
3. Bend at the hips only, keeping knees locked at roughly 20 degree angle.
4. Think "big butt" when you are driving upward.
5. Lower to point in which you can longer maintain spinal posture.

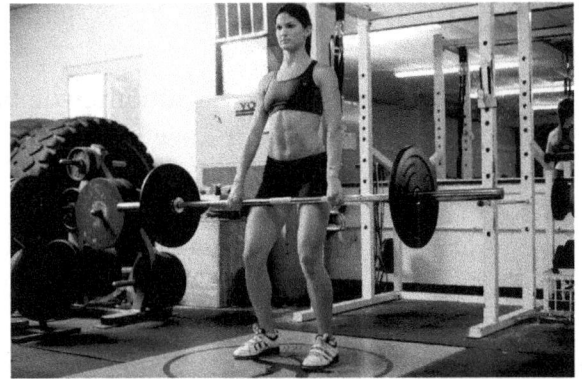

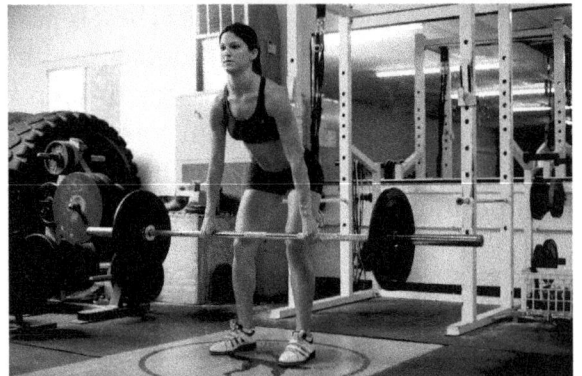

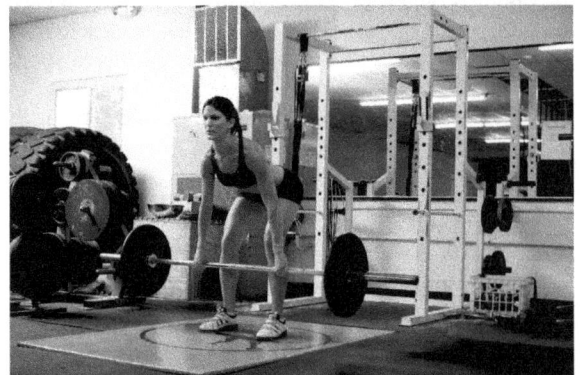

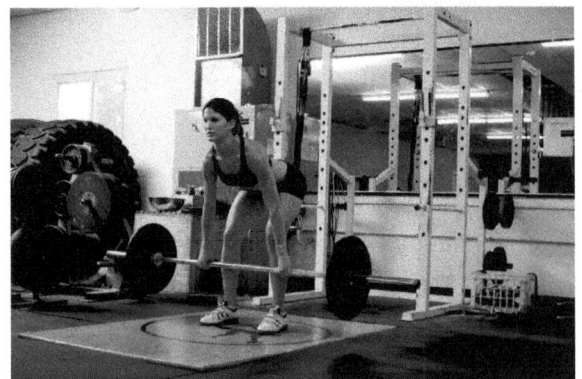

Rotational Low Back Extension

Exercise Prerequisites: Use caution if you have neck, knee, or low back pain.

Movement: Set up on either 45 degree or conventional back extension machine, with the Achilles tendons pressed firmly against the foot pad. With your forearms crossed or hands at your ears, assume a lordotic/neutral posture and begin lowering your torso by bending at the hips. At the same time, begin rotating opposite elbow downward toward your opposite knee maintaining back posture. At the bottom, the upper body should be rotated with the opposite side elbow across the body. The ascent begins with hip extension and unwinding of the torso. Extend until the body is back to the neutral starting position. Perform reps on one side, rest, then perform reps for the opposite side.

To add resistance to this exercise, use a dowel stick across the upper back with light weight loaded on one side only. Once you progress past the dowel, move onto light barbells and eventually proceed to Olympic barbell. A dumbbell can also be used to enhance the effect of this exercise. As you rotate downward, reach toward the ground below the opposite side knee. During the concentric motion, perform a dumbbell row at the same time, ending up in isometric row contraction with your torso parallel to the floor at the top.

Keys to Movement:

1. Position body in correct start position on conventional back extension machine.
2. Lower down, rotating opposite elbow toward opposite side knee.
3. At the bottom, the upper body should be rotated with opposite side elbow across the body.
4. Raise up by uncoiling and extending at the same time until you reach neutral starting position. Try not to hyperextend.

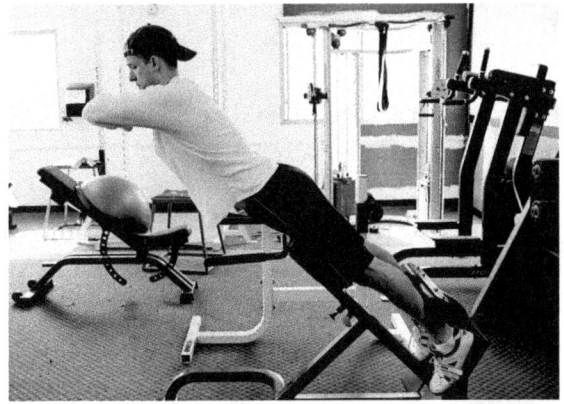

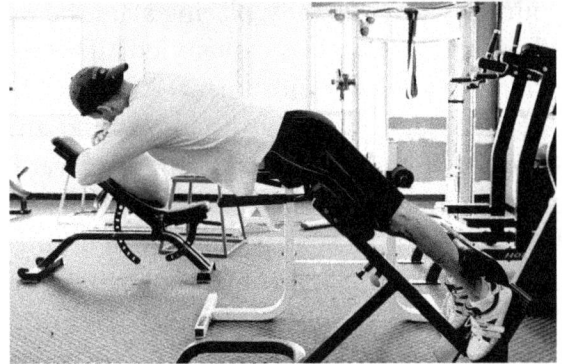

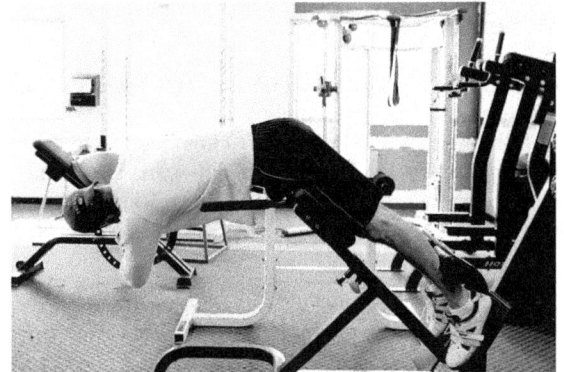

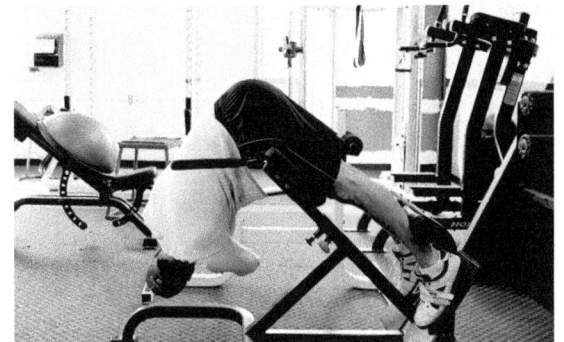

Rotational Plank

Exercise Prerequisites: Use caution if you have low back, neck, or shoulder pain

Movement: This exercise learned from spine and low back expert Dr. Stu McGill. Assume a plank position with your forearms parallel to each other (and perpendicular to the body) and feet spread wider than the hips. Keeping the body locked, with neutral spine, begin the movement by sliding your left elbow laterally, placing all of the weight on your right elbow and feet. Make sure your left hip does not move or rotate prior to the elbow movement. After you have slid the elbow laterally, begin rotating the hips, torso and feet at the same time. Drive the left elbow up and backward as you rotate. You should end up in a position similar to a side plank. Rotate the body back to the start position with both elbows on the floor and perform the same movement pattern on the opposite side.

Movement Mechanics:

1. Assume a plank position, but with forearms parallel to each other and perpendicular to the body.
2. Shift weight to one forearm without moving hip.
3. Rotate all the way until hip and shoulder are parallel to a wall.
4. Lower back to start position and perform on other side.

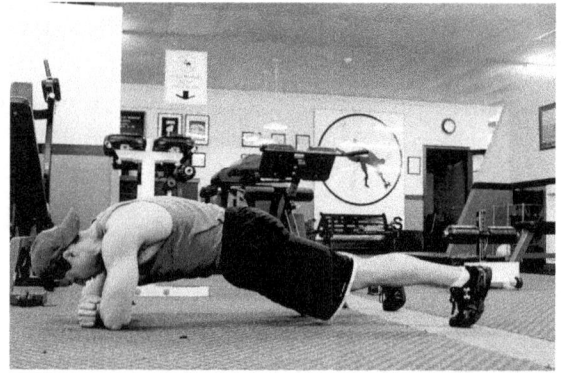

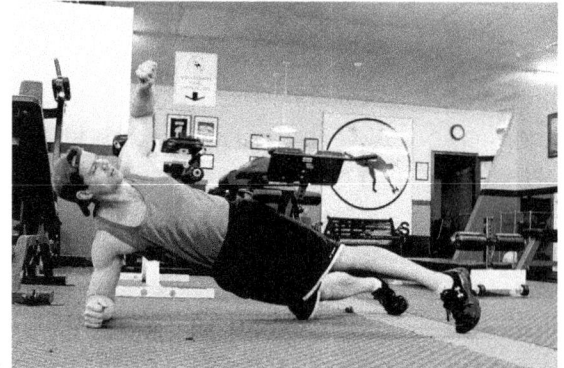

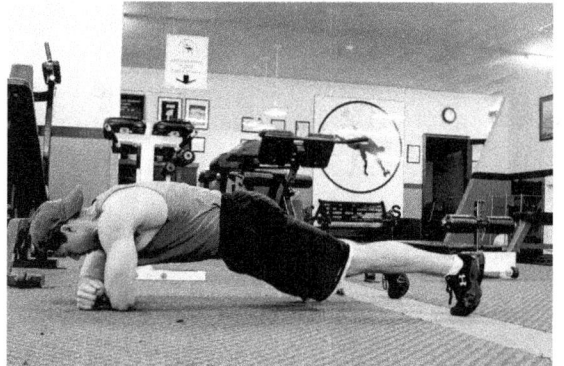

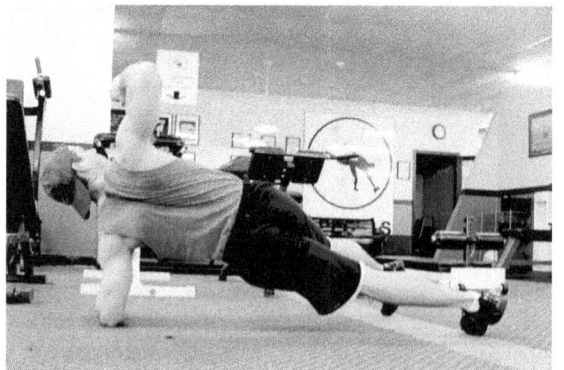

Seated Cable Row

Exercise Prerequisites: Use caution if you have neck, low back, shoulder, elbow, or wrist problems.

Movement: Sit on a seated cable row machine holding the cable handle in front of the body. With a slight bend in the knees arch your back into a lordotic/neutral posture, with your chest out, shoulders pulled back and down, and eyes straight ahead. Ensure that your shoulders/torso remains directly over the hips as there is a tendency to lean back during the rowing movement.
Pull the weight toward your sternum/belly button, activating the rear delt muscles, rhomboid and lat muscles. Try to focus on retracting your shoulder blades back and down during the movement. Try not to allow the shoulders to shrug upward as this may take away from the contraction of the mid back/ shoulder retractor muscles. Also try not to bounce or round the back during the movement. Slowly lower the weight back to start and perform next repetition.

Movement Mechanics:

1. Position body in correct starting position with slight bend at the knees, chest out, back arched, and shoulders directly over hips.
2. Initiate movement by retracting shoulders back and down while keeping the shoulders directly over hips.
3. Focus on pulling elbows back.
4. Try not to allow the shoulders to shrug upward or torso to lean backward.
5. Row until maximal contraction of shoulder blades.

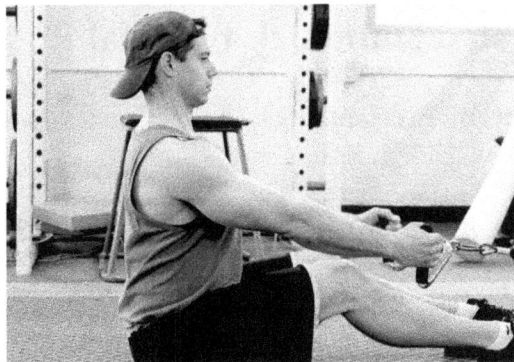

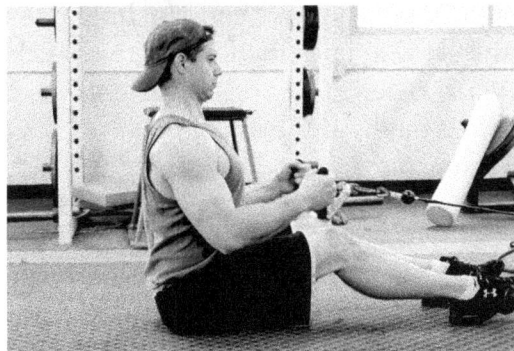

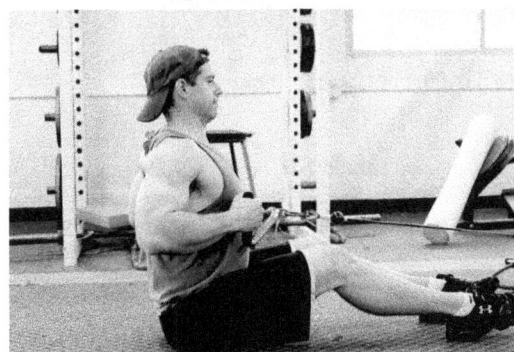

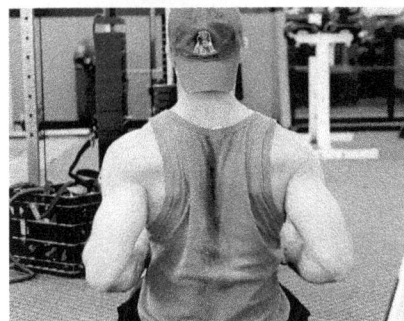

Seated Dumbbell External Rotator

Exercise Prerequisites: Use caution if you have neck, shoulder or low back pain.

Movement: This exercise, taught to me by Charles Poliquin and his Poliquin Institute staff, is an excellent exercise for increasing rotator cuff strength and shoulder stability. Sit on a bench with one foot on the bench and the other foot on the floor with both knees bent. Holding a dumbbell in the hand on the same side as the foot on the bench, place your elbow on your knee. Focus on keeping a 90 degree angle at the elbow throughout the entire movement. Lower the dumbbell down toward the inside of your thigh by internally rotating at the shoulder. Once you have reached full range of motion, externally rotate upward back to start position, keeping the angle at the elbow at roughly 90 degrees. Ensure that you keep the elbow in contact with knee throughout the movement.

Keys to Movement:

1. Keep torso upright throughout entire movement.
2. Ideally, you should have a 90 degree angle at the hips when positioning for the exercise.
3. Same side elbow on top of the knee that is on the bench.
4. Keep elbow in contact with knee throughout the movement.
5. Maintain 90 degree angle at the elbow throughout movement.

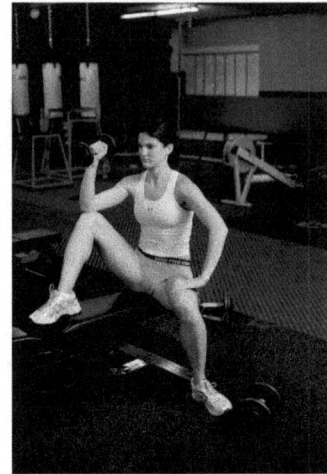

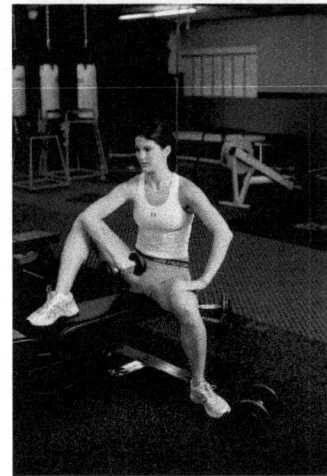

Single Arm Trap-3 Lift

Exercise Prerequisites: Use caution if you have neck, shoulder or low back pain.

Movement: Another excellent shoulder stabilizing exercise taught by Charles Poliquin and his staff at the Poliquin Institute. Hold a dumbbell in one hand with thumb pointing upward. Your other arm should rest with your forearm across a stable object and your torso at roughly a 45 degree angle. Rest your forehead on the forearm. Position your feet in a staggered stance, with foot on the same as the hand holding the dumbbell positioned behind. Maintaining a neutral or slightly arched posture, extend the arm holding the dumbbell downward until it is perpendicular to the floor. Retract the shoulder blade of that arm and raise your extended left arm at a 45 degree angle away from the head until the elbow passes the ear. Once the elbow passes the ear, reach outward and lower back to start.

Keys to Movement:

1. Torso is at roughly a 45 degree angle to the floor with forearm resting against a brace.
2. Feet staggered with foot on the side of the hand holding the dumbbell in back.
3. Retract shoulder blade keeping arm straight to start the movement.
4. Raise straight arm at 45 degree angle from the head until the elbow passes the ear.
5. Reach away as you lower.

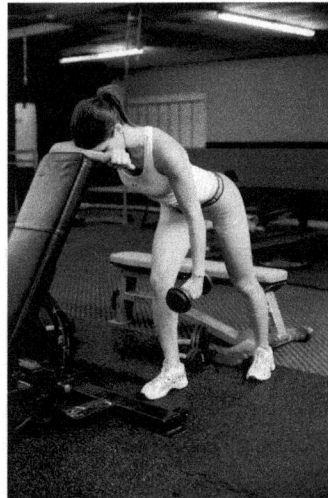

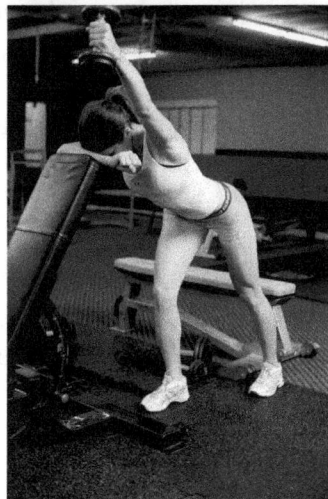

Side Bridge

Exercise Prerequisites: Use caution if you have knee, shoulder, neck, or low back pain.

Movement: As back problems can be common in school aged athletes, lateral strengthening of the quadratus lumborum and oblique musculature can aid in creating a healthy low back. Compressive loading resistance exercises including squats and deadlifts could potentially exacerbate any asymmetrical imbalances of the low back musculature if gone uncorrected. Conventional low back extension variations may not fix the imbalance as the overactive musculature may be preferentially recruited. The side lying bridge, a favorite of world renowned low back specialist Dr. Stuart McGill, puts emphasis on the oblique and Quadratus Lumborum musculature. This is practical for repairing and maintaining optimal low back health in athletes with muscular imbalances.

Lie on your side with your hand or elbow on a padded surface. With your legs and feet stacked, lift your hips off the ground, maintaining contact with the ground on your elbow/hand and feet only. Make sure to keep the hips completely extended and glutes contracted.

Keys to Movement:

1. Lie on your side with hand or elbow on padded surface.
2. With legs and feet stacked, raise your hips straight upward.
3. Try not to allow your top hip to rotate backward.

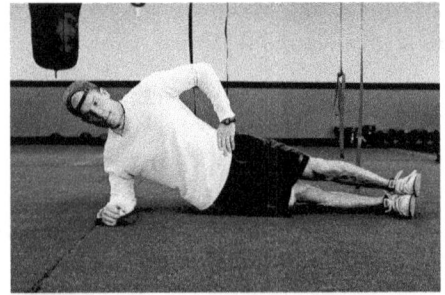

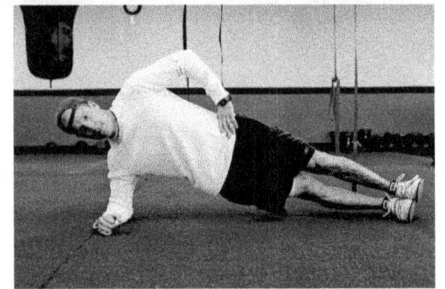

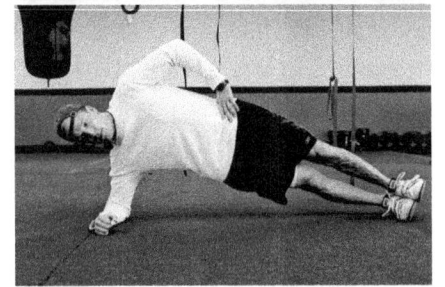

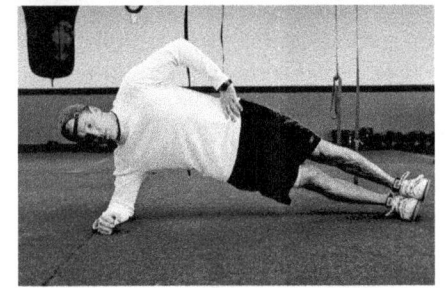

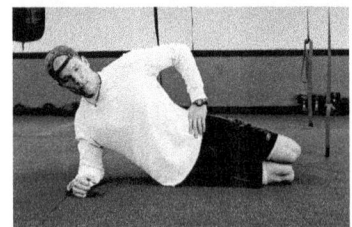

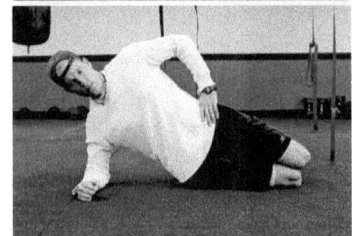

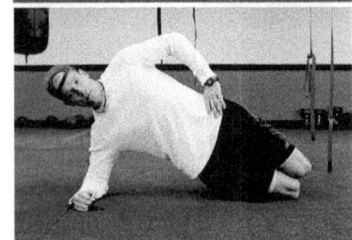

Snatch Variations

Exercise Prerequisites: Use caution if you have elbow, shoulder, wrist, neck, knee, or low back pain.

Movement:

Start Position:

Feet shoulder width apart with toes pointed slightly out. Feet should be flat on the ground.

Back arched or flat with bar directly over the instep of your foot.

Shoulders and knees out over or past the bar.

Hands out wide with elbows turned upward and hook grip on bar.

Head should be neutral, focusing on a point straight ahead.

1st Pull
- Maintaining neutral or arched back, the bar is raised by extending the knees, allowing the knees to come behind the bar.
- The shoulders remain over the bar.

2nd Knee Bend
- This occurs between knee and mid thigh, with a re-bending of the knees (this is the second knee bend of the double knee bend) creating a mild "unloading" effect.
- The body is basically re-aligned to position itself for greater vertical force production.
- The bar is pulled between mid and upper thigh

2nd Pull
- The hips are powerfully extended, with the bar making contact with upper thigh or hips
- The feet are plantar flexed pushing the toes and balls of the feet into the ground.
- The shoulders are shrugged toward the ears

The Catch
- The body drops under the bar into overhead squat or partial knee bend (power) overhead squat position while maintaining a neutral/lordotic posture
- Arms are locked out with active shoulders
- Feet flat on the ground.
- Eyes looking straight ahead with head neutral.

Variations:
1. "Hang" refers to variations in start ranging from below the knee, above the knee, mid thigh, etc..
2. Power Snatch refers to a catch that does not result in deep overhead squat, with the tops of the thighs above parallel. This exercise is more common in training and testing for sport as it reflects powerful pulling/triple extension rather than flexibility and front squat strength.
3. "From the blocks" refers to a start position directly off a measured box height.

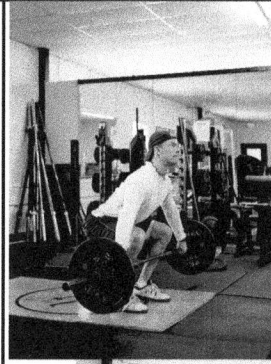

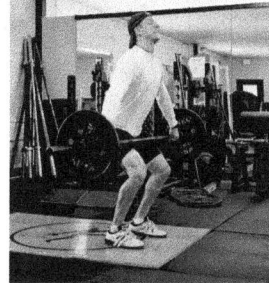

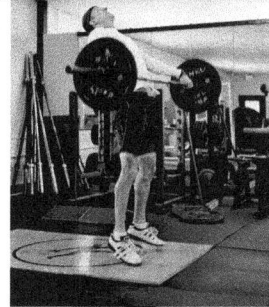

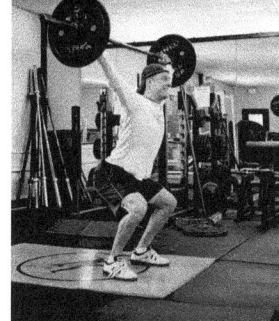

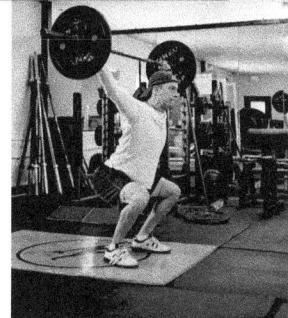

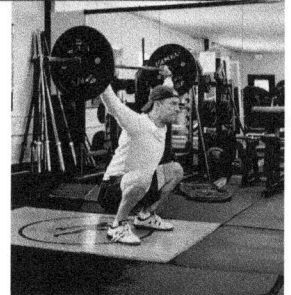

Split Squat Jumps

Exercise Prerequisites: Use caution if you have knee, ankle, or low back problems.

Movement: Position your body into bottom part of a lunge. Maintain torso upright with knees and feet pointing straight ahead. Drive straight up as high as you can off both legs, initiating movement from lead leg hip extensor musculature. Once you have reached peak jump height, scissor kick your legs and land softly with the opposite leg in front. Dip back down in to the lunge and jump again, emphasizing the lead leg hip extensors. Try to minimize ground contact time.

Keys to Movement:

1. Position legs into correct lunge position with torso upright.
2. Feet and knees pointing straight ahead.
3. Focus on driving through the lead leg hip extensors.
4. Keep hips square. Do not allow them to rotate throughout the movement.
5. Minimal ground contact time between jumps.

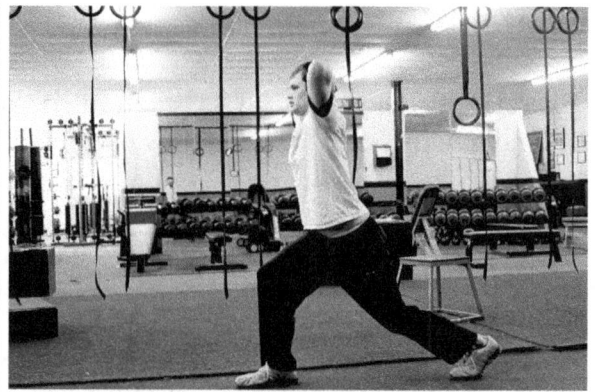

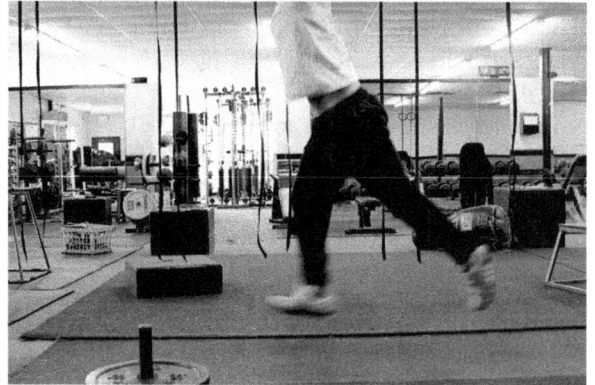

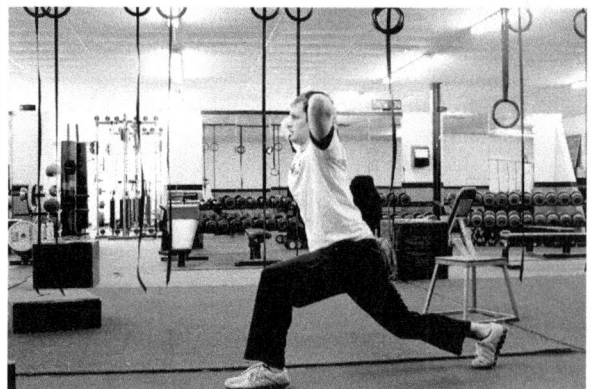

Standing Barbell Overhead Press

Exercise Prerequisites: Use caution if you have neck, knee, elbow, wrist, or low back pain.

Movement: Stand with feet parallel hip width or staggered stance. Hold barbell with pronated grip (palms forward) resting across upper chest/clavicle area. Begin with your upper arms pointing downward/slightly forward with triceps making contact with lats. Keeping the pelvis neutral, heels in contact with the floor, and eyes straight, begin pressing the bar straight overhead. Once the barbell has passed the top of your head, bring your head through the space between your arms (make sure not to hit your head with the bar). Continue pressing straight upward, until you have reached full extension of the arms and shoulders. Once you reach top position, slowly lower back to start.

Keys to Movement:

1. Keep torso upright throughout entire movement.
2. Do not allow heels to come off the ground.
3. Hold barbell in pronated grip.
4. Triceps in contact with lats at the beginning of the movement.
5. Bring your head through once the barbell has passed the top of your head.
6. Do not allow your back to hyperextend as you press overhead.
7. "Active" shoulders at the top.

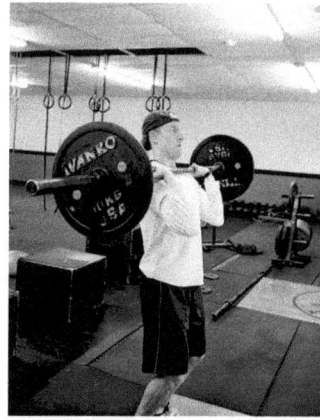

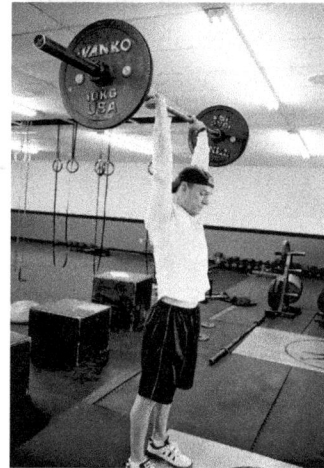

Standing Cable External Rotator

Exercise Prerequisites: Use caution if you have neck, shoulder, elbow, or low back pain.

Movement: Stand next to a cable column with your upper arm down by your side and elbow bent roughly 90 degrees. Make sure the elbow is kept directly below the shoulder throughout the movement. If it is allowed to abduct or adduct, the recruitment of the external rotator musculature may be altered. Keeping the upper arm locked in place, begin externally rotating the humerus trying to maintain the 90 degree angle at the elbow. The forearm is kept parallel to the floor throughout the movement. Rotate as far as your muscles/flexibility allows or until you break technique or elbow angle.

Keys to Movement:

1. Keep torso upright throughout entire movement.
2. Elbow is directly below the shoulder.
3. Maintain 90 degree angle at the elbow throughout the movement.

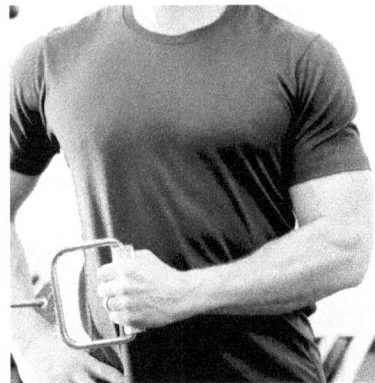

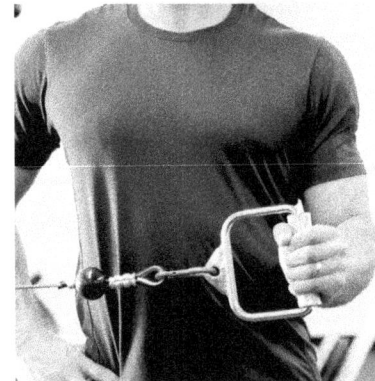

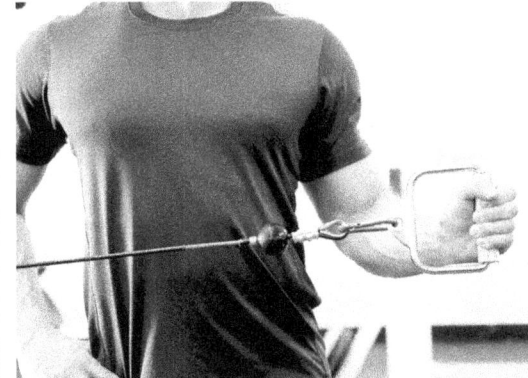

Standing Dumbbell Overhead Press

Exercise Prerequisites: Use caution if you have neck, knee, elbow, wrist, or low back pain.

Movement: Stand with feet parallel hip width or staggered stance. Hold the dumbbells with neutral or pronated grip (palms forward) slightly in front of or on the anterior delts. Begin with your upper arms pointing downward/slightly forward with triceps making contact with lats. Keeping the pelvis neutral, heels in contact with the floor, and eyes straight, begin pressing the dumbbells straight overhead. Once the dumbbells have passed the top of your head, bring your head through the space between your arms (make sure not to hit your head with the bar). Continue pressing straight upward, until you have reached full extension of the arms and shoulders. Once you reach top position, slowly lower back to start.

Keys to Movement:

1.   Keep torso upright throughout entire movement.
2.   Do not allow heels to come off the ground.
3.   Hold dumbbells in neutral or pronated grip throughout movement.
4.   Triceps in contact with lats at the beginning of the movement.
5.   Tuck your chin once the dumbbells have passed the top of your head.
6.   Do not allow your back to hyperextend as you press overhead.
7.   "Active" shoulders at the top.

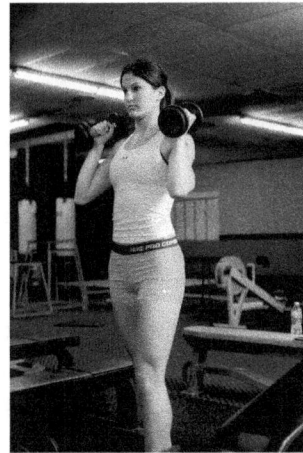

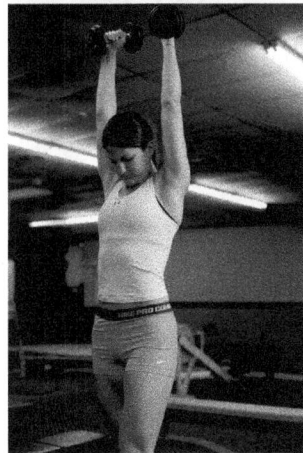

Standing Face Pull

Exercise Prerequisites: Use caution if you have elbow, shoulder, neck, wrist, or low back pain.

Movement: Adjust a cable column to roughly shoulder/chin height. Attach a triceps rope to the cable. Stand further than arm's length from the column with feet staggered. Grasp rope with pronated grip, arms extended and thumbs pointing toward the cable column. With arms parallel to the floor, begin by retracting the shoulder blades first. Initiate pull by pulling the elbows back and upward. Ensure that the elbows are higher than the hands throughout the movement. Pull back until your elbows are parallel to or behind your ears. Coach Charles Poliquin has an excellent exercise tutorial of this on his website www.charlespoliquin.com .

Keys to Movement:

1. Stand with feet staggered facing cable column.
2. Pronated grip on rope with thumbs forward.
3. Retract shoulder blades back first then pull elbows backward.
4. Try to keep your elbows higher you're your hands.
5. Keep elbows above ear height when pulling back.
6. Pull back until elbows are parallel to or behind ears.

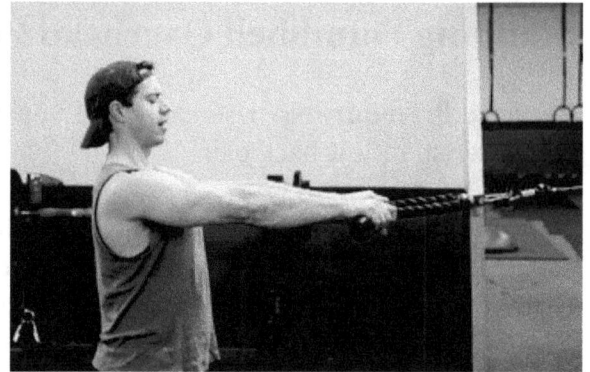

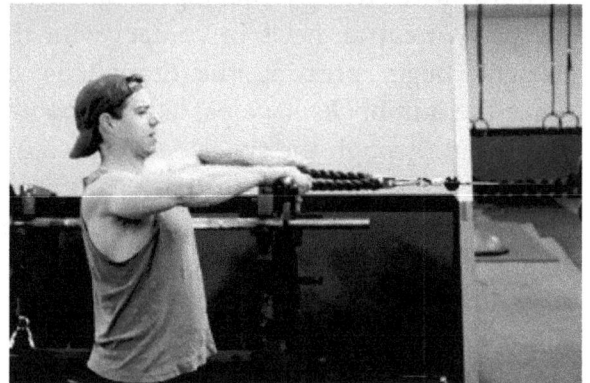

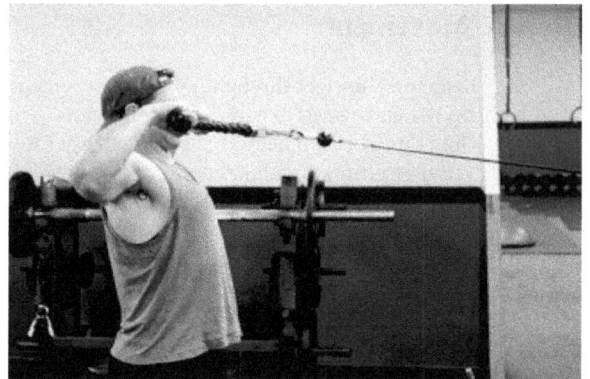

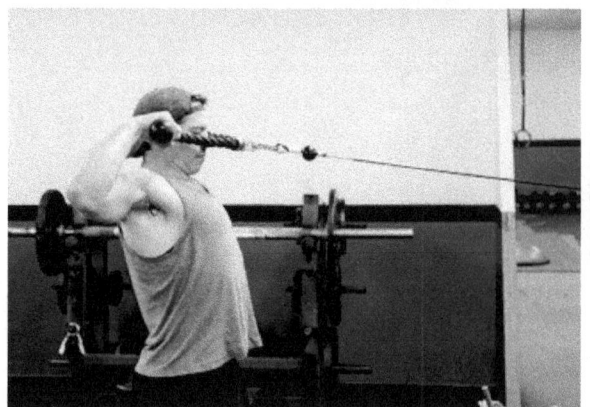

Step Forward Lunges

Exercise Prerequisites: Use caution if you have neck, knee, or low back pain.

Antagonistic Muscles to movement: Hamstrings as flexors of the knee.

Movement: Stand with your feet hip width apart, torso in neutral/slightly lordotic posture, with dumbbells held at your sides or barbell across the shoulders. Maintain upright posture throughout movement. With toes pointing straight ahead, take a large step forward. Lower the hips forward and downward maintaining upright posture with no minimal lean in the torso. Keeping the back leg as straight as possible, descend until the front leg hamstring comes in contact with the calf. Try not to lean forward or allow the front foot heel to come off the ground throughout the movement. As the hamstring comes in the contact with the calf, the knee may cross the toe plane. If the knees are healthy, this can help to strengthen the knee. Once you have lunged as deep as your flexibility/strength allows, initiate the return to start through the ball of the front foot. Perform all reps on one leg then perform on the opposite leg.

Keys to Movement:

1. Maintain upright posture throughout the movement.
2. Take a large step forward keeping the front heel in contact with the ground.
3. Focus on keeping the back leg as straight as possible to ensure maximal tension on front leg and stretching of back leg hip flexors.
4. Lower down until hamstring comes in contact with calf.
5. Begin the ascent by focusing on driving the shoulders/torso back and upward.
6. Do not allow the front heel to come off during the movement.
7. Try not to allow torso to lean over during the movement.

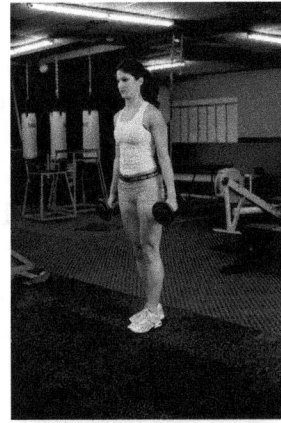

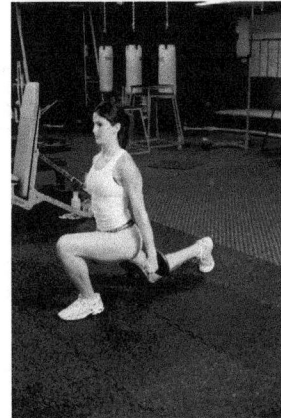

Suitcase Carries

Exercise Prerequisites: Use caution if you have knee, shoulder, neck, elbow, or low back pain.

Movement: Stand beside a dumbbell, barbell, kettlebell, or farmer carry implement. Lift the weight in one hand only, keeping the torso locked upright, and walk a pre-determined distance. After you have completed your predetermined distance, perform on the alternate side.

Keys to Movement:

1. Lift weight on one side of the body with proper deadlift technique.
2. Keep torso in rigid upright posture.
3. Walk pre-determined distance.

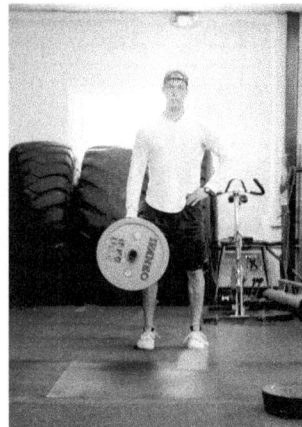

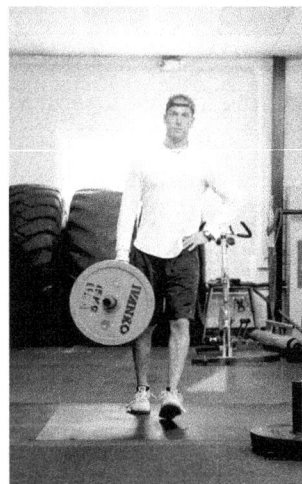

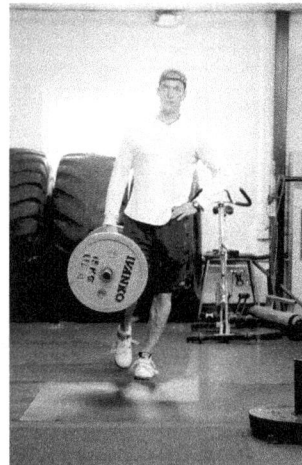

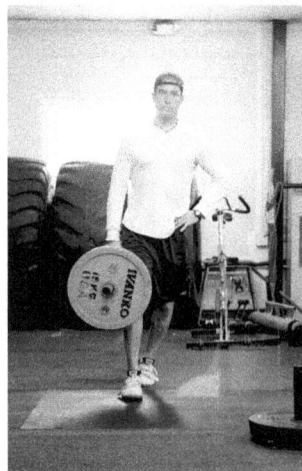

Swiss Ball Hamstring Curls

Exercise Prerequisites: Use caution if you have neck, knee, or low back pain.

Movement: Lie flat on your back on the floor with your heels hip width apart on the top of a Swiss ball. Put your hands down by your sides with arms straight. Begin by bridging the hips upward, maintaining shoulders in contact with the ground. Keeping a straight line between the shoulders, hips, and knees, curl your heels toward your glutes. The ball will roll toward your glutes as you do this. Once you have reached a comfortable flexion of the knees lower slowly back to start. To correct structural imbalances about the hamstrings, you can adjust foot positioning by pointing the toes inward, outward, or neutral. Another option is to plantar flex the foot to minimize gastroc assistance.

Keys to Movement:

1. Lie flat on your back on the floor with heels hip width apart on top of a Swiss ball.
2. Extend hips, bringing glutes off the ground.
3. Make sure you have a straight line between shoulders, hips, and knees throughout the entire movement.
4. Curl heels toward your glutes.
5. Adjusting foot positioning can aid in correcting structural imbalances about the hamstring musculature.

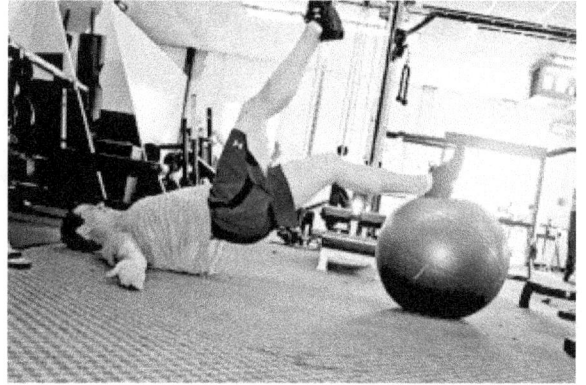

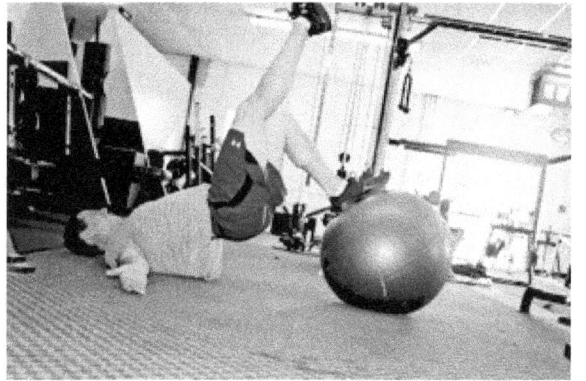

Swiss Ball Stir the Pot

Exercise Prerequisites: Use caution if you have knee, shoulder, elbow, neck, or low back pain.

Movement: Another exercise learned from low back and spine expert Dr. Stu McGill. Position your elbows on a Swiss ball with toes on the floor and body locked into a plank position. Contract your glutes and quads and begin "stirring the pot" or drawing out the letters of the alphabet with your elbows. Stop as soon as you feel stress or strain about the low back or once there is a breakdown in the quality of movement.

Keys to Movement:

1. With elbows directly below your shoulder on a Swiss ball, lock your body into rigid neutral plank position with glutes contracted.
2. Move elbows in "stirring the pot" fashion or draw letters of the alphabet with your elbows.

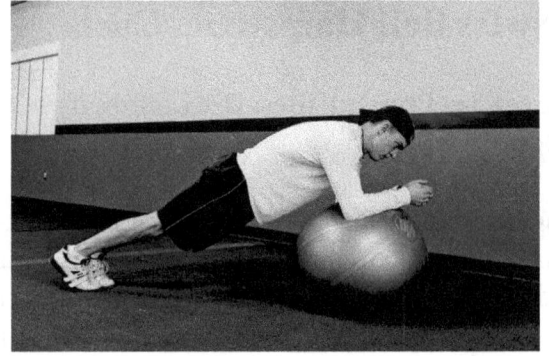

Two Arm Trap-3 Lift

Exercise Prerequisites: Use caution if you have neck, shoulder or low back pain.

Movement: Lie face down on a 45 degree incline bench with your chin resting on the top of the bench. Hold dumbbells in your hands with thumb pointing upward. Maintaining a neutral posture, extend your arms downward so they are perpendicular to the floor. To start the movement, retract the shoulder blades back and down. With scapular retraction, raise your extended arms at a 45 degree angle relative to the head until your elbows pass your ears. Once your elbows pass your ears, reach outward and lower back to start.

Keys to Movement:

1. Lie face down on a 45 degree incline bench.
2. Retract shoulder blades keeping arms straight.
3. Raise straight arms at 45 degree angles relative to the head until the elbows pass the ears.
4. Reach away as you lower.

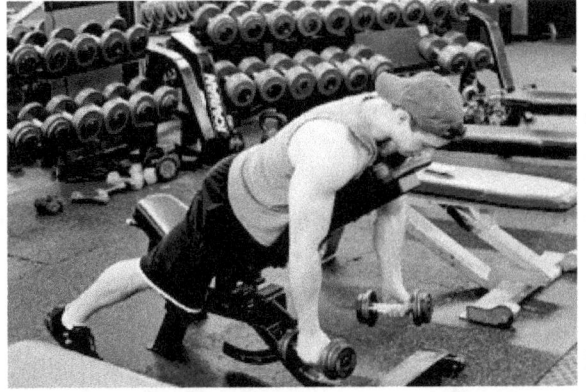

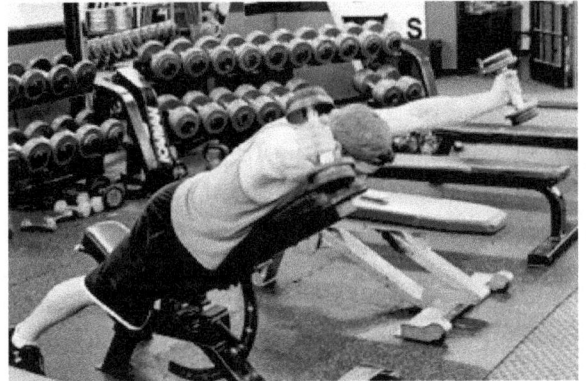

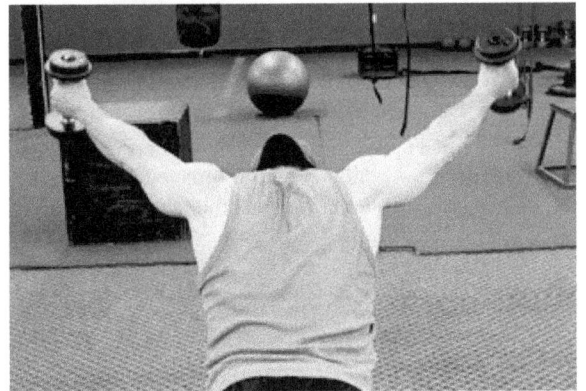

Walking Lunges

Exercise Prerequisites: Use caution if you have neck, knee, or low back pain.

Antagonistic Muscles to movement: Hamstrings as flexors of the knee.

Movement: Stand with feet hip width apart and torso upright. Hold dumbbells at your sides or a barbell across the back of your shoulders or in front squat position. Try to keep torso in upright posture throughout movement. With toes pointing straight ahead take a large step forward. Lower the hips forward and down toward the ground. Trying to keep the back leg as straight as possible, descend until the lunging leg hamstring comes in contact with the calf. It is important not to lean forward or allow the front foot heel to come off the ground during the lunge. Once you have lowered as far as your strength/flexibility allows, begin to extend the front leg knee and hip by driving through the heel, pulling your body back to the original start position. Lunge out on the other leg.

Keys to Movement:

1. Keep torso upright throughout entire movement.
2. Do not allow front foot heel to come off the ground.
3. Keep lunging knee pointing in the same direction as the toes.
4. If the knees are healthy, lunge down and forward until hamstring touches the calf.
5. Try to keep back leg as straight as possible during the lunge

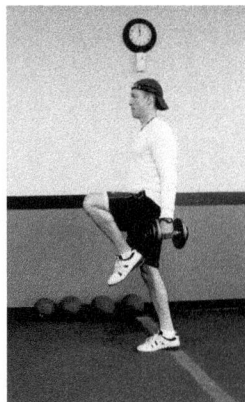

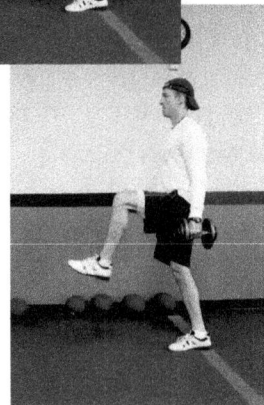

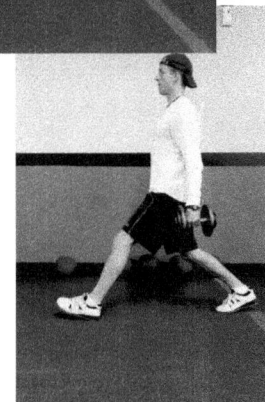

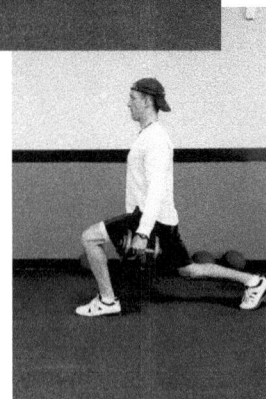

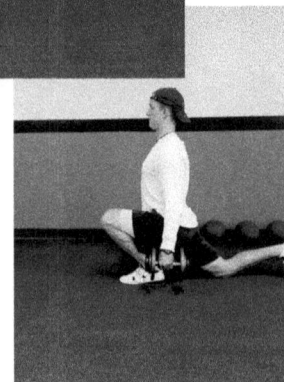

Wall Facing Squat

Exercise Prerequisites: Use caution if you have low back, knee, or neck pain.

Antagonistic Muscles to movement: Hamstrings as flexors of the knee.

Movement: Stand with your toes against a wall in a conventional squat starting position. Toes can point outward roughly 15-20 degrees if you prefer. With your hands on top of your head begin to squat allowing your knees to touch the wall. Squat as low as you can while maintaining weight on your heels and feet in contact the wall. Be careful not to fall backward. A spotter with their hand placed in the middle of your back can help in increasing range of motion while minimizing the risk of falling. Try to ensure that the knees point in the same direction as the toes throughout the entire movement.

Keys to Movement:

1. Stand with toes touching the wall, pointing outward roughly 15-20 degrees.
2. Ensure that the knees point in the same direction as the toes as you squat down.
3. Allow the knees to touch the wall.
4. Squat as low as you can, maintaining posture and technique.
5. A spotter with hand placed in middle of the back can aid in increasing range of motion without falling backward.
6. Keep heels in contact with the ground throughout the movement.

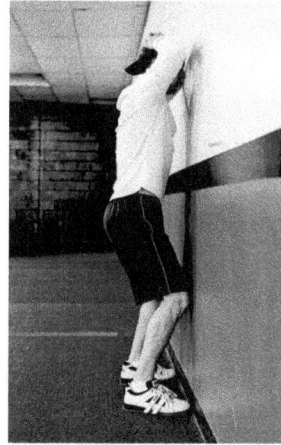

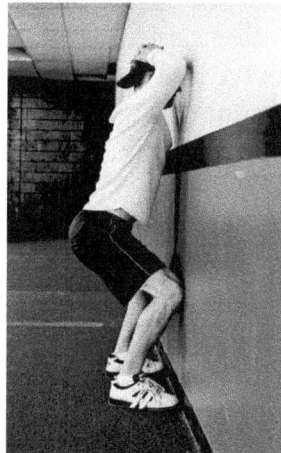

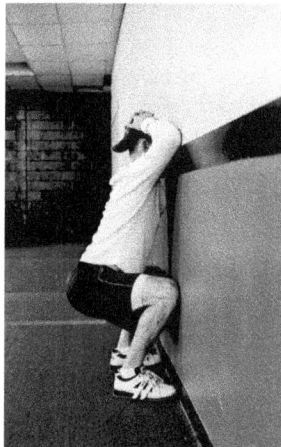

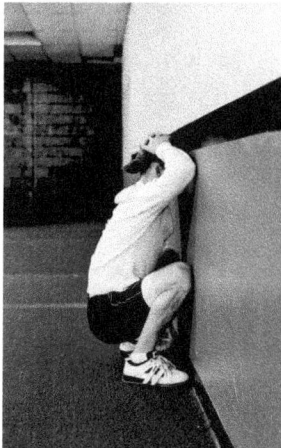

Wall Series

Exercise Prerequisites: Use caution if you have shoulder, neck, or low back pain.

Movement: Sit with your back and butt flat against a wall, with your legs in butterfly stretch position. Hold a dowel rod just above your head, with elbows bent at 90 degree angles pressed firmly against the wall. Keeping your butt, back, and head flat against the wall, press the dowel rod overhead. Try to to keep your elbows and hands in contact with the wall throughout the movement.

The second exercise in the wall series begins in the same position as above, but this time you will rotate the dowel rod down toward your chest while keeping the upper arms parallel to the floor. Once you reach your chest, rotate the dowel rod back to the wall.

Keys to Movement:

1. Sit with your butt and back flat against the wall.
2. Roughly 90 degree angle at elbows with hands and elbows against the wall
3. Press overhead maintaining elbows and hands in contact with the wall.

Same start position.
1. Keep upper arm parallel to the floor.
2. Maintain contact with elbows and upper arms against the wall.
3. Rotate down toward chest.
4. Rotate upward overhead until hands touch the wall.

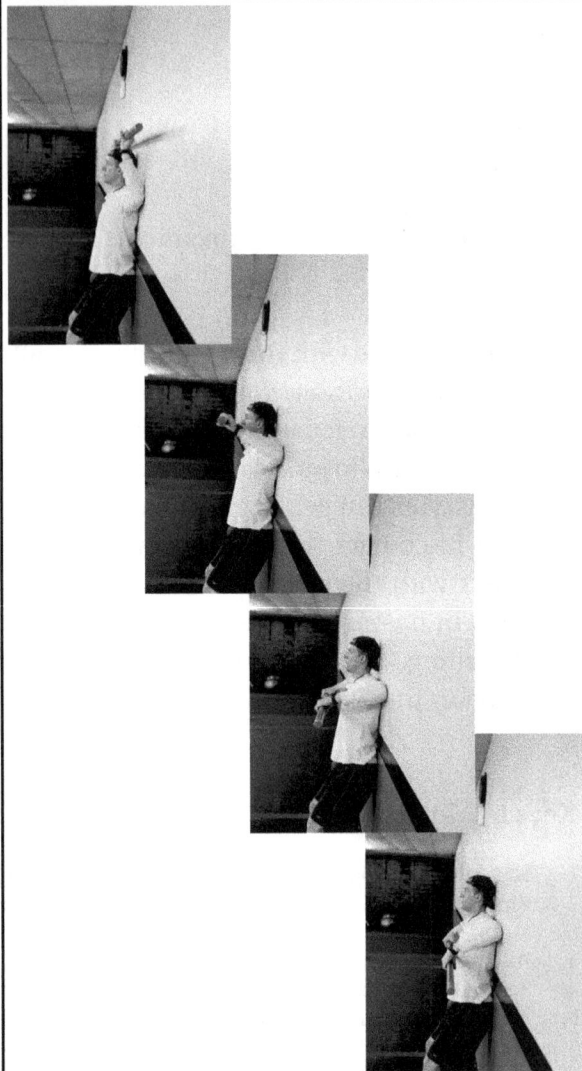

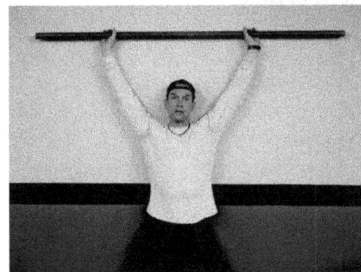

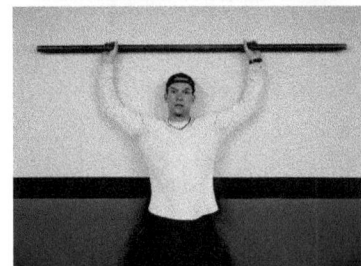

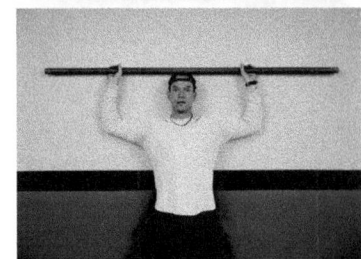

Wide Pull-ups

Exercise Prerequisites: Use caution if you have elbow, shoulder, neck or low back pain.

Movement: Grasp a pull-up bar with hands pronated, about 6-12' wider than the shoulders. Hang from the bar, with arms, hips and shoulders in extension. Initiate the movement by retracting shoulder blades back and down. Pull your body straight upward trying not to allow your shoulders to internally rotate as you pull upward.

Pinch your shoulder blades back and raise until the upper portion of the chest comes in contact with the bar.

Lower slowly, retracing the same pattern until you reach the full extension starting position.

If you cannot perform a regular pull-up, you can use the assistance of a partner or a band around the knee or foot.

Movement Mechanics:

1. Pronated grip with hands 6-12" wider than the shoulders.
2. Begin in dead hang position.
3. Retract shoulders back and down during the movement.
4. Focus on pulling the elbows back and down.
5. Try not to allow the shoulders to internally rotate,
6. Pull up until upper part of chest comes in contact with the bar.
7. Lower down until full extension in the elbows and shoulders.

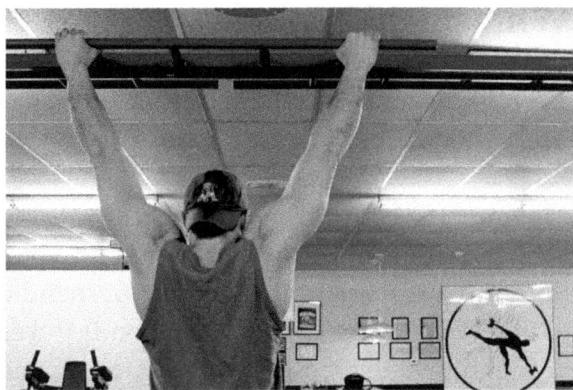

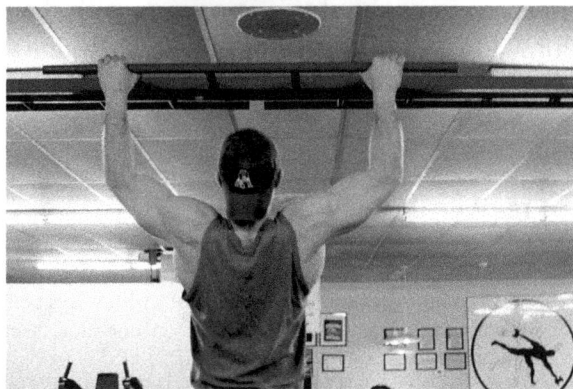

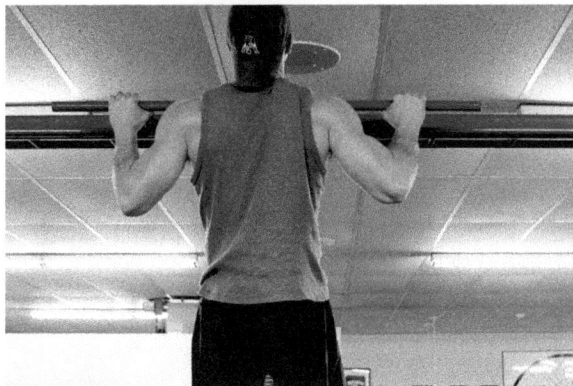

Windshield Wipers

Exercise Prerequisites: Use caution if you have knee, shoulder, neck, shoulder, or low back pain.

Movement: Lie flat on your back with arms anchored in a "T" position out to your sides. With your back flat on the floor, lift your legs until they are perpendicular to the floor with feet above the hips. A variation is to keep the knees bent at roughly 90 degrees with the lower leg parallel to the floor. Keeping your shoulders in contact with the floor, rotate at the hips, lowering the legs to one side. Rotate back to start, and then perform on the opposite side, similar to the movement of a windshield wiper.

Keys to Movement:

1. Lie flat on your back with arms anchored in a "T" position.
2. Keep thighs perpendicular to the floor with knees bent or straight.
3. Rotate both legs toward the floor on one side, keeping the opposite side shoulder in contact with the ground.
4. Rotate back to start.

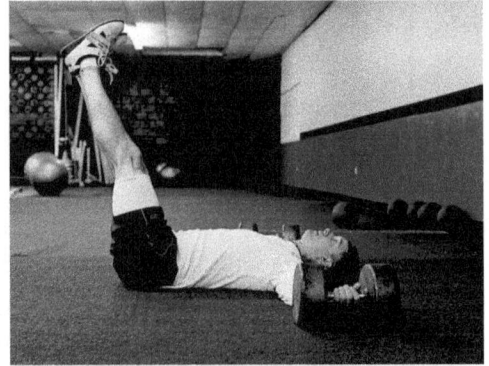

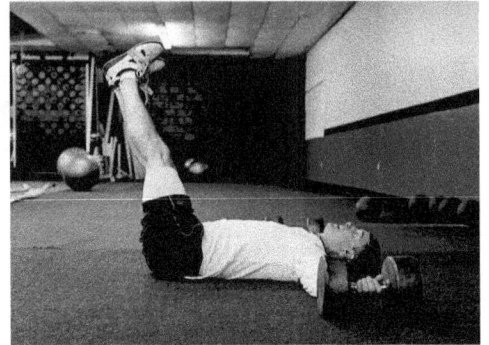

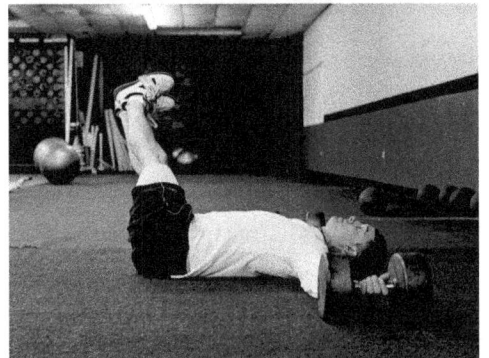

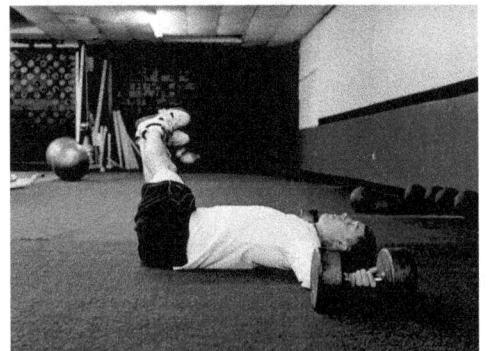

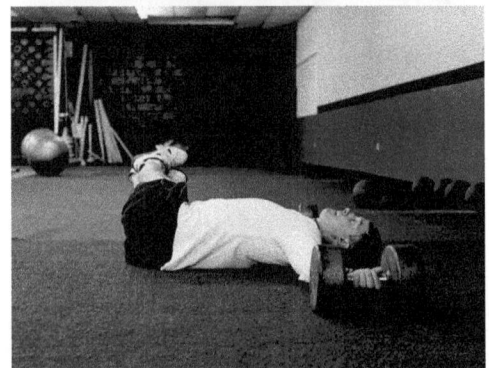

W, Y, T, L

Exercise Prerequisites: Use caution if you have shoulder, neck, elbow, or low back pain.

Movement: Lie face down on a bench. For each of these, picture looking down from the ceiling at your body for the relative position of your arms to your body. The movement should draw parallels to the letter associated with the exercise.

W: Lie face down on a bench with your elbows directly by your sides and forearms parallel to the floor and elbows bent roughly 45-90 degrees relative to your upper arm. Your thumbs should be pointing upward. Keeping your head down, externally rotate your upper arms bringing your forearms upward. Squeeze your shoulder blades together, forming the letter W with your upper arms and forearms. Lower back to start.

Y: Lie face down on a bench with your arms extended past your head at a 45 degree angle relative to your head. With your thumbs pointing upward, retract your shoulder blades, and raise your extended arms until your elbows pass your ears. Try to maintain the upper arms at a 45 degree angle relative to your head throughout the movement.

T: Lie face down on a bench with your arms extended out to your sides. With your thumbs up, raise your extended arms from the floor. Pinch your shoulder blades and raise until your upper arms are parallel to the floor. Ensure that your thumbs are pointing upward and arms extended throughout the movement.

L: Lie face down on a bench with elbows bent 90 degrees and upper arms extended out to the sides. The upper arms should be parallel to the floor, aiming for roughly a 90 degree angle at the armpit. The forearms should be perpendicular to the floor at the start of the movement. Maintaining the angle at the elbows and armpit, externally rotate the upper arms, raising the forearms until they are roughly parallel to the floor.

Keys to Movement:

1. Lie face down on a bench.
2. Focus on complete range of motion.
3. Watch for deviations in upper arm positioning relative to the torso.

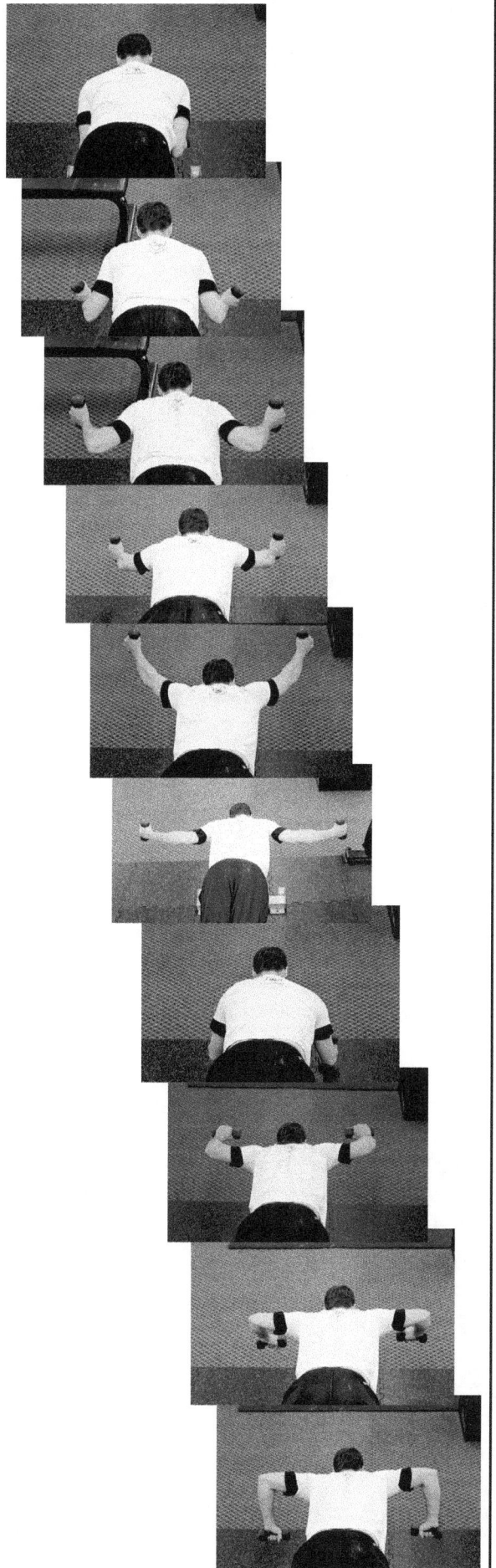

REFERENCES

CHAPTER I

1. Ames B, Shigenaga M, Hagen T. **Oxidants, antioxidants, and the degenerative diseases of aging.** *Proceedings of the National Academy of Sciences USA.* 90(17); Pp 7915-7922. 1993

2. Athar M, Back J, Kopelovich L, Bickers D, Kim A. **Multiple molecular targets of resveratrol: Anti-carcinogenic mechanisms.** *Archives of Biochemistry and Biophysics.* 486(2); Pp 95-102. 2009.

3. Ballie-Hamilton P. **Chemical toxins: a hypothesis to explain the global obesity epidemic.** *Journal of Alternative and Complimentary Medicine.* 8(2); Pp 185-192. 2002.

4. Banerjee A, Mandal A, Chanda D, Chakraborti S. **Oxidant, antioxidant and physical exercise.** *Molecular and Cellular Biochemistry.*253(1-2); Pp 307-312. 2003.

5. Baria G. **Endogenous oxidative stress: relationship to aging, longevity and caloric restriction.** *Aging Research Reviews.* 1(3); Pp 397-411. 2002..

6. Bartke A, Chandrashekar V, Dominici F, Turyn D, Kinney B, Steger R, Kopchick J. **Insulin-like growth factor 1 (IGF-1) and aging: controversies and new insights.** *Biogerentology.* 4(1); Pp 1-8. 2003.

7. Barzilai N, Bartke A. **Biological approaches to mechanistically understand the health y life span extension achieved by calorie restriction and modulation of hormones.** *The Journals of Gerentology.* 62(2); Pp 187-191. 2009.

8. Bendich A, Langseth L. **The health effects of vitamin C supplementation: a review.** *Journal of American College of Nutrition.* 14(2); Pp 124-136.1995.

9. Biewenga G, Haenen G, Bast A. **The pharmacology of the antioxidant lipoic acid.** *General Pharmacology.* 29(3); Pp 315- 331. 1997.

10. Block G et al. **Vitamin C treatment reduces elevated C-reactive protein.** *Free Radical Biology and Medicine.* 46(1); Pp 70-77. 2009.

11. Brown-Borg H. **Hormonal regulation of aging and life span.** *Trends in Endocrinology and Metabolism.* 14(4); Pp 151-153. 2003.

12. Clarke M, Burnett J, Croft K. **Vitamin E in human health and disease.** *Critical Reviews in Clinical Laboratory Sciences.* 45(5); Pp 417-450. 2008.

13. Dhanasekaran M, Ren J. **The emerging role of coenzyme Q-10 in aging, neurodegeneration, cardiovascular disease, cancer and diabetes milletus.** *Current Neurovascular Research.* 2(5); Pp 447- 459. 2005

14. Dirks Naylor A. **Cellular effects of resveratrol in skeletal muscle.** *Life Sciences.* 84(19-20); Pp 637-640. 2009

15. Elobeid M, Allison D. **Putative environmental-endocrine disruptors and obesity: a review.** *Current Opinon in Endocrinology, Diabetes, and Obesity.* 15(5); Pp 403-408. 2008.

16. Fremont L. **Biological effects of resveratrol.** *Life Sciences.* 66(8); Pp 663-673. 2000.

17. Fusco D, Colloca G, Lo Monaco M, Cesari M. **Effects of antioxidant supplementation on the aging process.** *Journal of Clinical Interventions in Aging.* 2(3); Pp 377-387. 2007.

18. Ginter E. **Chronic vitamin C deficiency increases the risk of cardiovascular diseases.** *Bratislava Medical Journal.* 108(9); Pp 417-421. 2007

19. Gredilla R, Baria G. **Minireview: the role of oxidative stress in relation to caloric restriction and longevity.** *Endocrinology.* 140(9); Pp 3717-3717. 2005.

20. Grun F, Blumberg B. **Environmental obesogens: organotins and endocrine disruption via nuclear receptor signaling.** *Endocrinology.* Pp 146. 2006.

21. Holzenberger M. **The GH/IGF-I axis and longevity.** *European Journal of Endocrinolgy.* 151(1); Pp 23-27. 2004

22. Johnston C, Meyer C, Srilakshmi J. **Vitamin C elevates red blood cell glutathione in healthy adults.** *American Journal of Clinical Nutrition.* 58(1) Pp 103-105.

23. Kagan V, Serbinova E, Forte T, Scita G, Packer L. **Recycling of vitamin E in human low density lipoproteins**. *Journal of Lipid Research*. 33(3); Pp 385-397. 1992

24. Keys A, Taylor H, Grande F. **Basal metabolism and age of adult men**. *Metabolism*. 22; Pp 579-587. 1973

25. Lenaz G, Fato R, Formiggini G, Genova M. **The role of Coenzyme Q in mitochondrial electron transport**. *Mitochondrion*. June 7. Pp S8-S33. 2007.

26. Liu Y, Schubert D. **The specificity of neuroprotection by antioxidants**. *Journal of Biomedical Sciences*. 16(1); Pp 98. 2009.

27. Maternak M, Panici J, Bonkowski M, Hughes L, Bartke A. **Insulin sensitivity as a key mediator of growth hormone actions on longevity**. *The Journals of Gerentology*. 64(4); Pp 516-521. 2009.

28. Maxwell S. **Prospects for the use of antioxidant therapies**. *Drugs*. 49(3); Pp 345-361. 1995.

29. Moini H, Packer L, Saris N. **Antioxidant and prooxidant activities of alpha-lipoic acid and dihydrolipoic acid**. *Toxicology and Applied Pharmacology*. 182(1); Pp 84-90. 2002.

30. Murray L, Reilly J, Choudhry M, Durnin J. **A longitudinal study of changes in body composition and basal metabolism in physically active elderly men**. *European Journal of Applied Physiology and Occupational Physiology*. 72(3); Pp 215-218. 1996

31. Newbold R, Padilla-Banks E, Jefferson W, Heindel J, **Effects of endocrine disruptors on obesity**. *The Journal of Andrology*. 31(2); Pp 201-208. 2008.

32. Nohl H, Kozlov A, Staniek K. Gille L. **The multiple functions of coenzyme Q**. *Bioorganic Chemistry*. 29(1); Pp 1-13. 2001.

33. Padmalayam I, Hasham S, Saxena U, Pillarisetti S. **Lipoic acid synthase (LASY): a novel role in inflammation, mitochondrial function, and insulin resistance**. *Diabetes*. 58(3); Pp 600-608. 2009

34. Piers L, Soares M, McCormick L, O'dea K. **Is there evidence for an age-related reduction in metabolic rate**. *Journal of Applied Physiology*. 85(6); Pp 2196-2204. 1998.

Pollan M. *In Defense of Food*. Penguin Press HC. 2008.

35. Rennie M. **Anabolic resistance: the effects of ageing, sexual dimorphism, and immobilization on human muscle protein turnover**. *Applied Physiology, Nutrition, and Metabolism*. 34(3); Pp 377-381. 2009.

36. Rocha-Gonzalez H, Ambriz-Tututi M, Granados-Soto V. **Resveratrol: a natural compound with pharmacological potential in neurodegenerative diseases**. *CNS Neuroscience and Therapeutics*. 14(3); Pp 234-247. 2008..

37. Sen C, Khanna S, Roy S. **Tocotrienols: Vitamin E beyond tocopherols**. *Life Sciences*. 78(18); Pp 2088-2098. 2006

38. Sies H, Stahl W, Sundquist A. **Antioxidant functions of vitamins. Vitamin E and C, beta-carotene, and other carotenoids**. *Annals of New York Academy of Sciencs*. 669; Pp 7-20. 1992.

39. Soares M, Piers L, O'dea K, Collier G. **Plasma leptin concentrations, basal metabolic rates and respiratory quotients in young and older adults**. *International Journal of Obesity and Related Metabolic Disorders*. 24(12); Pp 1592-1599. 2000.

40. Troen B. **The biology of aging**. *Mt Sinai Journal of Medicine*. 70(1); Pp 3-22. 2003.

41. Van den Beld A, de Jong F, Grobbe D, Pols H, Lambert S. **Measures of bioavailable serum testosterone and estradiol and their relationships with muscle strength, bone density, and body composition in elderly men**. *Journal of Clinical Endocrinology and Metabolism*. 85(9); 3276-3282. 2000.

42. Willet W. **Dietary fat plays a major role in obesity: no**. *Obesity Reviews*. 3(2); Pp 59-68. 2002.

43. Willet W, Leibel R. **Dietary fat is not a major determinant of body fat**. *The American Journal of Medicine*. 113(9B); Pp 47-59. 2002

Chapter 3

1. Baillie-Hamilton PF. **Chemical toxins: a hypothesis to explain the global obesity epidemic.** *Journal of Alternative and Complementary Medicine.* 8(2); Pp 185-192. 2002.

2. Elobeid MA, Allison DB. **Putative environmental-endocrine disruptors and obesity: a review.** *Current Opinion in Endocrinology, Diabetes, and Obesity.* 15(5). Pp 403-408. 2008.

3. Grün F, Blumberg B. **Environmental obesogens: organotins and endocrine disruption via nuclear receptor signaling.** *Endocrinology.* Pp 146. 2006

4. Hovinga ME, Sowers M, Humphrey HE. **Environmental exposure and lifestyle predictors of lead, cadmium, PCP and DDT levels in Great Lakes fish eaters.** *Archives of Environmental Health.* 48(2). Pp 98-104. 1993

5. Hanrahan LP, Falk C, Anderson HA, Draheim L, Kanarek MS, Olson J. **Serum PCB and DDE levels of frequent Great Lakes sport fish consumers-a first look. The Great Lakes Consortium.** *Environmental Research.* 80(2); Pp S26-S37. 1999

6. Newbold RR, Padilla-Banks E, Jefferson WN, Heindel JJ. **Effects of endocrine disruptors on obesity.** *Journal of Andrology.* 31(2). Pp 201-208. 2008.

7. Newbold RR, Padilla-Banks E, Jefferson WN. **Environmental estrogens and obesity.** *Molecular and Cellular Endocrinology.* 304 (1-2); Pp 84-89. 2009

8. O'Dea K. **Diabetes in Australian aborigines: impact of the western diet and lifestyle.** *Journal of Internal Medicine.* 232(2); Pp 103-117. 1992

9. O'Dea K. **Westernization, insulin resistance and diabetes in Australian aborigines.** *The Medical Journal of Australia.* 1991 Aug 19;155(4):258-64.

10. O'Dea K. **Westernization and non-insulin-dependent diabetes in Australian Aborigines.** *Ethnicity and Disease.* 1991 Spring;1(2):171-87..

11. O'Dea K, Spargo RM, Akerman K. **The effect of transition from traditional to urban lifestyle on the insulin secretory response in Australian Aborigines.** *Diabetes Care.* 1980 Jan-Feb;3(1):31-7.

12. O'Dea K. **Cardiovascular disease risk factors in Australian aborigines.** *Clinical and Experimental Pharmacology and Physiology.* 1991 Feb;18(2):85-8.

13. O'Dea K. **Marked improvement in carbohdrate and lipid metabolism in diabetic Australian aborigines after temporary reversion to traditional lifestyle.** *Diabetes.* 1984 Jun;33(6):596-603.

14. Parkinson A. *Basic body detoxification and cleansing.* Canton MS. 2007.

15. Puotinen C. *Herbs for Detoxification.* New Canaan CT. 1999.

16. Trankina ML, Beitz DC, Trenkle AH. **Effects of in vitro runnel on metabolic activity in subcutaneous adipose tissue and skeletal muscle from steers.** *Journal of Animal Sciences.* 60(3); Pp 652-658. 1985.

17. Winston D, Maimes S. *Adaptogens: Herbs for strength and stamina.* Rochestor VT. 2007

Chapter 4

1. Balkovetz D. **Tight junction claudins and the kidney in sickness and in health.** *Biochem et Biophysica Acta.* 1788(4); Pp 858-863. 2009.

2. Benard A, Desreaumeaux P, Huglo D, Hoorelbeke A, Tonnel A, Wallaert B. **Increased intestinal permeability in bronchial asthma.** *Journal of Allergy and Clinical Immunology.* 97(6); Pp 1173-1178. 1996.

3. Bengmark S. **Gut microbial ecology in critical illness: Is there a role for prebiotics, probiotics, and synbiotics.** *Current Opinions in Critical Care.* 8(2); Pp 145-151. 2002.

4. Boirivant M, Strober W. **The mechanism of action of probiotics.** *Current Opinion in Gastroenterology.* 23(6); Pp 679-692. 2007.

5. Furness J, Kunze W, Clerc N. **Nutrient tasting and signaling mechanism in the gut: II: The intestine as a sensory organ: neural, endocrine, immune responses.** *American Journal of Physiology.* 277(5); Pp 922-928. 1999.

6. Galmiche J, Janssens J. **The pathophysiology of gastro-oesophageal reflux disease: an overview.** *Scandanavian Journal of Gastroenterology: Supplement.* 211; Pp 7-18. 1995.

7. Grevet EH, Tietzmann MR, Shansis FM, Hastenpflugl C, Santana LC, Forster L, Kapczinskil F, Izquierdo I. **Behavioural effects of acute phynylalanine and tyrosine depletion in healthy male volunteers.** *Journal of Psychopharmacology.* 16(1); Pp 51-55. 2002.

8. Groschwitz K, Hogan S. **Intestinal barrier function: molecular regulation and disease pathogenesis.** *Journal of Allergy and Clinical Immunology.* 124(1); Pp 3-20. 2009.

9. Hollander D. **Intestinal permeability, leaky gut, and intestinal disorders.** *Current Gastroenterology Reports.* 1(5); Pp 410-416. 1999.

10. Horvath K, Perman J. **Autistic disorder and gastrointestinal disease.** *Current Opinions in Pediatrics.* 14(5); Pp 583-587. 2002.

11. Kahrilas P. **Gastroesophageal reflux disease.** *JAMA.* 276(12); Pp 983-988. 1996

12. Kapadia C. **Gastric atrophy, metaplasia, and dysplasia: a clinical perspective.** *Journal of Clinical Gastroenterology.* 36(5); Pp 29-36. 2003.   **B12 Deficiency, Cancer, and other problems associated with stomach problems.**

13. Kassarijan Z, Russel R. **Hypochlorydria: a factor in nutrition.** *Annual Review of Nutrition.* 9; Pp 271-285. 1989.

14. Kondoh M, Yoshida T, Kakutani H, Yagi K. **Targeting tight junction proteins-significance for drug development.** *Drug Discovery Today.* 13(3-4); Pp 180-186. 2008.

15. Koop H. **Review Article: metabolic consequences of long-term inhibition of acid secretion by omeprazole.** *Alimentary Pharmacology and Therapeutics.* 6(4); Pp 399-406. 1992.

16. Leyton M, Young SN, Pihl RO, Etezadi S, Lauze C, Blier P, Baker GB, Benkelfat C. **Effects on mood of acute phenylalanine/tyrosine depletion in healthy women.** *Neuropsychopharmacology.* 22(1); Pp 52-63. 2000.

17. Lindström E, Chen D, Norlén P, Andersson K, Håkanson R. **Control of gastric acid secretion: the gastrin-ECL cell-parietal cell axis.** *Comparative Biochemistry and Physiology Part A: Molecular and Integrative Physiology.* 128(3); Pp 505-514. 2001.

18. Liu Z, Li N, Neu J. **Tight junctions, leaky intestines, and pediatric diseases.** *Acta Paediatrica.* 94(4); Pp 386-393. 2005.

19. Madora J, Nash S, Moore R, Atisook K. **Structure and function of the intestinal epithelial barrier in health and disease.** *Monographs in Pathology.* 31; Pp 306-324. 1990.

20. Maes M, Kubera M, Leunis J. **The gut-brain barrier in major depression: intestinal mucosal dysfunction with an increased translocation of LPS from gram negative enterobacteria (leaky gut) plays a role in the inflammatory pathophysiology of depression.** *Neuroendocrinology Letters.* 29(1); Pp 117-124. 2008.

21. Malby E. **The digestion of beef proteins in the human stomach.** *The Journal of Clinical Investigation.* 13(2); Pp 193-207. 1934.

22. Murphy M, Eastham E, Nelson R, Pearson A, Laker M. **Intestinal permeability in Crohn's disease**. *Archives of Disease in Childhood*. 64(3); Pp 321-325. 1989.

23. Purohit V, Bode C, Bode C, Brenner D, Choudhry M, Hamilton F, Kang J, Keshavarzian A, Rao R, Sartor B, Swanton C, Turner J. **Alcohol, Intestinal Bacterial Growth, Intestinal Permeability to Endotoxin, and Medical Consequences**. *Alcohol*. 42(5); Pp 349-361. 2008.

24. Rao R. **Oxidative stress-induced disruption of epithelial and endothelial tight junctions**. *Frontiers in Bioscience*. 13; Pp 7210-7226. 2008.

25. Silva M. **Intestinal dendritic cells and epithelial barrier dysfunction in Crohn's disease**. *Inflammatory Bowel Diseases*. 15(3); Pp 436-453. 2009.

26. Smecuol E, Bai J, Vazquez H, Kogan Z, Cabanne A, Niveloni S, Pedreira S, Boerr L, Maurino E, Meddings J. **Gastrointestinal permeability in celiac disease**. *Gastroenterology*. 112(4); Pp 1129-1136. 1997.

27. Tabrez S, Roberts I. **Malabsorption and malnutrition**. *Primary Care*. 28(3); Pp 505-522. 2001.

28. Van de Laar M, can der Korst J. **Food intolerance in rheumatoid arthritis. I. A double blind, controlled trial of the clinical effects of elimination of milk allergens and azo dyes**. *Annals of the Rheumatic Diseases*. 51(3); Pp 298-302. 1992.

29. Vilioen M, Panzer A, Willemse N. **Gastro intestinal hyperpermeability: a review**. *East African Medical Journal*. 80(6); Pp 324-330. 2003.

30. Watson W, Sullivan S, Corke M, Rush D. **Globus and headache: common symptoms of the irritable bowel syndrome**. *The Canadian Medical Association Journal*. 118(4); Pp 387-388. 1978.

31. Wood RJ, Serfaty-Lacrosniere C. **Gastric acidity, atrophic gastritis, and calcium absorption**. *Nutrition Reviews*. 50(2); Pp 33-40. 1992.

CHAPTER 5

1. Ahima R, Prabakaran D, Mantzoros C, Qu D, Lowell B, Maratos-Flier E, Flier J. **Role of leptin in the neuroendocrine response to fasting**. *Nature*. 382(6588); Pp 250-252. 1996.

2. Baghaei F, Rosmond R, Westberg L, Hellstrand M, Landen M, Eriksson E, Holm G, Bjorntorp P. **The lean woman**. *Obesity Research*. 10(2); Pp 115-121. 2002

3. Bain J. **The many faces of testosterone**. *Journal of Clinical Interventions in Aging*. 2(4); Pp 567-576. 2007.

4. Berger A. **Resistin: a new hormone that links obesity with type 2 diabetes**. *The British Medical Journal*. 322(7280); Pp 193. 2001.

5. Berggren J, Hulver M, Houmard J. **Fat as an endocrine organ: influence of exercise**. *Journal of Applied Physiology*. 99(2); Pp 757-764. 2005.

6. Bertoli S, Magni P, Krogh V, Ruscica M, Dozio E, Testolin G, Battezzati A. **Is ghrelin a signal of decreased fat-free mass in elderly subjects?** *European Journal of Endocrinology*. 155(2); Pp 321-330. 2006.

7. Bjorntorp P. **Hormonal control of regional fat distribution**. *Human Reproduction*. 12(1); pp 21-25. 1997.

8. Bjorntorp P. **The regulation of adipose tissue distribution in humans**. *International Journal of Obesity and Related Metabolic Disorders*. 20(4); Pp 291-302. 1996.

9. Bjorntorp P. **Adipose tissue distribution and function**. *International Journal of Obesity*. 15(2); Pp 67-81. 1991.

10. Bjorntorp P. **Growth hormone, insulin-like growth factor-I and lipid metabolism: interactions with sex steroids**. *Hormone Research*. 46(4-5); Pp 188-191. 1996.

11. Bjorntorp P. **Regional obesity and NIDDM**. *Advances in Experimental Medicine and Biology*. 334; Pp 279-285. 1993.

12. Bjorntorp P. **Regional fat distribution—implications for type II diabetes**. *International Journal of Obesity and Related Metabolic Disorders*. 16(4); Pp 19-27. 1992.

13. Bjorntorp P. **Metabolic implications of body fat distribution**. *Diabetes Care*. 14(12); Pp 1132-1143. 1991.
14. Bjorntorp P. **Adipose tissue distribution and function**. *International Journal of Obesity*. 15(2); Pp 67-81. 1991
15. Britton R, Koyes G, Orrego H, Kalant H, Phillips M, Khanna J, Israel Y. **Suppression of antithyroid drugs of experimental hepatic necrosis after ethanol treatment. Effect on thyroid gland or on peripheral deiodination.** *Toxicology and Applied Pharmacology*. 51(1); Pp 145-155. 1979.
16. Buteau-Lozano H, Velasco G, Cristofari M, Balaquer P, Perrot-Applanat M. **Xenoestrogens modulate vascular endothelial growth factor secretion in breast cancer cells through an estrogen receptor dependent mechanism.** *The Journal of Endocrinology*. 196(2); Pp 399-412. 2008.
17. Chan J, Heist K, Depaoli A, Veldhuis J, Mantzoros C. **The role of falling leptin levels in the neuroendocrine and metabolic adaptation to short-term starvation in healthy men.** *Journal of Clinical Investigation*. 111(9); Pp 1409-1421. 2003.
18. Daly W, Seegers C, Rubin D, Dobridge J, Hackney A. **Relationship between stress hormones and testosterone with prolonged endurance exercise.** *European Journal of Applied Physiology*. 93(4); Pp 375-380. 2005.
19. Davis D, Bradlow H, Wolff M, Woodruff T, Hoel D, Anton-Culver H. **Medical hypothesis: xenoestrogens as preventable causes of breast cancer.** *Environmental Health Perspectives*. 101(5); Pp 372-377. 1993.
20. Deng R. **Therapeutic effect of guggul and its constituent guggulsterone: cardiovascular benefits.** *Cardiovasc Drug Rev*. 25(4); Pp 375-390. 2007.
21. Doerge DR, Sheehan DM. **Goitrogenic and estrogenic activity of soy isoflavones.** *Environmental Health Perspectives*. 110; Pp 349-53. 2002
22. Duick D, Wahner H. **Throid axis in patients with Cushing's syndrome.** *Archives of Internal Medicine*. 139(7); Pp 767-772. 1979.
23. Dyck D. **Dietary fat intake, supplements, and weight loss.** *Canadian Journal of Applied Physiology*. 25(6); Pp 495-523. 2000.
24. Elobeid M, Allison D. **Putative environmental-endocrine disruptors and obesity: a review.** *Current Opinion in Endocrinology, Diabetes, and Obesity*. 15(5); Pp 403-408. 2008.
25. Epel E, McEwen B, Seeman T, Mathews K, Castellazzo G, Brownell K, Bell J, Ickovics J. **Stress and body shape: stress induced cortisol secretion is consistently greater among women with central fat.** *Psychosomatic Medicine*. 62(5); Pp 623-632. 2000.
26. Epel E, Moyer A, Martin C, Macary S, Cummings N, Rodin J, Rebuffe-Scrive M. **Stress induced cortisol, mood, and fat distribution in men.** *Obesity Research*. 7(1); Pp 9-15. 1999.
27. Flier J, Harris M, Hollenberg A. **Leptin, nutrition, and the thyroid: the why, the wherefore, and the wiring.** *The Journal of Clinical Investigation*. 105(7); Pp 859-861. 2000.
28. Frankish H, Dryden S, Hopkins D, Wang Q, Williams G. **Neuropeptide Y, the hypothalamus, and diabetes: insights into the central control of metabolism.** *Peptides*. 16(4); Pp 757-771. 1995.
29. Frisch H. **Growth hormone and body composition in athletes.** *Journal of Endocrinological Investigation*. 22(5); Pp 106-109. 1999.
30. Goodman H, Gorin E, Schwartz Y, Tai L, Chipkin S, Honeyman T, Frick G, Yamaguchi H. **Cellular effects of growth hormone on adipocytes.** *Clinical Journal of Physiology*. 34(1); Pp 27-44. 1991.
31. Gordon G, Altman K, Southren A, Rubin E, Lieber C. **Effect of alcohol (ethanol) administration on sex-hormone metabolism in normal men.** *New England Journal of Medicine*. 295(15); Pp 793-797. 1976.
32. Gordon G, Vittek J, Ho R, Rosenthal W, Southren A, Lieber C. **Effect of chronic alcohol use on hepatic testosterone 5-alpha-A-ring reductase in the baboon and in the human being.** *Gastroenterology*. 77(1); Pp 110-114. 1979.
33. Gregory J. **Metabolic effects of stopping growth hormone: body composition and energy expenditure.** *Journal of Pediatric Endocrinology and Metabolism*. 15(5); Pp 1347-1350. 2002.
34. Gupta A, Gupta R, Lai B. **Effect of Trigonella foenum-graecum (fenugreek) seeds on glycaemic control and insulin resistance in type 2 diabetes mellitus: a double blind placebo controlled study.** *Journal of the Association of Physicians of India*. 49. Pp 1057-1061. 2001.
35. Holmang A, Bjorntorp P. **The effects of cortisol on insulin sensitivity in muscle.** *Acta Physiologica Scandinavica*. 144(4); Pp 425-431. 1992.
36. Hutley L, Prins J. **Fat as an endocrine organ: relationship to the metabolic syndrome.** *The American Journal of Medical Sciences*. 330(6); Pp 280-289. 2005.

37. Hwa J, Ghibaudi L, Compton D, Fawzi A, Strader C. **Intracerebroventricular injection of leptin increases thermogenesis and mobilizes fat metabolism in ob/ob mice.** *Hormone and Metabolic Research.* 28(12); Pp 659-663. 1996.

38. Jackson M, Ahima R. **Neuroendocrine and metabolic effects of adipocytes-derived hormones.** *Clinical Science (Lond).* 110(2); Pp 143-152. 2006.

39. Jang M, Mistry A, Swick A, Romsos D. **Leptin rapidly inhibits hypothalamic neruopeptide Y secretion and stimulates corticotrophin-releasing hormone secretion adrenalectomized mice.** *Journal of Nutrition.* 130(11); Pp 2813-2820. 2000.

40. Jaworski K, Sarkaki-Nagy E, Duncan R, Ahmadian M, Sook Sui H. **Regulation of triglyceride metabolism. IV. Hormonal regulation of lipolysis in adipose tissue.** *American Journal of Gastrointestinal and Liver Physiology.* 293(1) Pp G1-G4. 2007.

41. Johannsson G, Karlsson C, Lonn L, Marin P, Bjorntrop P, Sjorstrom L, Carlsson B, Carlsson L, Bengtsson B. **Serum leptin concentrations and insulin sensitivity in men with abdominal obesity.** *Obesity Research.* 6(6); Pp 416-421. 1998.

42. Kolaczynski J, Ylikahri R, Harkonen M, Koivisto V. **The acute effect of ethanol on counterregulatory response and recovery from insulin-induced hypoglycemia.** *Journal of Clinical Endocrinology and Metabolism.* 67(2); Pp 384-388. 1988

43. Kraemer W, Marchitelli L, Gordon S, Harman E, Dziados J, Mello R, Frykman P, McCurry D, Fleck S. **Hormonal and growth factor responses to heavy resistance exercise protocols.** *Journal of Applied Physiology.* 69(4); Pp 1442-1450. 1990.

44. Kusminski C, McTernan P, Kumar S. **Role of resistin in obesity, insulin resistance and type II diabetes.** *Clinical Science (Lond).* 109(3); Pp 243-256. 2005.

45. Kvist H, Hallgren P, Jonsson L, Pettersson P, Sjoberg C, Sjostrom L, Bjorntorp P. **Distribution of adipose tissue and muscle mass in alcoholic men.** *Metabolism.* 42(5); Pp 569-573. 1993.

46. Lazar M. **Resistin and obesity associated metabolic diseases.** *Hormone and Metabolic Research.* 39(10); Pp 710-716. 2007.

47. Marcus C, Bolme P, Micha-Johansson G, Margery V, Bronnegard M. **Growth hormone increase the lipolytic sensitivity for catecholamines in adipocytes from healthy adults.** *Life Sciences.* 54(18); Pp 1335-1341. 1994.

48. Marin P, Rosmond R, Bengtsson B, Gustafsson C, Holm G, Bjorntorp P. **Growth hormone secretion after testosterone administration to men with visceral obesity.** *Obesity Research.* 2(3); Pp 263-270. 1994

49. Marin P et al. **Androgen treatment of abdominally obese men.** *Obesity Research.* 1(4); Pp 245-251. 1993.

50. Marin P, Kvist H, Lindstedt G, Sjostrom L, Bjorntorp P. **Low concentrations of insulin-like growth factor-I in abdominal obesity.** *International Journal of Obesity and Related Metabolic Disorders.* 17(2); Pp 83-89. 1993.

51. Marin P, Bjorntorp P. **Endocrine-metabolic pattern and adipose tissue distribution.** *Hormone Research.* 39(3); Pp 81-85. 1993.

52. Marin P, Krotkiewski M, Bjorntorp P. **Androgen treatment of middle aged, obese men: effects on metabolism, muscle and adipose tissues.** *European Journal of Medicine.* 1(6); Pp 329-336. 1992.

53. McTernan P, Kusminski C, Kumar S. **Resistin.** *Current Opinion in Lipidology.* 17(2); Pp 170-175. 2006.

54. Meinhardt U, Nelson A, Hansen J, Birzniece V, Clifford D, Leung K, Graham K, Ho K. **The effects of growth hormone on body composition and physical performance in recreational athletes: a randomized trial.** *Annals of Internal Medicine.* 152(9); Pp 568-577. 2010.

55. Mistry A, Swick A, Romsos D. **Leptin rapidly lowers food intake and elevates metabolic rates in lean and ob/ob mice.** *Journal of Nutrition.* 127(10); Pp 2065-2072. 1997.

56. Nass R, Pezzoli S, Oliveri M, Patrie J, Harrell F, Clasey J, Heymsfield S, Bach M, Vance M, Thorner M. **Effects of an oral ghrelin mimetic on body compositin and clinical outcomes in healthy older adults: a randomized trial.** *Annals of Internal Medicine.* 149(9); Pp 601-611. 2008.

57. Nestler J, Clore J, Strauss J, Blackard W. **The effects of hyperinsulinemia on serum testosterone, progesterone, dehydroepiandrosterone sulfate, and cortisol levels in normal women and in a woman with hyperandrogenism, insulin resistance, and acanthosis nigricans.** *Journal of Clinical Endocrinology and Metabolism.* 64(1); Pp 180-184. 1987.

58. Nishiyama S, Futagoishi-Suginohara Y, Matsukura M, Nakamura T, Higashi A, Shinohara M, Matsuda I. **Zinc supplementation alters thyroid hormone metabolism in disables patients with zinc deficiency.** *Journal of American College of Nutrition.* 13(1); Pp 62-67. 1994.

59. Nussey S, Whitehead S. *Endocrinology: an integrated approach.* Informa Healthcare. 2001.

60. Pantanetti P, Carrapa G, Mantero F, Boscaro M, Faloia E, Venarucci D. **Adipose tissue as an endocrine organ? A review of recent data related to cardiovascular complications of endocrine dysfunctions.** *Clinical and Experimental Hypertension.* 26(4); Pp 387-398. 2004.

61. Pasarica M, Zachweija J, Dejonge L, Redman S, Smith S. **Effect of growth hormone on body composition and visceral adiposity in middle aged men with visceral obesity.** *Journal of Clinical Endocrinology and Metabolism.* 92(11); Pp 4265-4270. 2007.

62. Popovic V, Duntas L. **Leptin TRH and ghrelin: influence on energy homeostasis at rest and during exercise.** *Hormone and Metabolic Research.* 37(9); Pp 533-537. 2005.

63. Rebuffe-Scrive M, Marin P, Bjorntorp P. **Effect of testosterone on abdominal adipose tissue in men.** *International Journal of Obesity.* 15(11); Pp 791-795. 1991

64. Rice D, Brannigan R, Campbell R, Fine S, Jack L, Nelson J, Regan-Klich J. **Men's health, low testosterone, and diabetes: individualized treatment and a multidisciplinary approach.** *Diabetes Education.* 34(5); Pp 97-112. 2008.

65. Richelson B. **Action of growth hormone in adipose tissue.** *Hormone Research.* 48(5); Pp 105-110. 1997.

66. Rogers R, Barnes M, Hermann G. **Leptin "gates" thermogenic action of thyrotropin-releasing hormone in the hindbrain.** *Brain Research.* 1295; Pp 135-141. 2009.

67. Rubello D, Sonino N, Casara D, Girelli M, Busnardo B, Boscaro M. **Acute and chronic effects of high glucocorticoid levels on hypothalamic-pituitary-thyroid axis in man.** *Journal of Endocrinological Investigation.* 15(6); Pp 437-441. 1992.

68. Ruz M, Codoceo J, Galgani J, Munoz L, Gras N, Muzzo S, Leiva L, Bosco C. **Single and multiple selenium-zinc-iodine deficiencies affect rat thyroid metabolism and ultrastructure.** *Journal of Nutrition.* 129(1); Pp 174-180. 1999.

69. Schwartz M, Baskin D, Bukowski T, Kujiper J, Foster D, Lasser G, Prunkard D, Porte D, Woods S, Seeley R< Weigle D. **Specificity of leptin action on elevated blood glucose levels and hypothalamic neuropeptide Y gene expression in ob/ob mice.** *Diabetes.* 45(4); Pp 531-535. 1996

70. Seidell J et al. **Androgenicity in relation to body fat distribution and metabolism in 38-year old women—the European Fat Distribution Study.** *Journal of Clinical Epidemiology.* 43(1); Pp 21-34. 1990.

71. Seidell J, Bjorntorp P, Sjostrom L, Sannerstedt R, Krotkiewski M, Kvist H. **Regional distribution of muscle and fat mass in men—new insight into the risk of abdominal obesity using computed tomography.** *International Journal of Obesity.* 13(3); Pp 289-303. 1989.

72. Tena-Sempere M, Pinilla L, Gonzalez L, Diequez C, Casanueva F, Aguilar E. **Leptin inhibits testosterone secretion from adult rat testis in vitro.** *Journal of Endocrinology.* 161(2); Pp 211-218. 1999.

73. Toni R, Malaguti A, Castorina S, Roti E, Lechan R. **New paradigms in neuroendocrinology: relationships between obesity, systemic inflammation and the neuroendocrine system.** *Journal of Endocrinological Investigation.* 27(2); Pp 182-186. 2004.

74. Tripathi Y, Tripathi P, Malhotra O, Tripathi S. **Thyroid stimulatory action of (Z)-guggulsterone: a mechanism of action.** *Planta Medica.* 54(4); Pp 271-277. 1988.

75. Tripathi Y, Malhotra O, Tripathi S. **Thyroid stimulating action of Z-Guggulsterone Obtained from Commiphora Mukul.** *Planta Medica.* 50(1); Pp 78-80. 1984.

76. Vilimaki M, Harkonen M, Eriksson C, Yikahri R. **Sex hormones and adrenocortical steroids in men acutely intoxicated with ethanol.** *Alcohol.* 1(1); Pp 89-93. 1984.

77. Wahrenberg H, Engfeldt P, Arner P, Wennlund A, Ostman J. **Adrenergic regulation of lipolysis in human adipocytes: findings in hyper- and hypothyroidism.** *Journal of Clinical Endocrinology and Metabolism.* 63(3); Pp 631-638. 1986.

78. Wallerius S, Rosmond R, Liung T, Holm G, Bjorntorp P. **Rise in morning saliva cortisol is associated with abdominal obesity in men: a preliminary report.** *Journal of Endocrinological Investigation.* 26(7); Pp 616-619. 2003.

79. Weinberg J. **Neuroendocrine effects on prenatal alcohol exposure.** *Annals of the New York Academy of Sciences.* 697. Pp 86-96. 1993.

80. Wetherill Y, Fisher N, Staubach A, Danielson M, de Vere White R, Knudsen K. **Xenoestrogen action in prostate cancer: pleiotropic effects dependent on androgen receptor status.** *Cancer Research.* 65(1); Pp 54-65. 2005.

81. White T, Ozel B, Jain J, Stanczyk F. **Effects of transdermal and oral contraceptives on estrogen-sensitive hepatic proteins.** *Contraception.* 74(4); Pp 293-296. 2006.

82. Willoughby D, Taylor L. **Effects of sequential bouts of resistance exercise on androgen receptor expression.** *Medicine and Science in Sports and Exercise.* 36(9); Pp 1499-1506. 2004.

83. Xu S, De Pergola G, Bjorntorp. **Testosterone increases lipolysis and the number of beta-adrenoceptors in male rat adipocytes.** *Endocrinology.* 128(1); Pp 379-382. 1991.

84. Zhu H, Xiao X, Zheng J, Zheng S, Dong K, Yu Y. **Growth-promoting effect of bisphenol A on neuroblastoma in vitro and in vivo.** *Journal of Pediatric Surgery.* 44(4); Pp 672-680. 2009.

Chapter 6

1. Berkemeyer S, Vormann J, Gunther A, Rylander R, Frassetto L, Remer T. **Renal net acid excretion capacity is comparable in prepubescence, adolescence, and young adulthood but falls with aging.** *Journal of the American Geriatrics Society.* 56(8); Pp 1442-1448. 2008.

2. Berkemeyer S. **Acid-base balance and weight gain: are there crucial links via protein and organic acids in understanding obesity?** *Medical Hypotheses.* 73(3); Pp 347-356. 2009.

3. Dawson-Hughes B, Harris S, Ceglia L. **Alkaline diets favor lean tissue mass in older adults.** *American Journal of Clinical Nutrition.* 87(3); Pp 662-665. 2008

4. Dormandy T. **Body pH.** *Lancet.* 1(7440); Pp 755-759. 1966.

5. Eaton S, Eaton S (3rd). **Paleolithic vs modern diets: selected pathophysiological implications.** *European Journal of Nutrition.* 39(2); Pp 67-70. 2000.

6. Eaton S. **The ancestral human diet: what was it and should it be a paradigm for contemporary nutrition.** *Proceedings of the Nutrition Society.* 65(1); Pp 1-6. 2006.

7. Frassetto L, Schlotter M, Mietus-Snyder M, Morris R, Sebastian A. **Metabolic and physiologic improvements from consuming a paleolithic, hunter-gatherer type diet.** *European Journal of Clinical Nutrition.* 63(8); Pp 947-955. 2009.

8. Frassetto L, Morris R, Sellmeyer D, Todd K, Sebastian A. **Diet, evolution and aging--the pathophysiologic effects of the post-agricultural inversion of the potassium-to-sodium and base-to-chloride ratios in the human diet.** *European Journal of Nutrition.* 40(5); Pp 200-213. 2001.

9. Frassetto L, Morris R, Sebastian A. **Effect of age on blood acid-base composition in adult humans: role of age-related renal functional decline.** *American Journal of Physiology.* 271(1); Pp 1114-1122. 1996.

10. Jonsson T, Ahren B, Pacini G, Sundler F, Wierup N, Steen S, Sioberg T, Ugander M, Frostegard J, Goransson L, Lindeberg S. A **Paleolithic diet confers higher insulin sensitivity, lower C-reactive protein and lower blood pressure than a cereal-based diet in domestic pigs.** *Nutrition and Metabolism (Lond).* 2(3); Pp 39. 2006.

11. Jonsson T, Granfeldt Y, Ahren B, Branell U, Palsson G, Hansson A, Soderstrom M, Lindeberg S. **Beneficial effects of a Paleolithic diet on cardiovascular risk factors in type 2 diabetes: a randomized cross-over pilot study.** *Cardiovascular Diabetology.* 16(8); Pp 35. 2009.

12. Remer T. **Influence of nutrition on acid-base balance: metabolic aspects.** *European Journal of Nutrition.* 40(5); Pp 214-220. 2001

13. Remer T. **Influence of diet on acid-base balance.** *Seminars in Dialysis.* 13(4); 221-226. 2000.

14. Remer T, Manz F. **Potential renal acid load of foods and it's influence on urine PH**. *Journal of the American Dietetics Association.* 95(7); Pp 791-797. 1995.

15. Remer T, Berkemeyer S, Rylander R, Vormann J. **Muscularity and adiposity in addition to net acid excretion as predictors of 24-h urinary pH in young adults and elderly.** *European Journal of Clinical Nutrition.* 61(5); Pp 605-609. 2007.

16. Sebastian A, Frassetto L, Sellmeyer D, Merriam R, Morris R. **Estimation of the net acid load of the diet of ancestral preagricultural Homo sapiens and their hominid ancestors.** *American Journal of Clinical Nutrition.* 76(6); Pp 1308-1316. 2002.

17. Sebastian A, Frassetto L, Sellmeyer D, Morris R. **The evolution-informed optimal dietary potassium intake of human beings greatly exceeds current and recommended intakes.** *Seminars in Nephrology.* 26(6); Pp 447-453. 2006.

Chapter 7

1. Adler A, Boyko E, Schraer C, Murphy N. **Lower prevalence of impaired glucose tolerance and diabetes associated with daily seal oil or salmon consumption among Alaska Natives.** *Diabetes Care.* 17(12); Pp 1498-1501. 1994.

2. Aschner J, Aschner M. **Nutritional aspects of manganese homeostasis.** *Molecular Aspects of Medicine.* 26(4-5); Pp 353-362. 2005.

3. Barbagallo M, Dominguez L, Resnick L. **Magnesium metabolism in hypertension and type 2 diabetes mellitus.** *American Journal of Therapeutics.* 14(4); Pp 375-385. 2007.

4. Bhatnagar D, Durrington P. **Omega-3 fatty acids: their role in the prevention and treatment of atherosclerosis related risk factors and complications.** *International Journal of Clinical Practice.* 57(4); Pp 305-314. 2003.

5. Blanc P, Boussuges A. **Cardiac Beriberi.** *Arch Mal Coeur Vaiss.* 93(4); Pp 371-379. 2000.

6. Canner P, Berge K, Wenger N, Stamler J, Friedman L, Prineas R, Fridewald W. **Fifteen year mortality in Coronary Drug Project patients: long term benefit with niacin.** *Journal of the American College of Cardiology.* 8(6); Pp 1245-1255. 1986.

7. Carney H. **Wound healing with low vitamin C level.** *Annals of Surgury.* 123(6); Pp 1111-1119. 1946.

8. Chariot P, Bignani O. **Skeletal muscle disorders associated with selenium deficiency in humans.** *Muscle Nerve.* 27(6); Pp 662-668. 2003.

9. Clarke M, Burnett J, Croft K. **Vitamin E in human health and disease.** *Critical Reviews in Clinical Laboratory Sciences.* 45(5); Pp 417-450. 2008.

10. Delange F. **The disorders induced by iodine deficiency.** *Thyroid.* 4(1); Pp 107-128. 1994.

11. Deruelle F, Baron B. **Vitamin C: is supplementation necessary for optimal health?** *The Journal of Alternative and Complimentary Medicine.* 14(10); Pp 1291-1298. 2008.

12. Galland L. **Magnesium and immune function: an overview.** *Magnesium.* 7(5-6); Pp 290-299. 1988.

13. Ganji S, Kamanna V, Kashyap M. **Niacin and cholesterol: role in cardiovascular disease (review).** *The Journal of Nutritional Biochemistry.* 14(6); Pp 298-305. 2003.

14. Genead M, Fishman G, Lindeman M. **Fundus white spots and acquired night blindness due to vitamin A deficiency.** *Documenta Ophthalmologica.* 119(3); Pp 229-233. 2009.

15. Ginter E. **Chronic vitamin C deficiency increases the risk of cardiovascular diseases.** *Bratisl Lek Listy.* 108(9); Pp417-421. 2007.

16. Harding A. **Vitamin E and the nervous system**. *Critical Reviews in Neurobiology*. 3(1); Pp 89-103. 1987.

17. Harris WS. **Dietary fish oil and blood lipids.** *Current Opinions in Lipidology*. 7(1); Pp 3-7. 1996.

18. Hellmann H, Mooney S. **Vitamin B6: a molecule for human health?** *Molecules*. 15(1); Pp 442-459. 2010.

19. Hodges R, Ohlson, Bean W. **Pantothenic acid deficiency in man.** *Journal of Clinical Investigation*. 37; Pp 1642-1657. 1958.

20. Hordyiewska A, Pasternak K. **Magnesium role in cardiovascular diseases**. *Ann Univ Mariae Curie Sklodowska Med*. 59(2); Pp 108-113. 2004.

21. Houston D et al. **Association between vitamin D status and physical performance: the InCHIANTI study**. *The Journals of Gerontology*. 62(4); Pp 440-446. 2007

22. Hyas A, Juul S, Bech P, Nexo E. **Vitamin B6 level is associated with symptoms of depression**. *Psychotherapy and Psychosomatics*. 73(6); Pp 340-343. 2004.

23. Kagan V, Serbinova E, Forte T, Scita G, Packer L. **Recycling of vitamin E in human low density lipoproteins**. *The Journal of Lipid Research*. 33(3); Pp 385-397. 1992.

24. Johnston C, Corte C, Swan P. **Marginal vitamin C status is associated with reduced fat oxidation during submaximal exercise in young adults.** *Nutrition and Metabolism (Lond)*. 3; Pp 35. 2006.

25. Johnston C, Meyer C, Srilakshmi J. **Vitamin C elevates red blood cell glutathione in healthy adults**. *American Journal of Clinical Nutrition*. 58(1) Pp 103-105. 1993

26.

27. Ju J, Picinich S, Yang Z, Zhao Y, Suh N, Kong A, Yang C. **Cancer preventative activities of tocopherols and tocotrienols.** *Carciongenesis*. 31(4); Pp 533-542. 2009.

28. Kagan V, Serbinova E, Forte T, Scita G, Packer L. **Recycling of vitamin E in human low density lipoproteins**. *The Journal of Lipid Research*. 33(3); Pp 385-397. 1992

29. Kamanna V, Kashyap M. **Mechanism of action of niacin**. *The American Journal of Cardiologoy*. 101(8); Pp 20-26. 2008

30. Kohrle J, Gardner R. **Selenium and thyroid**. *Best Practice and Research: Clinical Endocrinology and Metabolism*. 23(6); Pp 815-827. 2009.

31. Koller L, Exon J. **The two faces of selenium deficiency and toxicity—are similar in animals and man**. *Canadian Journal of Veterinary Research*. 50(3); Pp 297-306. 1986.

32. Laires M, Monteiro C, Bicho M. **Role of cellular magnesium in health and human disease**. *Frontiers in Bioscience*. 9; Pp 262-276. 2004.

33. Lambert D et al. **Crohn's disease and vitamin B12 metabolism**. *Digestive Diseases and Sciences*. 41(7); Pp 1417-1422. 1996.

34. Larsson S, Giovannucci E, Wolk A. **Folate and risk of breast cancer: a meta-analysis.** *Journal of the National Cancer Institute*. 99(1); Pp 64-76. 2007.

35. Lips P. **Vitamin D physiology.** *Progress in Biophysics and Molecular Biology*. 92(1); Pp 408. 2006

36. Lonsdale D. **A review of the biochemistry, metabolism and clinical benefit of thiamine and its derivatives.** *Evidence Based Complementary and Alternative Medicine*. 3(1); Pp 49-59. 2006.

37. MacDonald A, Forsyth A. **Nutritional deficiencies and the skin**. *Clinical and Experimental Dermatology*. 30(4); Pp 388-390. 2005.

38. Maier J. **Low magnesium and atherosclerosis: an evidence based link**. *Molecular Aspects of Medicine*. 24(1-3); Pp 137-146. 2003.

39. Maroon J, Bost J. **Omega-3 fatty acids (fish oil) as an anti-inflammatory: an alternative to nonsteroidal anti-inflammatory drugs for discogenic pain.** *Surgical Neurology*. 65(4); Pp 326-331. 2006.

40. Mathieu C, Gysemans C, Giulietti A, Bouillon R. **Vitamin D and diabetes**. *Diabetologia*. 48(7); Pp 1247-1257. 2005.

41. Medrano M, Sierra M, Almazan J, Olalla M, Lopez-Abente G. **The association of dietary folate, B6, B12 with cardiovascular mortality in Spain: an ecological analysis**. *American Journal of Public Health.* 90(10); Pp 1636-1638. 2000.

42. Moat S et al. **Folate, homocysteine, endothelial function and cardiovascular disease**. *The Journal of Nutritional Biochemistry.* 15(2); Pp 64-79. 2004.

43. Montrone M, Martorelli D, Rosato A, Dolcetti R. **Retinoids as critical modulators of immune functions: new therapeutic perspectives for old compounds**. *Endocrine, Metabolic and Immune Disorders- Drug Targets.* 9(2): Pp 113-131. 2009.

44. Mori T. **Omega-3 fatty acids and hypertension in humans**. *Clinical and Experimental Pharmacology and Physiology.* 33(9); Pp 842-846. 2006.

45. Mustacich D, Bruno R, Traber M. **Vitamin E**. *Vitamins and Hormones.* 76;Pp 1-21. 2007.

46. Novakovic P, Stempak J, Sohn K, Kim Y. **Effects of folate deficiency on gene expression in the apoptosis and cancer pathways in colon cancer cells**. *Carcinogenesis.* 27(5); Pp 916-924. 2006.

47. Omenn G, Beresford A, Motulsky A. American Heart Association, Inc. **Preventing coronary heart disease**. *Circulation.* 97; Pp 421-424. 1998.

48. Pittas A, Laskowski U, Kos L, Saltzman E. **Role of vitamin D in adults requiring nutrition support**. *The Journal of Parenteral and Enteral Nutrition.* 34(1); Pp 70-78. 2010.

49. Prasad A. **Zinc: an overview**. *Nutrition.* 11(1); Pp 93-99. 1995.

50. Prasad A. **Clinical manifestations of zinc deficiency**. *Annual Review of Nutrition.* 5; Pp 341-363. 1985.

51. Prasad A, Mantzoros C, Beck F, Hess J, Brewer G. **Zinc status and serum testosterone levels of healthy adults**. *Nutrition.* 12(5); Pp 344-348. 1996. .

52. Prasad A. **Zinc in human health: effect of zinc on immune cells**. *Molecular Medicine.* 14(5-6); Pp 353-357. 2008.

53. Rayman M. **Selenium in cancer prevention: a review of the evidence and mechanism of action**. *Proceedings of the Nutrition Society.* 64(4); Pp 527-542. 2005.

54. Rose D, Connolly J. **Omega-3 fatty acids as cancer chemopreventive agents**. *Pharmacology and Therapeutics.* 83(3); Pp 217-244. 1999.

55. Rude R, Singer F, Gruber H. **Skeletal and hormonal effects of magnesium deficiency**. *Journal of the American College of Nutrition.* 28(2); Pp 121-141. 2009.

56. Ryan-Harshman M, Aldoori W. **Vitamin B12 and health**. *Canadian Family Physician.* 54(4); Pp 536-541. 2008.

57. Sen C, Khanna S, Roy S. **Tocotrienols: Vitamin E beyond tocopherols**. *Life Sciences.* 78(18); Pp 2088-2098. 2006

58. Shearer M, Newman P. **Metabolism and cell biology of Vitamin K**. *Journal of Thrombosis and Haemostasis.* 100(4); Pp 530-547. 2008.

59. Sies H, Stahl W, Sundquist A. **Antioxidant functions of vitamins. Vitamin E and C, beta-carotene, and other carotenoids**. *Annals of the New York Academy of Sciences.* 669; Pp 7-20. 1992

60. Simopoulos A. **Omega-3 fatty acids in inflammation and autoimmune diseases**. *The Journal of the American College of Nutriton.* 21(6); Pp 495-505. 2002.

61. Solomons N, Rosenberg I, Sandstead H, Vo-Khachu K. **Zinc deficiency in Crohn's disease**. *Digestion.* 16(1-2); Pp 87-95. 1977.

62. Strain J, Dowey L, Ward M. Pentieva K, McNulty H. **B-vitamins, homocysteine metabolism and CVD**. *Proceedings of the Nutrition Society.* 63(4); Pp 597-603. 2004.

63. Swaminathan R. **Magnesium metabolism and its disorders**. *The Clinical Biochemist Reviews.* 24(2); Pp 47-66. 2003.

64. Tahiliani A, Beinlich C. **Panothenic acid in health and disease**. *Vitamins and Hormones.* 46; Pp 165-228. 1991

65. Trump D, Deeb K, Johnson C. **Vitamin D: Considerations in the Continued Development as an agent for cancer prevention and therapy.** *The Cancer Journal.* 16(1); Pp 1-9. 2010.
66. Wood R. **Manganese and birth outcome.** *Nutrition Reviews.* 67(7); Pp 416-420. 2009.
67. Zimmerman M, Jooste P, Pandav C. **Iodine-deficiency disorders.** *Lancet.* 372(9645); Pp 1251-1262. 2008.

Chapter 8

1. Achten J, Gleeson M, Jeukendrup A. **Determination of exercise intensity that elicits maximal fat oxidation.** *Medicine and Science in Spors and Exercise.* 34(1); Pp 92-97. 2002

2. Achten J, Jeukendrup A. **Optimizing fat oxidation through exercise and diet.** *Nutrition.* 20(7-8); Pp 716-727. 2004.
3. Ahtiainen J, Pakarinen A, Alen M, Kraemer W, Hakkinen K. **Short vs. long rest period between the sets in hypertrophic resistance training influence on muscle strength, size, and hormonal adaptations in trained men.** *Journal of Strength and Conditioning Research.* 19(3); Pp 572-582. 2005.
4. Allred C, Ju Y, Allred K, Chang J, Helferich W. **Dietary genistin stimulates growth of estrogen-dependent breast cancer tumors similar to that observed with genistein.** *Carcinogenesis.* 22(10); Pp 1667-1673. 2001.
5. Burns J, Keenan AM, Redmond AC. **Factors associated with triathlon-related overuse injuries.** *Journal of Orthopaedic and Sports Physical Therapy.* 33(4); Pp 177-84. 2003.
6. Crist D, Peake G, Egan P, Waters D. **Body composition response to exogenous GH during training in highly conditioned adults.** *Journal of Applied Physiology.* 65(2); Pp 579-584. 1988.
7. Cosca DD, Navazio F. **Common problems in endurance athletes.** *American Family Physician.* 76(2); Pp 237-44. 2007.

8. Egermann M, Brocai D, Lill CA, Schmitt H. **Analysis of injuries in long-distance triathletes.** *International Journal of Sports Medicine.* 24(4); Pp 271-6. 2003

9. Folland J, Williams A. **The adaptations to strength training: morphological and neurological contributions to increased strength.** *Sports Medicine.* 37(2); Pp 145-168. 2007

10. Gabriel D, Kamen G, Frost G. **Neural adaptations to resistive exercise: mechanisms and recommendations for training practices.** *Sports Medicine.* 36(2); Pp 133-149. 2006

11. Goto K, Ishii N, Sugihara S, Yoshioka T, Takamatsu K. **Effects of resistance exercise on lipolysis during subsequent submaximal exercise.** *Medicine and Science in Sports and Exercise.* 39(2); Pp 308-315. 2007.
12. Hackney A, Szczepanowska E, viru A. **Basal testicular testosterone production in endurance-trained men is suppressed.** *European Journal of Applied Physiology.* 89(2); Pp 198-201. 2003.

13. Hakkinen K, Pakarinen A. **Acute hormonal responses to two different fatiguing heavy resistance protocols in male athletes.** *Journal of Applied Physiology.* 74(2); Pp 882-887. 1993.

14. Hunter G, Weinsier R, Bamman M, Larson D. **A role for high intensity exercise on energy balance and weight control.** *International Journal of Obesity and Related Metabolic Disorders.* 22(6); Pp 489-493. 1998.

15. Izquierdo M, Ibanez J, Hakkinen K, Kraemer W, Ruesta M, Gorostiaga E. **Maximal strength and power, muscle mass, endurance and serum hormones in weightlifters and road cyclists.** *Journal of Sports Sciences.* 22(5); Pp 465-478. 2004.
16. Kraemer W. ***Endocrine responses to resistance exercise.*** *Medicine and Science in Sports and Exercise.* 20(5); Pp 152-157. 1988

17. Kraemer W, Ratamess N. **Hormonal responses and adaptations to resistance exercise and training.** *Sports Medicine.* 35(4); Pp 339-361. 2005

18. Krivickas LS. **Anatomical factors associated with overuse sports injuries.** *Sports Medicine.* 24(2); Pp 132-46. 1997.

19. Lehmann MJ, Lormes W, Opitz-Gress A, Steinacker JM, Netzer N, Foster C, Gastmann U. **Training and overtraining: an overview and experimental results in endurance sports.** *The Journal of Sports Medicine and Physical Fitness.* 37(1); Pp 7-17. 1997.

20. Lehman WL Jr. **Overuse syndromes in runners.** *American Family Physician.* 29(1); Pp 157-61. 1984.

21. Lindegaard B, Hansen T, Hvid T, van Hall G, Plomgaard P, Ditlevsen S, Gerstoft J, Pedersen BK. **The effect of strength and endurance training on insulin sensitivity and fat distribution in human immunodeficiency virus-infected patients with lipodystrophy.** *The Journal of Clinical Endocrinology & Metabolism.* 93(10); Pp 3860-9. 2008.

22. Linnamo V, Pikarinen A, Komi P, Kraemer W, Hakkinen K. **Acute hormonal responses to submaximal and maximal heavy resistance and explosive exercises in men and women.** *Journal of Strength and Conditioning Research.* 19(3); Pp 566-571. 2005.

23. MacDougall J, Sale D, Elder G, Sutton J. **Muscle ultrastructural characteristics of elite powerlifters and bodybuilders.** *European Journal of Applied Physiology and Occupational Physiology.* 48(1); Pp 117-126. 1982.

24. Meinhardt U, Nelson A, Hansen J, Birzniece V, Clifford D, Leung K, Graham K, Ho K. **The effects of growth hormone on body composition and physical performance in recreational athletes: a randomized trial.** *Annals of Internal Medicine.* 152(9); Pp 568-577. 2010.

25. O'Toole ML. **Prevention and treatment of injuries to runners.** *Medicine and Science in Sports and Exercise.* 24(9 Suppl); Pp S360-3. 1992.

26. Ranallo R, Rhodes E. **Lipid metabolism during exercise.** *Sports Medicine.* 26(1); Pp 29-42. 1998.

27. Renström P, Johnson RJ. **Overuse injuries in sports. A review.** *Sports Medicine.* 2(5); Pp 316-33. 1985

28. Rosmond R, Dallman MF, Björntorp P. **Stress related cortisol secretion in men; relationships with abdominal obesity and endocrine metabolic and hemodynamic abnormalities.** *Journal of Clinical Endocrinology and Metabolism.* 83(6); Pp 1853-1859. 1998.

29. Roy D, Colerangle J, Singh K. **Is exposure to environmental or industrial endocrine disrupting estrogen-like chemicals able to cause genomic instability.** *Frontiers in Bioscience.* 6(3); Pp 913-921. 1998.

30. Smith R, Rutherford O. **Spine and total body bone mineral density and serum testosterone level in male athletes.** *European Journal of Applied Physiology and Occupational Physiology.* 67(4); Pp 330-334. 1993

31. Taunton JE, Ryan MB, Clement DB, McKenzie DC, Lloyd-Smith DR, Zumbo BD. **A retrospective case-control analysis of 2002 running injuries.** *British Journal of Sports Medicine.* 36(2) Pp 95-101. 2002.

32. Timmons B, Araujo J, Thomas T. **Fat utilization enhanced by exercise in cold environment.** *Medicine and Science in Sports and Exercise.* 17(6); 673-678. 1985.

33. Treff G, Steinacker J. **Molecular, cellular and physiological responses to resistance training.** *Med Monatsschr Pharm.* 32(4); Pp 129-136. 2009.

34. Urhausen A, Kindermann W. **Behavior of testosterone, sex hormone binding globulin (SHBG), and cortisol before and after a triathlon competition.** *International Journal of Sports Medicine.* 8(5); Pp 305-308. 1987

35. Wheeler G, Singh M, Pierce W, Epling W, Cumming D. **Endurance training decreases serum testosterone levels in men without change in lutenizing hormone pulsatile release.** *Journal of Clinical Endocrinology and Metabolism.* 72(J2); Pp 422-425. 1991.

Chapter 9

1. Anderson A, Meador K, McClure J, Makrozahapoulos D, Brooks D, Mirka G. **A biomechanical analysis of anterior load carriage.** *Ergonomics.* 50(12); Pp 2104-2117. 2007

2. Callaghan J, McGill S. Muscle activity and low back loads under external shear and compressive loading. *Spine (Phila, Pa 1976).* 20(9); Pp 992-998. 1995

3. Fatone C, Guescini M, Balducci S, Battistoni S, Settequattrini A, Pippi R, Stocchi L, Mantuano M, Stocchi V, De Feo P. **Two weekly sessions of combined aerobic and resistance exercise are sufficient to provide beneficial effects in subjects with Type 2 diabetes mellitus and metabolic syndrome.** *Journal of Endocrinological Investigation.* 33(7); Pp 489-495. 2010.

4. Hakkinen K, Pakarinen A, Alen M, Kauhanen H, Komi P. **Relationships between training volume, physical performance capacity, and serum hormone concentrations during prolonged training in elite weight lifters.** *International Journal of Sports Medicine.* 8(1); Pp 61-65.1987.

5. Hakkinen K, Pakarinen A, Alen M, Kauhanen H, Komi P. **Neuromuscular and hormonal responses in elite athletes to two successive strength training sessions in one day.** *European Journal of Applied Physiology and Occupational Physiology.* 57(2); Pp 133-139. 1988.

6. Hakkinen K, Pakarinen A, Alen M, Kauhanen H, Komi P. **Daily hormonal and neuromuscular responses to intensive strength training in 1 week.** *International Journal of Sports Medicine.* 9(6); Pp 422-428. 1988.

7. Hakkinen K, Pakarinen A, Alen M, Kauhanen H, Komi P. **Neuromuscular and hormonal adaptations in athletes to strength training in two years.** *Journal of Applied Physiology.* 65(6); Pp 2406-2412. 1988.

8. Hakkinen K, Pakarinen A, **Acute hormonal responses to two different fatiguing heavy-resistance protocols in male athletes.** *Journal of Applied Physiology.* 74(2); Pp 882-887. 1993

9. Hakkinen K, Kallinen M. **Distribution of strength training volume into one or two daily session and neuromuscular adaptations in female athletes.** *Electromyography and Clinical Neurophysiology.* 34(2); Pp 117-124. 1994.

10. Hakkinen K, Komi P, Alen M, Kauhanen H. **EMG, muscle fibre and force production characteristics during a 1 year training period in elite weight lifters.** *European Journal of Applied Physiology and Occupational Physiology.* 56(4); pp 419-427. 1987.

11. Hamlyn N, Behm D, Young W. **Trunk muscle activation during dynamic weight-training exercises and isometric instability activities.** *Journal of Strength and Conditioning Research.* 21(4); Pp 1108-1112. 2007

12. Hartman M, Clarke B, Bembens D, Kilgore J, Bemben M. **Comparisons between twice-daily and once daily training sessions in male weightlifters.** *International Journal of Sports Physiology and Performance.* 2(2); Pp 159-169. 2007.

13. Henriksen E. Invited review: **Effects of acute exercise and exercise training on insulin resistance.** *Journal of Applied Physiology.* 93(2); Pp 788-796. 2002

14. Huang S, Czech M. **The GLUT 4 Glucose Transporter.** *Cell Metabolism Review.* 5; Pp 237-252. 2007.

15. Izquierdo M, Ibanez J, Hakkinen K, Kraemer W, Ruesta M, Gorostiaga E. **Maximal strength and power, muscle mass, endurance, and serum hormones in weightlifters and road cyclists.** *Journal of Sports Sciences.* 22(5); Pp 465-478. 2004.

16. Izquierdo M, Ibanez J, Gonzalez-Badillo J, Hakkinen K, Ratamess N, Kraemer W, French D, Eslava J, Altadill A, Asiain X, Gorostiaga E. **Differential effects of strength training leading to failure versus not to failure on hormonal responses, strength, and muscle power gains.** *Journal of Applied Physiology* 100(5); Pp 1647-1656. 2006

17. Kirwan J, del Aguila L. **Insulin signaling, exercise and cellular integrity.** *Biochemical Society Transactions.* 31(6); Pp 1281-1285. 2003

18. Kraemer W, Fry A, Warren B, Stone M, Fleck S, Kearney J, Conroy B, Maresh C, Weseman C, Triplett, et al. **Acute hormonal responses in elite junior weightlifters.** *International Journal of Sports Medicine.* 13(2); Pp 103-109. 1992.

19. Maynar M, Timon R, Gonzalez A, Olcina G, Toribio F, Maynar J, Caballero M. **SHBG, plasma, and urinary androgens in weight lifters after strength training.** *Journal of Physiology and Biochemistry.* 66(2); Pp 137-142. 2010.

20. Mazzetti S, Douglass M, Yocum A, Harber M. **Effect of explosive versus slow contractions and exercise intensity on energy expenditure.** *Medicine and Science in Sports and Exercise.* 39(8); Pp 1291-1301. 2007.

21. McGill S, McDermott A, Fenwick C. **Comparison of different strongman events: trunk muscle activation and lumbar spine motion, load, and stiffness.** *Journal of Strength and Conditioning Research.* 23(4); Pp 1148-1161. 2009

22. Yaspelkis B. **Resistance training improves insulin signaling and action in skeletal muscle.** *Exercise and Sport Sciences Reviews.* 34(1); Pp 42-46. 2006.

Chapter 10

1. Berry M, Russo A, Wishart J, Tonkin A, Horowitz M, Jones K. **Effect of solid meal on gastric emptying of, and Glycemic and cardiovascular responses to liquid glucose in older subjects.** *American Journal of Physiology – Gastrointestinal and Liver Physiology.* 284(4); Pp 655-662. 2003.

2. Bird S., Tarpenning K., Marino F. **Independent and combined effects of liquid carbohydrate/essential amino acidingestion on hormonal and muscular adaptations following resistance training in untrained men.** *European Journal of Applied Physiology*; 97(2): pp 225-238. 2006

3. Chromiak J., Smedley B., Carpenter W., Brown R., Koh Y., Lamberth J., JoeL., Abadie B., Altorfer G. **Effect of a 10-week strength training program and recovery drink on boy composition, muscular strength and endurance, andanaerobic power and capacity.** *Nutrition*; 20(5): pp 420-427. 2004

4. Ebbeling C, Leidig M, Feldman H, Lovesky M, Ludwig D. **Effects of low Glycemic load vs low fat diet in obese young adults: a randomized trial.** *JAMA.* 297(19); Pp 2092-2102. 2007.

5. Fry R, Morton A, Garcia-Webb P, Crawford G, Keast D. **Biological responses to overload in endurance sports.** *European Journal of Applied Physiology and Occupational Physiology.* 64(4); Pp 335-344. 1992.

6. Gomez-Merino D, Chennauol M, Drogou C, Bonneau D, Guezenner C. **Decreases in serum leptin after prolonged physical activity in men.** *Medicine and Science in Sports and Exercise.* 34(10); Pp 1594-1599. 2002.

7. Kindermann W, Schnabel A, Schmitt W, Biro G, Cassens J, Weber F. **Catecholamines, growth hormone, cortisol, insulin, and sex hormones in anaerobic and aerobic exercise.** *European Journal of Applied Physiology and Occupational Physiology.* 49(3); Pp 389-399. 1982.

8. Periera M, Swain J, Goldfine A, Rifai N, Ludwig D. **Effects of low Glycemic load diet on resting energy expenditure and heart disease risk factors during weight loss.** *JAMA.* 292(20); Pp 2482-2490. 2004.

9. Riccardi G, Rivellese A, Giacco R. **Role of Glycemic index and Glycemic load in healthy state, in prediabetes, and in diabetes.** *American Journal of Clinical Nutrition.* 87(1); Pp 269-274. 2008.

10. Shikany J, Thomas S, Henson C, Reddon D, Heimburger D. **Glycemic index and glycemic load of popular weight loss diets.** *MedGenMEd.* 25;8(1); Pp 22. 2006.

11. Sullivan A. **The he hormone.** The *New York Times Magazine.* 2007

12. Thomas D, Elliot E, Baur L. **Low Glycemic index or low Glycemic load diets for overweight and obesity.** *Cochrane Database Systematic Reviews.* 18(3); CD005105. 2007.

13. Urhausen A, Gabriel H, Kinderman W. **Blood hormones as markers of training stress and overtraining.** *Sports Medicine.* 20(4); Pp 251-276. 1995.

14. Uusitalo A, Huttunen P, Hanin Y, Uusitalo A, Rusko H. **Hormonal responses to endurance training and overtraining in female athletes.** *Clinical Journal of Sports Medicine.* 8(3); Pp 178-186. 1998.

15. Willms B, Werner J, Holst J, Orskov C, Creutzfeldt W, Nauck M. **Gastric emptying, glucose responses, and insulin secretion after a liquid test meal: effects of exogenous glucagon-like peptide-1 (GLP-1)-(7-36) amide in type 2 (noninsulin-dependent) diabetic patients.** *Journal of Clinical Endocrinology and Metabolism.* 81; Pp 327-332. 1996

CHAPTER 11

1. Allred CD, Ju YH, Allred KF, Chang J, Helferich WG. **Dietary genistin stimulates growth of estrogen-dependent breast cancer tumors similar to that observed with genistein.** *Carcinogenesis.* 2001 Oct;22(10):1667-73.

2. Anderson A, Meador K, McClure J, Makrozahapoulos D, Brooks D, Mirka G. **A biomechanical analysis of anterior load carriage.** *Ergonomics.* 50(12); Pp 2104-2117. 2007.

3. Anderson J, Johnstone B, Newell-Cook M. **Meta-Analysis of the effects of soy protein intake on serum lipids.** *New England Journal of Medicine.* 333 (5); Pp 276-282. 1995

4. Aude Y, Agatston A, Lopez-Jiminez F, Lieberman E, Marie A, Hansen M, Rojas G, LamasG, Hennekens C. **The National cholesterol education program diet vs a diet lower in carbohydrates and higher in protein and monounsaturated fat: a randomized trial.** *The Archives of Internal Medicine.* 164(19); Pp 2141-2146. 2004

5. Asmus HG, Braun J, Krause R, Brunkhorst R, Holzer H, Schulz W, Neumayer HH, Raggi P, Bommer J. **Two year comparison of sevelamer and calcium carbonate effects on cardiovascular calcification and bone density.** *Nephrology Dialysis Transplantation.* 20(8); Pp 1653-1661. 2005.

6. Bell S, Sears B. **A proposal for a new national diet: a low glycemic load diet with a unique macronutrient composition.** *Metabolic Syndrome and Related Disorders.* 1(3); Pp 199-2008. 2003.

7. Braun J, Asmus HG, Holzer H, Brunkhorst R, Krause R, Schulz W, Neumayer HH, Raggi P, Bommer J. **Long-term comparison of a calcium-free phosphate binder and calcium carbonate-phosphorus metabolism and cardiovascular calcification.** *Clinical Nephrology.* 62(2); Pp 104-115. 2004.

8. Caterisano A, Moss R, Pellinger T, Woodruff K, Lewis V, Booth W, Khadra T. **The effect of back squat depth on the EMG activity of 4 superficial hip and thigh muscles.** *Journal of Strength and conditioning Research.* 16(3); Pp 428-432. 2002.

9. Chandler T, Wilson G, Stone M. The **effect of the squat exercise on knee stability.** *Medicine and Science in Sports and Exercise.* 21(3). Pp 299-303. 1989.

10. Doerge DR, Sheehan DM. **Goitrogenic and estrogenic activity of soy isoflavones.** *Environmental Health Perspectives.* 2002 Jun;110 Suppl 3:349-53.

11. Gross L, Li L, Ford E, Liu S. **Food pyramid increased consumption of refined carbohydrates and the epidemic of type 2 diabetes in the United States: an ecologic assessment.** *American Journal of Clinical Nutrition.* 79(5); Pp 774-779. 2004

12. Hamlyn N, Behm D, Young W. **Trunk muscle activation during dynamic weight-training exercises and isometric instability activities.** *Journal of Strength and Conditioning Research.* 21(4); Pp 1108-1112. 2007.

13. Jakobsen MU, Bysted A, Andersen NL, Heitmann BL, Hartkopp HB, Leth T, Overvad K, Dyerberg J. **Intake of ruminant trans fatty acids and risk of coronary heart disease-an overview.** *Atherosclerosis Supplements.* 7(2); Pp 9-11. 2006.

14. Johannsen H, Lind T, Jakobsen B, Kroner K. **Exercise-induced knee joint laxity in distance runners.** *British Journal of Sports Medicine.* 23(3); Pp 165-168. 1989

15. Klein K. **The deep squat exercise as utilized in weight training for athletes and its effects on the ligaments of the knee.** *American Journal of Physical Medicine and Rehabilitation.* 15; Pp 6-11. 1961.

16. Lindegaard B, Hansen T, Hvid T, van Hall G, Plomgaard P, Ditlevsen S, Gerstoft J, Pedersen BK. **The effect of strength and endurance training on insulin sensitivity and fat distribution in human immunodeficiency virus-infected patients with lipodystrophy.** *The Journal of Clinical Endocrinology & Metabolism.* 93(10); Pp 3860-9. 2008.

17. Luz J, Pasin VP, Silva DJ, Zemdegs JC, Amaral LS, Affonso-Silva SM. **Effect of food restriction on energy expenditure of monosodium glutamate induced obese rats.** *Annals of Nutrition and Metabolism.* 56(1); Pp 31-35. 2009.

18. McGill S, McDermott A, Fenwick C. **Comparison of different strongman events: trunk muscle activation and lumbar spine motion, load and stiffness.** *Journal of Strength and Conditioning Research.* 23(4); Pp 1148-1161. 2009.

19. Meyers E. **Effect of selected exercise variables on ligament stability and flexibility of the knee.** *Research Quarterly.* 42(4); Pp 411-422. 1971.

20. Mozaffarian D, Aro A, Willet W. **Health effects of trans-fatty acids: experimental and observational evidence.** *European Journal of Clinical Nutrition.* 63; Pp S5-21. 2009.

21. Nestle M. **The ironic politics of obesity.** *Science.* 299(5608); Pp 781. 2003.

22. NHANES data on the Prevalence of Overweight Among Children and Adolescents: United States, 2003–2006. CDC National Center for Health Statistics, Health E-Stat.

23. (http://www.cdc.gov/nchs/products/pubs/pubd/hestats/overweight/overwght_child_03.htm)

24. O'Dea K. **Westernization, insulin resistance and diabetes in Australian aborigines.** *The Medical Journal of Australia.* 155(4); Pp 258-64. 1991.

25. O'Dea K. **Cardiovascular disease risk factors in Australian aborigines.** *Clinical and Experimental Pharmacology and Physiology.* 18(2); Pp 85-8. 1991.

26. O'Dea K. **Diabetes in Australian aborigines: impact of the western diet and life style.** *Journal of Internal Medicine.* 232(2); Pp 103-17. 1992.

27. O'Dea K. **Westernization and non-insulin-dependent diabetes in Australian Aborigines.** *Ethnicity and Disease.* 1(2); Pp 171-87. 1991.

28. O'Dea K. **Obesity and diabetes in "the land of milk and honey".** *Diabetes/Metabolism Reviews.* 8(4); Pp 373-88. 1992.

29. O'Dea K, Spargo RM, Akerman K. **The effect of transition from traditional to** *Diabetes Care.* 3(1); Pp 31-37. 1980.

30. O'Dea K. **Marked improvement in carbohydrate and lipid metabolism in diabetic Australian aborigines after temporary reversion to traditional lifestyle.** *Diabetes.* 33(6); Pp 596-603.

31. Ogden CL, Carroll MD, Flegal KM. **High Body Mass Index for Age Among US Children and**
Adolescents, 2003–2006. *JAMA* 2008;299:2401–2405

32. Oza Frank R, Cheng Y, Naravan K, Gregg E. **Trends in nutrient intake among adults with Diabetes in the United States: 1998-2004.** *Journal of American Dietetic Association.* 109(7); Pp 1173-1178. 2009.

diabetes in the United States: 1988-2004. *Journal of American Dietetic Association.* 109(7); Pp 1173-1178. 2009.

33. Pischon T, Giovannucci E, Hankinson S, Ma J, Rifai N, Rimm E Wu T. **Fructose, glycemic load, and quantity and quality of carbohydrates in relation to plasma C-peptide concentrations in US women.** *American Journal of Clinical Nutrition.* 80(4); Pp 1043-1049. 2004.

34. Panariello R, Backus S, Parker J. **The effect of the squat exercise on anterior-posterior knee translation in professional football players.** *American Journal of Sports Medicine.* 22(6); Pp 768-773. 1994

35. Pollan M. *In Defense of Food.* Pp 50. London, En. 2008.

36. Reinberg S. **Rate of diabetes cases doubles in 10 years.** CDC. US NEWS. October 30, 2008

37. Rosenkvist, H., and A. Hansen. **The antimicrobial effect of organic acid sourdough and nisin against** *Bacillus subtilis*Bacillus subtilis **and** *Bacillus licheniformis*Bacillus licheniformis **isolated from wheat bread.** *Journal of Applied Microbiology.* 85:621-631. 1998

38. Reuters. **Obese Americans now outweigh the merely overweight.** January 9, 2009

39. Steiner M, Grana W, Chilag K, Schelberg-Karnes E. **The effect of exercise on anterior-posterior knee laxity.** *American Journal of Sports Medicine.* 14(1); Pp 24-29. 1986.

40. Thuvander A, Oskarsson A. **Effects of subchronic exposure to Caramel Colour III on the immune system in mice.** *Food and Chemical Toxicology.* 32(1); Pp 7-13. 1994.

41. Tuohy PG. **Soy infant formula and phytoestrogens.** *Journal of Pediatrics and Child Health.* 2003 Aug;39(6):401-5.

42. Wikipedia.co; Food Pyramid Controversy.

43. Willett W. **Trans fatty acids and cardiovascular disease-epidemiological data.** *Atherosclerosis Supplements.* 7(2); Pp 5-8. 2006.

44. Xiong J, Branigan D, Li M. **Deciphering the MSG controversy.** *International Journal of Clinical and Experimental Medicine.* 2(4); Pp 329-336. 2009.

45. Zung A, Glaser T, Kerem Z, Zadik Z. **Breast development in the first 2 years of life: an association with soy-based infant formulas.** *Journal of Pediatric Gastroenterology and Nutrition.* 2008 Feb;46(2):191-5.

About The Author

With over 16 years of practical experience as a coach and educator, Jason Shea has earned a reputation as a strength coach and body composition specialist capable of training athletes and trainees at the highest levels. As the owner of APECS (www.apec-s.com) and CrossFit Tri-Valley (www.crossfit-trivalley.com) Jason has earned the distinguished honor of being recognized as one of less than a dozen PICP Level IV International Strength Coaches in the U.S. His clientele has included professional, college, high school, and Olympic hopeful athletes as well as Fortune 500 business executives, SWAT Teams, military personnel, state and local firefighters, and more than 40 local high school, club, and college teams.

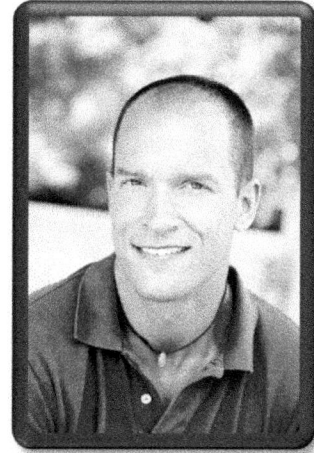

He has been strength coach to 2 High School Super Bowl Teams, 5 State Champion Lacrosse Teams, numerous State and New England Champion wrestlers and track athletes, Boston Globe Players of the year in Football, Volleyball, Wrestling, Lacrosse, and Soccer, over 25 High School and College league MVP's from all sports, College and high school league all-stars in nearly every sport, and league champion teams in high school sports including Football, Field Hockey, Soccer, Basketball, Hockey, Baseball, Field Hockey, Lacrosse, Wrestling, and Softball.

Jason holds a Bachelor's Degree in Exercise Science and a Master's in Human Movement. He has been certified through various organizations including the USAW, NASM, NSCA, ISSA, ACE, and PICP. Not one to rest on his laurels, Jason has traveled throughout the US and Europe to learn the most effective techniques in training, soft tissue, nutrition, and body composition taught by the Poliquin Strength Institute and PICP Certification Program.

Along with his role as Head Strength Coach at APECS and CrossFit Tri-Valley Jason is also the Massachusetts Statewide Health and Wellness Coordinator for the Municipal Police Training Committee. In this role he is responsible for academy certification and dissemination of continuing education for municipal police officers teaching at the Municipal Police Academies in Massachusetts.

The success of his business and clientele has led to current positions as Adjunct Professor in the Sport Fitness department at Dean College, consulting Strength Coach to the highly successful Dean College Football and Soccer Teams, Performance Director for the Speed and Power Academy at Franklin High School, Strength and Conditioning Coach to the nationally ranked Boston Irish Wolfhounds Rugby Team, columnist for the Metrowest Daily News, and the opportunity to co-author Law Enforcement articles with world renowned strength coach Charles Poliquin. He has also been a featured lecturer on strength and conditioning topics for various organizations including local colleges, corporation and high schools, Blue Chip Football Camps, and club teams in all sports.

Most important to Jason is the time he spends with his inspirations; son Ayden, daughter Bryn, and beautiful wife Wendy.

www.ingramcontent.com/pod-product-compliance
Lightning Source LLC
Chambersburg PA
CBHW080016280326
41934CB00015B/3365